THE U.S. HEALTH SYSTEM
Origins and Functions
5th Edition

Delmar Staff
Business Unit Director: *William Brottmiller*
Product Development Manager: *Marion Waldman*
Development Editor: *Robin Irons*
Executive Marketing Manager: *Dawn F. Gerrain*
Channel Manager: *Tara S. Carter*
Executive Production Manager: *Karen Leet*
Project Editor: *Maureen M. E. Grealish*
Production Coordinator: *Nina Lontrato*
Art/Design Coordinator: *Jay Purcell*

Library of Congress Cataloging-in-Publication Data

Raffel, Marshall W.
    The U.S. health system : origins and functions / Marshall W. Raffel, Camille K. Barsukiewicz.—5th ed.
        p. cm.
    Includes bibliographical references and index.
    ISBN 0-7668-0714-2 (alk. paper)
    1. Medical care—United States. 2. Public health—United States. I. Barsukiewicz, Camille K. II. Title.

RA395.A3 R33 2001
362.1'0973—dc21 2001028360

THE U.S. HEALTH SYSTEM
Origins and Functions

Fifth Edition

Marshall W. Raffel, Ph.D.

Professor Emeritus of Health Policy and Administration
The Pennsylvania State University
University Park, Pennsylvania

Camille K. Barsukiewicz, Ph.D.

School of Urban Affairs and Public Policy
University of Memphis
Memphis, Tennessee

DELMAR

THOMSON LEARNING

Australia Canada Mexico Singapore Spain United Kingdom United States

This fifth edition is dedicated to Jennifer Godri, Craig Seland, and Darryl Seland.

CONTENTS

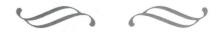

PREFACE

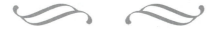

Whether you are considering a career in health administration, direct patient care, health policy and planning, or health care finance, an understanding of the varied and interconnected aspects of the U.S. healthcare delivery system is essential. Understanding is complicated by the rapid rate of change occurring in our healthcare system. Managed care, market forces, regulation, and technology development contribute to the rapid change.

Since the failure of comprehensive health care reform efforts of the mid-1990s, changes brought about by market forces, greater emphasis on data collection for outcomes measurement, increased cost constraints, integrated organizations, and incremental approaches to regulation have made understanding the healthcare system imperative not only in our professional lives, but in our role as health care consumers. Where once we were provided with a health insurance plan by our employer, we are now asked to choose among plans with varied benefits and varied costs to us. We may even be faced with the fact that our employer will no longer provide health insurance as one of our employment benefits. Where once we relied on our physicians' advice, we are now asked to evaluate, compare, and monitor alternatives to care.

Previous editions of this text have been rich in a historical approach to understanding health care delivery and applying that historical knowledge to current trends. This fifth edition has undergone extensive revisions in its format and content. Its primary purpose remains as a text for introductory courses in health care delivery systems. It retains some of its historical approach, while bringing broader attention to health care delivery and the unique challenges it faces in the United States today.

The text has been divided into three major sections, each important to the delivery of health care services. Part 1 focuses on the external health care environment. Chapter 1 provides an overview of the changes in health care delivery through an extensive case study of one hospital's growth into a multifaceted health care system. Chapter 2 discusses the cost of health care, trends in spending, some reasons for increasing costs, and attempts at containing costs.

Chapter 3 provides a background on how we pay for health care, including both historical and current trends in private health insurance and government programs. It discusses Medicare, Medicaid, managed care, and the phenomenon of the uninsured population in a system largely defined as an employment-based insurance system. Chapter 4 is an overview of physician training, licensing, and credentialing.

Part 2 focuses on the internal health care environment—the organizations and persons who deliver health care. Chapter 5 introduces other personnel that are key to the delivery of medical services, including personnel in areas that might be referred to as "alternative medicine."

The emphasis in Chapter 6 changes somewhat to health care organizations, beginning with ambulatory care, or outpatient services. Chapter 7 discusses acute inpatient care, primarily hospital care, and the dramatic market changes facing this segment of health care delivery.

Chapter 8 addresses the many facets of long-term care and the challenges brought about by an aging population. The section is brought to a close with a discussion of mental health services and systems in Chapter 9.

Changes in the health care environment are addressed in Part 3. Chapter 10 discusses the growing importance of information management and the application of technology to improve the quality of care.

Chapter 11 brings the text to a conclusion with a look toward innovative approaches that organizations take to address issues of quality of care and outcomes measurement, a look at what remains to be done, and the challenges we continue to face.

New with this edition also are the *Objectives* listed at the beginning of each chapter. The text is an overview of each of the areas presented and is not intended to be the last word in any area. As such, activities for further learning and questions for further debate (*Activity-Based Learning* and A Question of Ethics) are included in each chapter. Where possible, *In the Health Care Community* case studies appear at the end of the chapter. The case studies are based on actual visits to the facilities, input from the organizations, and/or historical documents. The instructor may include the case studies as practical examples, a springboard for discussion, or a comparison to cases in the local market.

While we have made an effort to include a comprehensive view of U.S. health care delivery, there is much room for further study. The text is not meant to be a study of health care policy; therefore, the "why" of many changes faced in health care delivery may require further inquiry. The health of the nation is not totally a result of medicine and health care delivery. Economics, culture, education, values, and many other factors determine the health of a nation. We hope that this overview stimulates further interest in the study of health care delivery in our nation and across the globe.

I would like to especially acknowledge Marshall and Norma Raffel and Delmar Publishers for giving me the opportunity to write the fifth edition of this book. Although different in its form from the first four editions, this new edition reflects the focus of the previous editions: the origins and functions of the U.S. health care system.

Special thanks also goes to the organizations who afforded me their time and attention so that I could prepare the case studies included in the text: the Baptist Memorial Health Care Corporation, the University of Tennessee Medical School, Lehigh Valley Eye Center and Lehigh Valley Ophthalmic Associates, the Memphis Jewish Home, Esse Health, Methodist Behavioral Health and Methodist Le Bonheur Children's Medical Center. Their willingness to include their stories adds an invaluable dimension to understanding the structure and delivery of health care in a wide variety of settings. Also, many thanks to my graduate assistants, Elizabeth Hearn and Kris Sanders, for their stamina in putting this project together.

Camille K. Barsukiewicz

CHAPTER

1

Introduction

Less than a decade ago the struggle with teaching health care systems to my students included what we might consider today to be an oxymoron; We neither focused on health nor were able to identify a true "system." Prior to the 1990s, little attention was paid to health and wellness, prevention, or treatment of chronic illness. The focus of health care providers was on cure and on "sick care" rather than health care. Care providers and organizations worked independently of one another in delivering services that they believed could achieve cure. There was no actual "system."

Because the approach to health care delivery was so disconnected, it was easy to design a textbook with each chapter focusing on a specific type of care provider—hospitals, doctors, nursing homes, and so on. Because of the specific methods of financing care and financing's impact on health care providers, the difficulty in designing a text came with the decision of the order of the topics, rather than the topics themselves.

Things have changed dramatically in the past decade. Greater attention is now paid to preventing disease and to wellness practices. Part of the prevention incentives come from managed care. Although managed care has been around in various forms since the early 1900s, its real growth began in the 1980s. (See the discussion of managed care in Chapter 3.) The failure of health care reform under the Clinton administration gave an added boost to managed care, which became the market's response to the lack of government reform.

The concept of managed care—case management for comprehensive care in the most efficient and effective way—is a sensible approach. Each consumer, whether healthy or sick, works with a primary care physician who establishes a long-term relationship with the patient. The primary care physician helps the patient to determine the appropriate provider of care and the appropriate setting for care when it is needed, and helps persons prevent illness through lifestyle changes. Unfortunately, the emphasis on case management has become cost management, and managed care has become controversial as a health care delivery system. However, it has been successful in moving the trends toward wellness and has been instrumental in the move toward integrated systems of care. (See the discussion of multihospital systems in Chapter 7.)

The integration has been in two major directions. Horizontal integration, in its most basic form, is an attempt to deliver similar services to a broader area, as in hospital mergers. Vertical integration, on the other hand, is an attempt to provide a wider range of services to the same population, as in a health care organization delivering physician services, hospital services, home care, and nursing-home care.

The new Healthy People 2010, launched by Health and Human Services Secretary Donna Shalala and Surgeon General David Satcher in January 2000, has two overarching goals:

1. To help individuals of all ages increase life expectancy and improve their quality of life
2. To eliminate health disparities among different segments of the population

Changes continue throughout provider organizations in the levels of financial commitment to health care, and in consumers' commitment to healthier lifestyles. While the term *health care system* is not quite the oxymoron that it was in the 1900s, it remains to be seen whether prevention can take precedence over the belief that every disease can be cured and whether integrated systems of health care delivery can provide more comprehensive and consistent care to all Americans. Although managed care has helped move attention to prevention and healthy lifestyles, it has not been the answer to eliminating health disparities among different segments of the population.

We begin the text with the story of a large health care system—from its beginnings as a hospital to its current position as an integrated system of care. The story will show how previously separate areas of health care delivery have come together; those separate areas will also be described in more detail in subsequent chapters. Part 1 (Chapters 2 through 4) is a view of the external environment of health care delivery including the cost of care, the financing of health care services, and the evolution of physician training. Part 2 (Chapters 5 through 9) contains an internal view of the health care environment through historical and current information regarding various providers of care. Part 3 (Chapters 10 and 11) focuses on some of the newer trends in the continually changing health care environment. Each chapter also includes a case study of a present-day organization—not to critique its management decisions or strategic plan, but to show the reader how various organizations cope or survive over the long term or how new organizations form to meet the demands of the times. Each chapter also asks the reader to consider difficult questions that do not always have one right answer. We call them "Questions of Ethics," but they are questions that pose difficult policy directions—for the organization, the consumer, or the nation. Somewhat more "hands-on" exercises are included in the "Activity-Based Learning" section of each chapter.

CASE STUDY 1.1: IN THE HEALTH CARE COMMUNITY

BAPTIST MEMORIAL HEALTH CARE CORPORATION*

Baptist Memorial Hospital was founded in 1912 in Memphis through collaboration of the Arkansas, Mississippi, and Tennessee Southern Baptist Conventions. What is currently the School of Medicine (University of Tennessee) donated land for construction of a teaching hospital. The original 150-bed hospital became a regional medical center and the cornerstone of the Baptist Memorial Health Care Corporation (BMHCC), a group of over thirty entities providing medical care to patients all across the mid-South. BMHCC now consists of sixteen hospitals, hospice and home health care services, a college of health sciences, rehabilitation services, various

(continues)

*Information for this case study was approved by BMHCC administration and includes material from interviews with three executives, organization brochures, the CD titled "The Past, Present & Future of Baptist Memorial Health Care," and from the website at www.bmhcc.org/services/home/index.asp.

(continued)

specialty clinics and services, and minor medical centers/clinics, and it is a well balanced study in the change in approach toward health care delivery in the United States today.

The mission of the hospital then, and the mission of the health care system today, remains the same: preaching, teaching, and healing in keeping with the threefold ministry of Christ. This mission has been retained in part by the fact that the organization has had only four CEOs in its eighty-eight–year history. A. E. Jennings became the first director in 1915 after he underwrote the indebtedness the hospital had incurred from caring for nonpaying patients in its first three years. He remained the director until his retirement in 1946.

Dr. Frank S. Groner took over the reins in 1946. Under his leadership, the emphasis was on education resulting in the establishment of high qualifications for medical staff privileges. The hospital grew in bed capacity and in services offered, while still maintaining its commitment to quality of care. Joseph H. Powell, who joined Baptist Memorial Hospital in 1954 as an administrative resident, became the third CEO in 1980, after Dr. Groner's retirement. Mr. Powell continued the organization's mission by developing the Minor Medical Centers, Baptist Trinity Home Care, and technology expansion for innovative information systems. His tenure ended with retirement in 1994.

BMHCC's leadership, now under the direction of Stephen Reynolds, is both a reflection and a reinforcement of the organization's mission. In a turbulent health care environment, BMHCC continues to re-evaluate the community's needs and adapt its services to those needs.

In Baptist Memorial's early inception, the tri-state Southern Baptist Conventions supported the hospital financially, but the hospital and BMHCC now operate independently of church funding. The rising costs of health care in the 1970s spawned an increase in government regulation of the industry (see Chapter 2 for more about the costs of health care). Each new effort at cost containment brought health care organizations to consider how integration and cooperation could bring cost efficiencies. For BMHCC, each decision to expand was based on the underlying question, What is best for the patients? A belief in not-for-profit service meant that any merger or lease agreement included a merger of mission as well as organizations. BMHCC made no effort to go out into communities to purchase other hospitals or services simply for the sake of expanding markets. BMHCC entered into discussions only with organizations that came to them for help. Any buyouts brought money to local foundations to be used for the good of the community.

Integration did not mean only expanding the number of hospitals by moving into new geographic locations. New services, within the hospital setting as well as outside the hospital setting, were incorporated into the organization as needs were identified by application of the overriding question: What is best for the patients?

The Growth of BMHCC

Although integration vertically and horizontally did not occur in a linear manner, it is best to describe the two aspects of integration separately. Horizontal integration is an attempt to provide the same services to a larger number of persons. Vertical integration can be described as an attempt to provide a greater variety of services to the same patient base or the immediate community. We begin with horizontal integration, the story of the expansion of the hospital system.

Baptist Memorial Hospital–Medical Center

The Baptist Memorial Hospital-Medical Center has grown in both size and service since its 1912 inception (see additional information on the history of hospitals in Chapter 7). In its downtown Memphis location, the medical center remains the cornerstone of BMHCC, providing care to over 40,000 patients annually. The medical center is particularly well

(continues)

(continued)

known for heart/lung transplants, as well as neuro-surgical, neurological, and orthopedic procedures. However, it offers a wide range of care to patients of every age and virtually any medical need. Its scope of services, its cutting-edge technology, its status as a teaching hospital, and its commitment to research attract respected specialists in all areas of medicine. Many "firsts" that took place at the medical center are described later in this chapter.

Memphis is expanding and its population growing to the east of the city. In an effort to take health care to the people, new centers were established. However, a continuing concern focuses on the proper use of the BMH-Medical Center. BMHCC is beginning the detailed planning for the medical center—both its physical structure and the best service mix for the downtown area. The planning process is complex and considers the future of both BMHCC and other health care providers in the central Memphis area serving a tristate area.

One consideration was to tear down the existing high-rise structure and replace it with a smaller neighborhood-based facility. Another option arose as area hospitals began negotiating the use of the large structure for an academic-based University Hospital Center. However, negotiations between the hospitals, the county, and BMHCC broke down and in November 2000 Baptist Memorial Hospital-Medical Center transferred its last patients to other facilities and closed its doors to patient care. The future of the facility is uncertain although some administrative functions and behavioral health still operate from the location.

Baptist Memorial Hospital-East

Baptist Memorial Hospital–East, which opened in 1979, was one of the first off-site expansion projects for Baptist Memorial Hospital. It is a 605-bed, tertiary care hospital providing acute care, inpatient and outpatient surgery, obstetric and pediatric care, emergency services, and a wide range of specialty care and ancillary services. BMH-East is currently undergoing an expansion project. A freestanding women's hospital will have 140 beds, including 40 neonatal intensive care beds. It will house the current women's services, such as ultrasound, mammography, osteoporosis screening, and specialty care for preterm and critically ill newborns.

An advanced facility for cardiac care at BMH-East will include areas for the treatment of outpatient cardiovascular disease, cardiovascular surgical suites, a heart observation suite, heart catheterization, intensive care beds, and other cardiac care beds. It will be attached to the current hospital but will have a distinct look and a prominent location at the main entrance to the BMH-East campus. The heart hospital is slated for completion in September 2001.

Looking at the services provided, it is easy to see why BMH-East is one of Tennessee's highest-volume hospitals. It has also received the Quality Award Leader #1 award from the National Research Council, recognizing that volume has not interfered with quality.

Other BMHCC Locations

The Baptist Memorial Health Care Corporation was formed in 1981. Since then, BMH-Medical Center and BMH-East have come to be known collectively as Baptist Metro. Other hospital locations of BMHCC are as follows:

- **BMH-Collierville** is a brand-new state-of-the-art facility that opened in May 1999 (see Chapter 11 for a more detailed story).
- **BMH-Germantown** is unlike any other of the Baptist facilities. Since 1994 it has provided a comprehensive array of both inpatient and outpatient rehabilitation services and includes 68 acute rehabilitation beds, 17 medical/surgical beds, 6 surgery suites focusing on orthopedic procedures, and an adjacent physicians' office building (see Chapter 8 for more on rehabilitation care).
- Carroll County General Hospital joined BMHCC and became **BMH-Huntingdon** in 1983, and

(continues)

(continued)

opened as a new 70-bed hospital in 1986. Located in rural West Tennessee, the facility has added a physicians' office building and a medical center and has expanded its health information management systems. BMH Huntingdon has improved quality care in the area by bringing in several physicians, including specialists in internal medicine, family practice, orthopedics, and so on.

- **BMH Lauderdale,** in Ripley, Tennessee, provides many services not usually found in a small city. This is a 70-bed acute care facility providing intensive care, surgery, outpatient services, outpatient rehabilitation, a senior-care unit for geriatric mental health services, state-of-the-art diagnostic services, and occupational health services, to name a few. The hospital also provides a home health care agency and hospice services.

- **BMH Tipton,** in Covington, Tennessee, joined the Baptist network in 1981. The hospital participates in a project sponsored by the Department of Family Medicine at the University of Tennessee, Memphis. The project's goal is to alleviate the shortage of family practice physicians in rural counties by providing hands-on training in rural health care for physicians (see Chapter 6 for more on rural health care).

- **BMH Union City** (Tennessee), formerly Obion County General Hospital, joined the Baptist network in 1982. In 1995 a construction project added patient rooms and tripled the size of the emergency room. Additional changes have included the expansion of behavioral health services, outpatient services, and obstetric services. New services added include a physicians' office building, radiation oncology, outpatient rehabilitation, and magnetic resonance imaging (MRI).

- **BMH Blytheville** and **BMH Osceola,** both located in Mississippi County, Arkansas, became part of the network in 1990. Both hospitals acquired new mammography and x-ray equipment. An 18-bed Adolescent Behavioral Health Unit opened at Osceola in 1995, and the 20-bed Senior Care geriatric behavioral health unit opened at Blytheville in 1994. Hospice and home health care

services are provided to both communities through Baptist Memorial Home Care.

- **BMH Forrest City** (Arkansas) joined the Baptist network in 1983 and opened a new 118-bed facility in 1986. In addition to providing acute and emergency care, this facility has a new 18-bed geriatric behavioral unit that provides care for elderly patients with psychiatric problems.

- **BMH Booneville** (Mississippi) joined the system in 1982. Since that time, facilities and services have undergone many updates and improvements. The Baptist Memorial Health Care Foundation helped to recruit physicians to the area and improve the quality of services available.

- **BMH Desoto** in Southaven, Mississippi, opened in 1988. Since then the population has boomed, and the hospital has responded with an expanded emergency room, a center for diagnostics, and the 120-bed Baptist Progressive Care Center, providing inpatient and outpatient rehabilitation services.

- **BMH Golden Triangle,** in Columbus, Mississippi, joined the Baptist network in 1993 and is the largest of the network's regional hospitals. A $44 million certificate of need for major construction and renovation was the largest project ever approved for a Mississippi hospital. The project included a new emergency room, a critical care unit, the region's first comprehensive cancer center, a cardiac care center, and an ambulatory care center.

- **BMH North Mississippi,** in Oxford, joined in 1989. Since then, it has undergone continuous renovation and construction and a tripling of its medical staff. Among its premier services are the Heart Care Center and the Sleep Disorders Center.

- **BMH Union County,** in New Albany, Mississippi, joined BMHCC in 1989 and underwent extensive renovations. Its Transitional Care Center opened in 1995 and provides recuperative care for patients who have been hospitalized and need additional rehabilitative care. The unit is designed especially for older adults needing further assistance before returning to assisted living, their home, or a nursing facility.

(continues)

(continued)

Integrated Services

New services, which might be described as vertical integration, became part of BMHCC over many years. Some are services that were a part of BMH's original mission and were incorporated later under BMHCC's formal structure. There are more services than can be presented here, but the following is an example of just how diversified health care services have become.

The Baptist Geriatric Assessment Center

The Baptist Geriatric Assessment Center, located at the BMH-Medical Center, is an assessment and treatment facility for adults sixty-five years or older who are experiencing symptoms of mental status changes, are a danger to themselves or to others, and cannot be treated as outpatients. The center, which opened January 1, 1997, offers a specialized treatment team of psychiatrists, primary care physicians, nurses, social workers, recreational therapists, and chaplains, who develop an individualized plan of care for each patient. During this ten-day assessment, the team, the patient, and the family make appropriate decisions for the future care of the patient (see Chapter 8).

Baptist Trinity Home Care & Hospice

Trinity Home Care was founded in 1974 and became part of BMHCC in the mid-1980s. Baptist Trinity Home Care & Hospice is a nonprofit home care, private-duty, supplemental staffing and hospice organization which primarily serves Shelby County, Tennessee, by way of three separate operational divisions.

The Home Health Agency provides registered nurses; certified nursing assistants; physical, speech, and occupational therapists; and social workers to care for clients in their homes. The Home Health Agency makes approximately 167,000 visits annually. Medicare, TennCare (Tennessee's Medicaid program), private insurance, or private payment may reimburse for these visits.

Health Care Services employs registered nurses, licensed practical nurses, and nursing assistants to provide two types of services. One is commonly known as *private duty*, in which the client is cared for in the home, nursing home, or hospital on an hourly, shift, or continuous basis. In these cases the Baptist Trinity employee works directly with the client, and reimbursement is by private payment or insurance to Baptist Trinity. The other type of service offered is *supplemental staffing*, in which a health care facility (hospital, clinic, or nursing home) contracts to use a Baptist Trinity employee as a member of its staff.

Hospice provides comprehensive services to terminally ill patients through an interdisciplinary team approach. Professionals who provide care through hospice include medical directors, registered nurses, nursing assistants, bereavement counselors, social workers, chaplains, and volunteers. Private insurance, private payment, Medicare, and TennCare reimburse for hospice.

Baptist Home Care & Hospice (regional) provides services in sixty counties in Arkansas, Tennessee, Mississippi, Alabama, Kentucky, and Missouri. Services provided include skilled nurses, speech and occupational therapists, nursing assistants, and medical social workers. In addition, hospice services are now available in all areas.

Baptist Home Medical Equipment provides high-tech respiratory and medical equipment for in-home use. With more than fifty years combined clinical experience in managing respiratory patients, credentialed therapists assess and coordinate patient care to ensure quality outcomes. Patient/caregiver education is provided upon delivery. Services and support are provided twenty-four hours a day.

Medical Alternatives provides a comprehensive menu of home infusion pharmacy services, including antibiotic therapy; pain management; total parenteral and enteral nutrition; and other injectable medications, supplies, and equipment to patients in

(continues)

(continued)

nonhospitalized environments. The team of professionals provides education training for patients and caregivers along with specialty infusion in-services for health care professionals.

Baptist & Physicians (Baptist Health Services Group)

Baptist & Physicians is a managed health care organization that offers an extensive network of providers to employers and payers, representing physicians and facilities throughout the mid-South. Established in the early 1980s, the Baptist Health Services Group became Baptist & Physicians in 1995, which has evolved into one of the nation's largest and most successful provider-sponsored managed care networks (see Chapter 3).

Baptist & Physicians currently provides services to approximately 2,500 physicians, 40 hospitals, and 125 ancillary facilities, as well as 5,000 employers, which represent over 700,000 covered lives. The Baptist & Physicians service area covers portions of three states—Arkansas, Tennessee, and Mississippi—extending 180 miles from Memphis.

Baptist & Physicians Preferred Provider Organization

This preferred provider organization (PPO) is a network of physicians, ancillary facilities, and hospitals that is actively marketed to payers and employers. It represents more than 2,500 primary care and specialty care physicians and 125 facilities. The Baptist & Physicians PPO is a fully owned corporation of BMHCC that serves over 5,000 employers.

Baptist & Physicians Integrated Delivery System

Baptist & Physicians Integrated Delivery System (B&P IDS) is a joint venture between BMHCC and affiliated Memphis-area physicians that was established as a platform for participation in managed care. B&P IDS serves as a vehicle for payer and provider risk contracting, and it administers the following support services: claims processing, marketing marketing services, provider network develop-

ment, product development, medical management, and provider credentialing, among others. Its network consists of more than 925 physicians, 6 inpatient facilities, and 50 ancillary facilities and it serves more than 150,000 covered lives.

Third-Party Administration Services

Baptist & Physicians has provided the following third-party administration services:

- Claims administration
- Coordination of quality initiatives
- Medical management
- Member services/eligibility
- Provider credentials management
- Provider relations
- Reporting

Workers' Compensation

CompTrac is a comprehensive workers' compensation program serving over 3,200 employers and more than 450,000 employees.

Baptist Memorial Health Care Foundation

Throughout the Baptist Memorial Health Care Corporation, many services are made possible or enhanced through financial assistance from the Baptist Memorial Health Care Foundation. Recent examples include a $3.1 million grant to the Baptist Cancer Institute, a grant to help fund a pediatric audiology center at Baptist Memorial Hospital-East, and support for the Baptist Heart Center, making possible the purchase of a new ventricular assist device to help patients with failing hearts who are awaiting transplants.

The charitable, nonprofit BMHC Foundation solicits and manages donations for a variety of projects, which include clinical research, new equipment, education, and indigent care. Donations may be earmarked for specific purposes or may be specified for use wherever the need is greatest, and

(continues)

(continued)

they may be made in the form of gifts, grants, or bequests—including stocks, trusts, or property. Often contributions are made to honor or memorialize an individual. Donors include employees, former patients, friends, community leaders, businesses, foundations, and organizations.

The BMHC Foundation receives no financial support from Southern Baptist Conventions, nor does it receive any tax support. Salaries of the foundation staff and most other administrative costs are paid from interest earned by the endowment fund and not from contributions to the foundation. One hundred percent of a donated gift goes toward its intended purpose.

The Baptist Cancer Institute

The Baptist Memorial Health Care System created the Baptist Cancer Institute (BCI), a comprehensive cancer program so strong that people throughout the mid-South will be aware of and reassured by the competence, excellence, and comprehensiveness of the program. BCI is committed to providing mid-South physicians, cancer patients, and their families the assurance and confidence that excellent, compassionate, state-of-the-art care is nearby.

As mentioned earlier, the Baptist Memorial Health Care Foundation made a $3.1 million grant to Baptist Memorial Hospital to support the creation of BCI. This major funding will catapult Baptist Memorial Hospital to the forefront as a national center for cancer treatment and research. Consequently, more people in the mid-South region and beyond can receive high-quality treatment without having to endure the added emotional and physical stress of traveling to another cancer center in a faraway city.

Baptist Memorial Hospital has already achieved excellence in many areas of cancer care. About 2,700 new cancer cases are seen each year, and the hospital follows over 70,000 patients in its registry. BMH provides diagnosis, surgery, and treatment to can-

cer patients. What BCI will seek to do is coordinate more effectively all aspects of current cancer services, as well as broaden the reach into areas that the hospital had not focused on in the past but are needed to make the cancer program more comprehensive. Those areas include clinical research, early detection, community awareness programs, and psychosocial services.

Baptist Memorial College of Health Sciences

Baptist Memorial College of Health Sciences is a private, coeducational, urban, specialized institution. The college focuses on the preparation of health care practitioners for the southern region. It seeks to attract diverse students who demonstrate a commitment to spiritual values and ethics, academic excellence, and lifelong professional development. The educational programs of the college provide quality postsecondary, baccalaureate, and continuing education in a Christian atmosphere in order to prepare health care professionals for the community-focused health care environment of the twenty-first century. Four-year baccalaureate degrees are available in nursing, respiratory care technology, and radiological sciences.

Firsts at Baptist

- A heart-valve operation was first performed in the mid-South at Baptist Memorial Hospital in the mid-1960s.
- Dr. H. Edward Garrett, Sr., is credited with performing the first open-heart surgery in the South. The procedure was performed at BMH in 1969.
- The first dual-chamber pacemaker implantation in the mid-South was performed at BMH in 1980.
- The first rate-responsive pacemaker implantation in the mid-South and the second in the United States was performed at BMH in 1985.
- The first single lung transplant in Memphis was performed at BMH in December 1991.

(continues)

(continued)

- In 1996, BMH was the first in the mid-South region to perform MIDCAB (minimally invasive direct coronary artery bypass), Heart Port, and cardiomyoplasty procedures (specialty cardiac services).
- As of 1996, BMH is the only hospital in Memphis designated as a Medicare-approved heart transplant center.

- BMH is the only health care provider in the mid-South that has been designated as a center for the Phase III Human Cardiomyoplasty Trial. Cardiomyoplasty is a procedure reserved for patients with end-stage congestive heart failure and for whom heart transplantation is not an option.
- In 1925, BMH was the first hospital to integrate a medical office building on its campus.
- In 1960, BMH was the first hospital to use a computer system.

CHAPTER

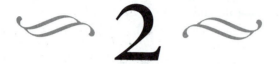

2

Health Care Costs

Chapter Objectives

After completing this chapter, the reader should have an understanding of:

- Trends in the cost of health care.
- Reasons for the rising cost of health care.
- Effects of the rising cost of health care.
- Reactions to the rising cost of health care.

INTRODUCTION

Health care cost containment has been the buzzword for over a decade in the United States. In order to understand why there is such a focus on cost containment, it is important to understand the costs associated with health care delivery. This chapter provides a background on the trends in health care costs, the causes of increases in costs, and the resources available to cover those costs.

Technological advances spawned the increased demand for medical care. The increased use of medical care, in turn, increased the cost of medical care. The technology and costs both caused major changes in the health care delivery system in the United States. Neither is the sole cause of change; together they are not the sole cause of change. Yet neither can be ignored as we move through this chapter and other considerations in this text.

TRENDS IN HEALTH CARE COSTS

If we placed a current dollar value on all goods and services produced by a country during any one year, the resulting sum would constitute what is known as the gross national product (GNP) or gross domestic product (GDP).[1] Economists have been able to use such figures as a rough index of a nation's economy, as an indication from one year to the next of the increasing or decreasing wealth in a society as measured by its productive capacity, and as a comparative measure of the economic vitality and productive

---

[1]The technical difference between the GNP and the GDP is as follows: The GNP measures what U.S. residents and corporations produced regardless of their location in the world and excludes the productivity of foreign-owned businesses in the United States; the GDP measures only the value of goods and services produced in the United States whether by U.S. or foreign-owned businesses. The figures are roughly comparable.

capacity of one country against another. The United States has historically used the GNP figure, but in late 1991 it began to switch to using the GDP. In the transition from GNP to GDP, one will find both figures used at different times for a number of years. The health sector has long accounted for one of the largest shares of the GDP in the United States as measured by the percentage of the GDP credited to it: the physicians, nurses, optometrists, dentists, therapists, and other health workers; and the hospitals, nursing homes, health insurance companies, community health agencies, public health departments, and support for medical research. The health sector has, over the years, captured a growing share of the GDP. In 1960, for example, national health expenditures constituted only 5.1 percent of the GDP. Since that time they have risen steadily, as shown in Table 2–1, to 13.5 percent in 1998 (Health Care Financing Administration, 2000). All indicators point to a continued rise.

Another important point is that the public (government) sector has, over the years, paid for an increasing share of all national health costs. In 1929, for example, only 13.6 percent of the total health expenditures were from tax sources. The 13.6 percent was for:

- the health services provided by the armed services, the Veterans Administration, and other federal government hospitals
- health services provided by state and local health departments
- care in state and local government general hospitals for psychiatric care and mental retardation

- limited monies provided by the federal government for medical research (mainly through grants)
- public health services for mothers and children

Since that time, government expenditures have risen to the point in 1998 at which government at all levels was responsible for 45.5 percent of all health expenditures. This percentage has been relatively constant since 1980 (see Table 2–1).

The rise in the government's share of the GNP for health care prior to the 1970s can be attributed to activities such as medical research; the Hill-Burton Construction Act, which for many years provided construction grant monies for hospitals and other health facilities; and such health services programs as crippled children's services, mental health, and other programs that, in their own way, added to the total public share. By 1970, we note a sharp rise in federal government expenditures. This was due largely to the implementation of Medicare and Medicaid. The growth in the public sector in subsequent years, for the most part, can be attributed to growth in the expenditures for these two programs.

By 1998, of all monies spent for health, 89 percent was for personal health care, which consists of the cost for hospital care, physician services, dental and other professional services, drugs, eyeglasses, nursing-home care, and related personal-care items (Table 2–2). Public health activities, research and construction of medical facilities, program administration, and the net cost of private health insurance

Table 2–1 National Health Expenditures Percent Distribution and Percent of Growth Domestic Product: Selected Calendar Years, 1960–1998

Item	1960	1970	1980	1985	1990	1995	1996	1997	1998
				Percent Distribution					
National health expenditures	100.0	100.0	100.0	100.0	100.0	100.0	100.0	100.0	100.0
Private	75.2	62.2	58.0	59.4	58.5	54.1	53.8	53.8	54.5
Public	25.0	38.0	42.0	40.6	40.5	45.9	46.2	46.2	45.5
				Percent of Gross Domestic Product					
National health expenditures	5.1	7.1	8.9	10.3	12.2	13.7	13.6	13.4	13.5

Source: Health Care Financing Administration, Office of the Actuary, National Health Statistics Group.

Table 2–2 National Health Expenditures, by Source of Funds and Type of Expenditure, 1998

	Total[1]	Private					Government				
		All Private Funds[2]	Consumer				Total[4]	Federal	State and Local	Medicare[5]	Medicaid
			Total[3]	Out-of-Pocket Payments	Private Health Insurance	Other					
				Amount in Billions							
National health expenditures	$1,149.1	$626.4	$574.4	$199.5	$375.0	$51.8	$522.7	$376.9	$145.8	—	—
Health services and supplies	1,113.7	613.4	574.6	199.5	375.0	38.8	500.4	360.4	140.0	$216.6	$170.6
Personal health care	1,019.3	574.5	536.5	199.5	337.0	37.9	444.9	343.6	101.3	210.5	159.6
Hospital care	382.8	149.9	130.9	12.8	118.0	19.1	232.9	187.4	45.5	123.9	60.8
Physician services	229.5	156.2	151.7	35.7	116.0	4.5	73.3	60.8	12.4	49.4	15.0
Dental services	53.8	51.5	51.3	25.8	25.5	0.2	2.3	1.3	1.0	0.1	2.0
Other professional services	66.6	52.4	47.4	27.2	20.2	5.0	14.2	11.2	3.0	9.2	1.7
Home health care	29.3	13.7	10.0	6.0	4.0	3.7	15.5	13.1	2.4	10.4	5.0
Drugs and other medical nondurables	121.9	103.1	103.1	55.4	47.8	—	18.8	10.7	8.1	1.2	15.5
Vision products and other medical durables	15.5	9.0	9.0	8.2	0.8	—	6.5	6.4	0.1	5.9	—
Nursing-home care	87.8	34.8	33.2	28.5	4.7	1.6	53.0	35.4	17.7	10.4	40.6
Other personal health care	32.1	3.8	—	—	—	3.8	28.3	17.1	11.2	—	19.0
Program Administration and net cost of private health insurance	57.7	38.9	38.0	—	38.0	0.9	18.8	12.6	6.2	6.1	11.0
Government public health activities	36.6	—	—	—	—	—	36.6	4.2	32.4	—	—
Research and construction	35.3	13.0	—	—	—	13.0	22.3	16.5	5.8	—	—
Research	19.9	1.6	—	—	—	1.6	18.3	15.5	2.8	—	—
Construction	15.5	11.5	—	—	—	11.5	4.0	1.0	3.0	—	—

Source: Health Care Financing Administration, Office of the Actuary, National Health Statistics Group.
[1]Total National Health Expenditures are the sum of all private funds and total government funds.
[2]All private funds are the total consumer funds plus other private funds.
[3]Total consumer payments are the sum of out of pocket payments plus private health insurance.
[4]Total government funds are the sum of federal and state/local funds.
[5]Medicare and Medicaid are paid by a combination of federal and state funds and are shown for illustration of spending only. They do not add up to or make up a portion of any other of the column totals.

(the difference between the premiums collected and the benefits paid) account for the remaining 11 percent.

MULTIPLE CAUSES OF INCREASED HEALTH CARE COSTS

Factors accounting for the health sector's increasing share of the nation's GDP can best be seen if we focus on personal health care expenditures, for this is where the big growth occurs. One factor in the rise in the health sector's share of the GNP is inflation—inflation that affects all sectors of the economy, as well as inflation that is specific to the health sector. Economy-wide inflation during the 1980s accounted for nearly half of the rise in personal health care costs. The cost of everything—food, electricity, telephones, gasoline, automobiles, and labor—rose. Health sector inflation stems from the introduction of new technology and the costs associated with its operation, the costs of equipment and drugs, and the rising cost of highly skilled professional personnel. As a labor-intensive sector and as a traditionally heavy employer of unskilled labor (as well as skilled labor), the health care sector is acutely sensitive to congressionally mandated raises in Social Security payroll deductions, to raises in the minimum wage, and to state or federal legislation mandating new employee benefits. Prior to the early 1990s, health care services added tens of thousands of workers nearly every month in medical offices, hospitals, home health care agencies, and so on. Growth in employment in these areas has slowed since 1992—both in numbers of persons employed and in wages paid compared to other business service areas (Engel, 1999).

Critics of the health field focus on inefficiencies that allegedly drive up costs unnecessarily. The economic pressures on the health sector since the mid-1980s have driven out the bulk of the inefficiencies that allegedly existed. Various attempts at effective cost control have included such payment mechanisms as diagnosis-related groups (discussed in more detail in Chapter 3), fixed fees, and capitation payments; and regulatory devices such as certificate of need programs, self-referral restrictions, and fraud and abuse legislation. Some of these efforts tend to suppress demand and decrease services. However, some may limit access for many who need care, thereby contributing to a lesser quality of care, and higher costs in the long run.

Inflation is not the only factor accounting for the health sector's increasing share of the GDP. Population increases contribute to increases in the use and intensity of services. There has been a continuing increase in our population, owing to a greater number of births than deaths and to more immigration than emigration. These increased numbers of people increase the basic demands on the health care system. The aging of our population also accounts for a significant share of these increased costs. People are living longer lives, but not necessarily healthy later years. Along with greater longevity comes a variety of acute and chronic debilitating diseases, the diagnosis and treatments for which are very costly.

As we look at the health sector and its rising costs, we note immediately that technological advances have been enormous: new drugs, which permit the more effective treatment of disease; organ transplants; new anesthetics that are safer and often more effective; new instrumentation, which permits the electronic monitoring of patients requiring intensive care and high-risk surgery; a variety of sophisticated diagnostic and therapeutic radiological devices (computed tomography [CT] scanners, magnetic resonance imaging [MRI] and cobalt therapy units, as well as diagnostic units that do exactly what other units do except with much less radiation exposure to the patient); autoanalyzers and an array of other laboratory equipment that allow faster, more accurate, and more sophisticated analyses; new metals and materials less toxic to the body; laser therapy and surgery; and so on.

The developmental costs of new pieces of equipment are typically high, and many require highly trained (and more costly) technicians to operate them. The very development of this new technology increases utilization and accompanying expenditures. New drugs and new anesthetics likewise frequently lead to expanded services and increased utilization and costs.

Hospitals and physicians often employ technology and use a greater number of diagnostic tests because of concern over an increase in malpractice claims. Often referred to as practicing defensive medicine, the substitution of tests for professional judgment may or may not always improve the overall quality of care, but it certainly increases costs.

There are some technological advances that increase costs but could be considered by some as unnecessary. For example, therapeutically, we could probably provide as effective care in hospitals by using the hand-cranked iron-posted beds of old instead of more expensive, electronically controlled beds in which the patient is able, by the push of a button, to raise and lower the head, the foot, and the knees. We could offer very plain rooms with multiple occupancy and few amenities. However, medical care is more than just treatment and medications, and both society and medicine have begun to realize the therapeutic benefit of a pleasant and caring environment (see Chapter 11). Medical necessity has been the definition used by health care payers, yet the comfort and caring that lead to healing are often not considered medical care.

Along with technological advances have come a number of other changes in the organization and utilization of health care services that have affected the overall cost picture. The number of patient visits to physician offices has increased. At the same time the number of hospital days has decreased, as has the average length of stay.

It is true, of course, that the way we paid for hospital care until the mid-1980s—reimbursement at cost or close to cost, or, frequently, payment of hospital charges that are above costs—encouraged expansion and did not encourage either provider or consumer economies. But this in itself should not be construed as inefficiency, though critics of the health sector are inclined to do so. In fact, the goals of health insurance and of many pieces of legislation—those that created Medicare, Medicaid, community and mental health centers, and others—were to facilitate access to care by removing the cost barriers, by assuring the hospitals through proper reimbursement that they would be able to provide all of the services necessary and of the highest quality. The enormous expansion of the National Institutes of Health (NIH) further encouraged the development of new technology. Although

mechanisms to pay the hospitals and other health care providers have changed to systems of negotiated rates and to prospective payment systems, the costs of delivering health care continue to rise.

Our population is an aging one, and the impact of this trend has been particularly significant on the overall cost picture. In 1995 there were approximately 33.5 million people of age 65 and over in the United States—about 12.8 percent of the population. After 2010, when the survivors of the Baby Boom start to enter this age group, its share of the population will begin to increase dramatically. By 2030, it is expected that 20 percent of the population will be in this age group. Large increases in the oldest of the elderly population because of longer life expectancy and the large number of people reaching the oldest ages are major causes of the higher numbers of elderly. The population aged 85 and over is the fastest-growing age group, although the population aged 100 years and over is also projected to grow substantially (U.S. Bureau of the Census, 1996).

The elderly are afflicted more than other age groups with a number of debilitating and degenerative conditions, such as heart disease and cancer, which make a heavy demand on health resources. Their conditions are more life threatening and complicated, and are often multiple. The results are longer lengths of stay in the hospital, use of more specialized hospital services, and attention of more personnel. In 1998, for example, while the average length of stay in short-stay hospitals for all patients was 4.6 days, for those 65 to 74 it was 6.2 days and for those 75 years and over it was 7.0 days (Centers for Disease Control and Prevention, 1999).

Because of advances in knowledge, surgical and anesthetic techniques, and monitoring devices, more and more elderly people can be successfully treated surgically than in years past. Consider the days of hospitalization in 1998 for an aging population:

- 611.0 days per 1,000 people for the total population
- 1,496.6 days per 1,000 people for those 65 to 74 years of age
- 2,160.8 days per 1,000 people for those 75 years and over (Centers for Disease Control and Prevention, 1999)

Considering the longer-than-average lengths of stay than in other age groups, higher surgical rates, and costs per hospital stay that average much more than the overall U.S. average, one can appreciate not only the continuing concern for the solvency of the Medicare health insurance trust fund but also the more fundamental policy question of whether we will be able to afford the continued allocation of resources at current growth rates.

Table 2–2 provides a detailed breakdown of the nation's health expenditures for 1998. The $1,019.3 billion for personal health care represents 89 percent of all monies spent that year on health. Personal health care, it should be noted, is the treatment and caring function of the health sector; it excludes public health activities, research, and construction of health facilities. Although planners are seeking to slow construction and to cut costs in other areas, the principal focus for cost containment is the personal care sector.

Hospital care accounts for $382.8 billion, or 37.6 percent, of all personal health care expenditures. Physician services come next, accounting for $229.5 billion, or 22.5 percent. Nursing-home care accounts for $87.8 billion, or 8.6 percent. These three components account for 69 percent of all personal health care expenditures, and it is these three elements that government seeks most urgently to address (see Figure 2–1). The other components of personal health care do not make a heavy demand on government resources;

therefore, the government has not paid much attention to these items. Drug and medical sundries consist of over-the-counter purchases; drugs that are provided in hospitals, nursing homes, and directly by physicians are charged to these categories. Prescription drugs are currently the focus of great concern. As new prescription drugs are developed for many conditions previously having no drug therapy, costs to consumers increase. Congress must consider adding a drug benefit because of the overwhelming costs to many seniors, while at the same time considering controlling overall health care costs. One should also note that the monies paid for salaries to hospital-based physicians appear as hospital costs, not physician services.

The first column of figures in Table 2–2 shows the total amount spent in a number of health categories. Who pays for each (the public or private sector) and how (consumer payments, health insurance, federal government, state/local government, or other groups) are shown for each category as we read across the table on each line. We might note that of the $382.8 billion spent on hospital care, about 3 percent, or $12.8 billion, was paid out of pocket because the patients had no health insurance or their benefits had been used up; because they had incurred extra charges for private rooms, telephone calls, and television rental; or because their insurance did not cover all of the charges. For the remaining costs (97 percent of the expenditures for hospital care), third parties (principally the insurance companies and government) made the payments.

Medicare accounted for 32.4 percent of all hospital expenditures, or $123.9 billion; Medicaid accounted for 15.9 percent, or $60.8 billion. Private health insurance was responsible for 30.8 percent, or $118 billion. These figures represent expenditures for hospital care, not hospital costs or hospital charges.

When we examine the physician services figures in Table 2–2, we find that patients paid $35.7 billion, or 15.6 percent, of the total $229.5 billion spent in that category. At first glance, this figure suggests how woefully inadequate health insurance is in this area. However, the figure includes copayments, or coinsurance payments, for care in physicians' offices, a type of care not usually covered by indemnity health

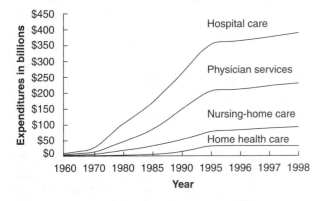

Figure 2–1 Health Expenditures, Percent Distribution and Percent of Loss Domestic Product: Selected Calendar Years, 1960–1998

insurance plans (fee for service). Many would argue that such first dollar coverage (i.e., insurance coverage for the total costs of visits to a physician's office) should not be part of any insurance package because it encourages frivolous visits to the physician, and under fee-for-service plans it encourages billing for extra visits by the physician. Under managed care plans, however, visits to the primary care physician are encouraged both for prevention of disease and early treatment, which helps avoid costly hospital care. Again, some of the out-of-pocket expenses represent payments toward deductibles or noncovered services (a more detailed explanation of insurance, Medicare, Medicaid, and managed care is provided in Chapter 3).

Under Medicare, after the deductible has been met, a physician who accepts *assignment* agrees to accept from Medicare 80 percent of what Medicare determines to be a reasonable fee, and the physician agrees to bill the patient only for the balance—that is, only 20 percent of the fee set by Medicare. In a growing number of states, state laws require physicians to accept assignment in all cases as a condition for retention of their license to practice medicine in that state. Federal legislation is lowering the amount that physicians may charge in nonassigned cases (115 percent of the approved amount). Nearly half of the Medicare population has taken out additional health insurance, which pays the deductible and the coinsurance (the 20 percent) portion of the allowed charges. These supplementary insurance policies also cover the deductible and coinsurance charges under the hospital portion of Medicare.

Another significant component of the sum paid directly by patients to physicians represents monies paid by non-Medicare patients for surgical and in-hospital medical care to cover charges over and above what the insurance company pays. Also in this category are payments by people who do not have health insurance.

Looking at nursing-home care in Table 2–2, in 1998, patients paid some 32.5 percent or $28.5 billion, of the total $87.8 billion spent in that category. Though the cost per day in a nursing home is substantially less than in a hospital, the length of stay is typically much longer, and the population in nursing homes is virtually all over sixty-five years of age. Medicare pays for skilled nursing care up to only 100 days, provided

that the patient had first spent three days in a hospital. After the twentieth day the patient has to pay a significant part of the cost. Many elderly people do not meet the initial hospitalization requirement. Other Medicare patients do not need skilled nursing care, but instead need custodial care, for which Medicare does not pay.

Though federal expenditures for nursing-home care under Medicare have been slight, under Medicaid they are substantial; the federal and state governments under the Medicaid program paid 46.2 percent of all nursing-home expenditures in 1998. Medicaid pays for intermediate and custodial care, but only after the nursing-home resident "spends down"—that is, uses any personal funds and assets available until he or she is poor enough to qualify for Medicaid funds.

Although hospital, physician, and nursing-home services make up 69 percent of health care expenditures, there are other areas that deserve attention. The rising cost of prescription drugs has gained much attention of late, particularly for senior citizens, who are often on fixed incomes and require continuing drug therapy for chronic ailments, and who are covered under Medicare, which does not cover prescription drugs. Drug coverage has been one of the primary legislative debates in the 1999–2000 congressional sessions. Another area to watch is the cost of "other professional services." As alternative medicine gains a foothold, many patients are seeking alternative treatments, and many third-party payers are willing to pay the cost of such treatment, which is often lower than the cost of traditional medical care. Included in these areas might be such services as chiropractic, massage therapy, herbal medicine, and acupuncture.

RESOURCES FOR HEALTH: ARE THERE ANY LIMITS?

The increase in health costs and the likelihood of continued increases raise the question of how much of the nation's resources should be allocated to the health sector. In 1998, 13.5 percent of the nation's GDP was spent in the health sector, a growing portion over the years. The increased spending has brought high-quality health care services to the population, contributing to its health and quality of life. But the increase in funds for health care services means less money available for other purposes.

To the extent that the consumer pays out of pocket for health care, the money cannot be spent for travel, clothes, food, transportation, entertainment, education, or a number of other things. Fortunately, the consumer has to pay for only about 17 percent of this cost directly by out-of-pocket payments (Figure 2–2). For the remainder, all citizens pay *indirectly* through taxes and in the prices paid for purchases, which usually include a component to cover the employers' contributions for employee health insurance (Moskowitz, 1999, p. 169). As the costs of health care go up and as the health care sector commands a growing percentage of the GDP, citizens pay one way or another. Although the population may feel that costs are getting out of hand, it is very likely that it is getting good value for its direct personal expenditures, as well as for its combined direct and indirect expenditures. People are nonetheless displeased when they have to spend more for insurance or out of pocket, because then other wants cannot be met. There is a certain public ambivalence about this issue. Although most Americans express concern over the rising cost of care, most still believe that the government should do more to increase access to care, and most still desire some form of universal health insurance, especially when confronted with the rising number of persons who are uninsured for health care. The philosophical desire for universal coverage is often offset by a fear of a government-controlled health care system.

Those most concerned over rising health care costs are business and industrial leaders, health insurance companies, government, those who cannot afford health insurance, and those who must purchase health insurance individually rather than as part of a group. Although the numbers have been decreasing in recent years, many large companies today pay all or part of the health insurance premiums for their employees. Company contributions are tax deductible as a bona fide business expense. In a very real sense, the company's contributions can also be viewed as nontaxable employee income. In order to increase its tax revenues, the federal government is increasingly seeking to limit the amount that business can deduct and also to tax some of these contributions as employee income. In any event, the cost of employer contributions must be recovered if the business or industry is to make a profit (see Figure 2–3). The costs are therefore built into the price of the product or service or hidden as a reduction in salaries paid to employees. The concern that employers have is that if costs continue to rise, or if the insurance benefits they pay for are expanded and cost more, the passed-on costs could jeopardize their competitive positions in the marketplace.

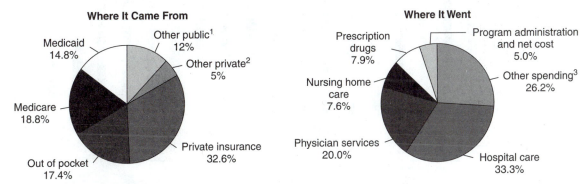

Where It Came From

- Medicaid 14.8%
- Other public[1] 12%
- Other private[2] 5%
- Medicare 18.8%
- Private insurance 32.6%
- Out of pocket 17.4%

Where It Went

- Prescription drugs 7.9%
- Program administration and net cost 5.0%
- Nursing home care 7.6%
- Other spending[3] 26.2%
- Physician services 20.0%
- Hospital care 33.3%

[1] "Other Public" includes programs such as workers' compensation, public health activity, Dept. of Defense, Dept. of Veterans, Indian Health Services, and State and local hospital and school health.
[2] "Other Private" includes industrial inplant, privately funded construction, and non-patient revenues including philanthropy.
[3] "Other Spending" includes dentist services, other professional services, home health, durable medical products, over-the-counter medicines and sundries, public health, research, and construction.
Source: Health Care Financing Administration, Office of the Actuary, National Health Statistics Group, from www.hcfa.gov/stats/nhc-oact/tables/chart.htm

Figure 2.2 The Nation's Health Dollar, 1998, Where It Came From; Where It Went.

Government, as well as others who are concerned with public policy, understands that as the health sector commands a greater share of the GDP, there will be less money in the economy for development in other sectors—improvements in public education, research, and defense, to cite just a few examples. Policy affects profitability and employment in these sectors as well as in health care. As suggested earlier, profitability is also affected if consumers cannot afford new products because of expenditures they make in the health area. Small wonder, then, that business and industrial executives are among the leaders in the drive to contain health care costs. The rise in health care costs is threatening to them.

In many cities and regions, businesses are joining together to review and define their own health plan needs. In a cooperative effort, they seek "bids" from local physician-hospital organizations (PHOs, explained more fully in Chapter 3) or commercial insurance plans for health care coverage as a group. Together, they are able to purchase more affordable health insurance, and the PHO or commercial insurer receives a larger base of clients for a given period (perhaps one or two years). Business coalitions such as these allow employers to have a greater say in defining the health plan while having leverage to control costs.

Commercial insurance companies are also unhappy about the rise in costs. As their payments rise, they must recover the costs through increased premiums from the insurance purchasers. When they raise their premiums, they run the risk of losing business to competitors, and they also get pressure from purchasers to do something about rising costs. The loss of business might entail not only health insurance but life and retirement policies as well. As nonprofit organizations, Blue Cross and Blue Shield face the additional problem of regulation by state insurance commissioners. They frequently have limits placed on the amounts they can pay in benefits and on how much they can charge for their policies; if the constraints make them less competitive, their insured may shift to the competition.

Federal, state, and local government combined paid 45.5 percent of all monies spent for health in 1998—32.8 percent federal, 12.7 percent state/local. In recent years these levels of government have sought to contain the rise in costs in several ways: through regulation (e.g., certificate of need and rate

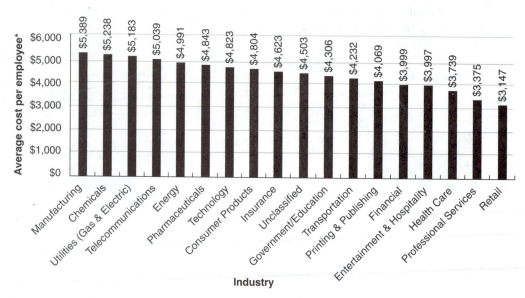

*Cost per employee represents employee claims and administration or insured premium, including managed care (HMO, POS, PPO) and indemnity.
Source: Moskowitz, D. (1999) Health Care Almanac & Yearbook, p. 169 New York: Faulkner & Gray, Inc.

Figure 2.3 Average Health Care Cost Per Employee, by Industry

control), by reducing their efforts in some areas (e.g., eliminating support for a variety of health education and health service programs), by shifting costs to the providers or to the consumers, by paying hospitals and physicians less, and by shifting the care of psychiatric patients from state psychiatric hospitals to noninstitutional and community services.

At the state level, the increases in Medicaid costs have outpaced increases in revenue in most states. The ability of a state under these circumstances to expand health services, improve education, or strengthen any of its other services is severely constrained. To trim costs, many states have moved Medicaid-eligible persons to managed care programs rather than cutting back on Medicaid eligibility and services or cutting back in other areas. Alternatively, states can raise taxes. But whatever a state does, except for securing federal action, it runs the risk of alienating voters. Legislators and governors can and have been voted out of office because of tax increases. Small wonder that federal solutions are sought; besides, the rapid rise in health care costs all started largely because of new federal initiatives.

At the federal level, the largesse began when the economy was booming and the population was expanding. In recent years, however, the economy has had its ups and downs, and the population is aging. The resulting drain on the Medicare trust fund has already been noted. A conservative ideology in the Reagan-Bush years deemphasized federal initiatives and actions in the health sector; the growing demands of other sectors precluded much action in the health area. The Clinton era, on the other hand, placed great emphasis on health care. A lengthy national debate resulted in a wide range of congressional proposals, from employer mandates to a single-payer universal health plan. A lack of consensus among competing interest groups, highly charged advertising to the public, and a very complicated (even unmanageable) proposal by the Clinton task force resulted in no action on the part of the government. Instead, market forces were allowed to take hold, resulting in a strong emphasis on managed care.

The health economist Uwe Reinhardt believes that the perceived cost crisis in health care is actually a moral crisis (Relman & Reinhardt, 1986). He points out that German and French firms pay a "larger share of the nation's health bill than do American firms." He notes that a government that spends billions of dollars in farm subsidies and other programs should be able to afford additional public health care expenditures. Reinhardt boldly describes "the dimension of the crisis before us: an apparent unwillingness of society's well-to-do to pay for the economic and medical maintenance of the poor. It is not an externally imposed economic or cost crisis; it is a moral crisis (p. 8)." Rather than face the real, troublesome issue directly, we try to "finesse" it by focusing on a symptom of the problem. The symptom is cost, and to deal with this is easier.

Increasing the share of the health sector spending denies the opportunity to fill other needs and wants. Finding the resources to permit health sector expansion requires other sectors to give up resources. The easy way out is to restrain the sector that is making the claim for additional resources.

The fight, and it is a fight, is over resources—over which sector of the economy gets a bigger piece of the pie. Ideology plays a role, as does propaganda. The health sector, we are told, is expanding too rapidly and commanding too great a share of the GDP, but on what basis is such an assertion made? Is there a right percentage? That the health sector commands more than most other nations means very little. The health sector is a major employer of both skilled and unskilled labor. Health workers pay taxes and spend money, thus fueling the nation's economy. As a heavy purchaser of supplies, drugs, and equipment, this sector generates employment in the firms that produce these goods, as well as in the construction industry because of the need for new buildings and for modernization of existing buildings. One cannot help but observe the relative ease with which a new weapons system is sold—a weapons system that may never be used—whereas the health system still has difficulty selling the need for new scanners, additional research dollars, more long-term care beds, and the community health and social services that would demonstratively be used to improve health and the quality of life in general, as well as contribute to the nation's economy.

There are inefficiencies and excesses in the health sector, but these exist in all sectors. They are not to be condoned, but should be dealt with as they are identified and as effective solutions are devised. In the battle for resources, however, the health sector has seen a great shift in societal values. The health sector now uses the language of business and economics—*cost effectiveness, marketing of services, vendor payments, multi-institutional management, corporate structure, risk management*, and the *health industry*—as though it were comparable to the automobile, banking, or airline industries. It uses businesslike language, speaking of *health sector competition, antitrust, mergers and acquisitions*, and *leveraging capital*. Health care has lost its beginnings as a social service, a societal need, and an altruistic undertaking.

Cunningham (1983) addressed this issue when he asked, "What has become of the underlying, care-before-cost philosophy—the system of motivating beliefs and concepts that created our hospitals and guided their activities for so many years? Given all the pressures of inflation, regulation, competition, and now the determination of government, insurers, and employers to cut down the amounts they are spending for health care, how could the direction of our ideas and convictions have shifted so far so fast?" (p. 88). He was concerned that the hospital has over-reacted to the pressures and that "the danger now is that there could be a confusion of means and ends; acceptance of the methods of commerce could lead to acceptance of the values of commerce" (p. 90).

Edwards, Garland, Bonazzola, and Crawshaw (1999) echoed these thoughts some fifteen years later in regard to the "I-Thou" and "I-It" attitude in the patient-physician relationship. The I-Thou attitude is one of true caring and valuing the other person. The I-It attitude regards the other person as a *thing* to be assessed, evaluated, and/or used. The authors describe the danger of a conversion of health care to business: "Unfortunately, a physician's I-Thou motivation to serve patients is susceptible to I-It conversion in response to strong and direct financial pressure from third-party payers. . . . Commercial concerns pressure doctors to see more patients, decreasing time available for each patient . . . severe time restriction is inefficient and dangerous as well as damaging to patient/physician rapport" (p. 22).

The health care sector certainly is not an island; it must coordinate with other sectors in society. In doing so, however, there is evidence to suggest that the health sector is failing to maintain and emphasize adequately the *value component* of its claim for resources, for it is the value element that can assist society in making a more balanced choice in the allocation of resources.

SUMMARY

Health care costs are increasing both in real dollars and in percent of the GDP. Economy-wide inflation, population increases, and technological advances all contribute to growth in health care spending. As additional monies are allocated to health care, other sectors of the economy do not have access to those same resources. The political dilemmas that flow from conflicting claims for use of the available monies are considerable. Though most consumers express concern over rising costs, they are insulated to a considerable extent because of their private health insurance, Medicare, Medicaid, and/or other government program protection. The principal groups that are most concerned in the clash over access to resources are business and industrial leaders, insurers, government, and those who would like to buy health insurance but cannot afford it.

Various tactics to reduce the cost of health care have been attempted, all with limited success. Price controls, reduced-payment schemes, shifting of responsibilities between and among responsible parties, and regulation have all been part of the cost containment efforts.

Most recently, competition in health care delivery has shifted the focus to outcomes analysis and treatment protocols to reduce variation in treatment. Outcomes analysis will allow health care providers to determine the highest quality of care at the lowest costs by comparing methods of treatment and eliminating ineffective, high-cost procedures and products. But outcomes analysis requires financial investment in computer technology and research personnel. Treatment protocols may be viewed by some as intrusive and a violation of both physician and patient autonomy.

The business of health care delivery, while focused on containing costs, must also emphasize quality care. Changes in the financing of health care discussed in Chapter 3, give us a better picture of the relationships among costs, quality, patient choice, and the debate over health care as a right or a privilege.

ACTIVITY-BASED LEARNING

Have you ever given much thought to the cost of health care services that you have received? Beyond the cost of your health insurance, have you ever inquired about the cost of a medical service before receiving that service?

- Consider a visit to your primary care physician. Do you pay only a flat fee (copay) at the time of the visit? What is the real charge for the visit? What does your insurance pay toward the visit? What is your reaction to the full cost? How difficult or easy would it be for you to pay the entire amount out of your pocket?
- Consider the possibility that your physician refers you to have an MRI or a mammogram. Would you call around to see how much that service costs before choosing the center where you would like to have the procedure done? If you did not (or do not) have insurance, how easy or difficult would it be for you to pay for the procedure?
- Is it even possible to find out the cost of an office visit or MRI or mammogram before making an appointment to have the procedure done? Try calling a local health care provider to find out the cost of an office visit or the cost of an MRI. Are you able to get a satisfactory answer? Would you be able to pay for the procedure? Try calling to find out the cost of a preventive screening exam. Would the cost of a colon cancer screening or a mammogram deter you from getting the service?

A QUESTION OF ETHICS

- Is health care delivery a business venture? How is it the same as any other business? How does it differ?

- How much is enough? Should we, as a society, really be concerned with how great a portion of our economy is focused on health care?
- In the last twenty to thirty years, we have achieved great advances in medical technology and the delivery of health care services. In the last twenty to thirty years, we have achieved great advances in computer technology and e-commerce. The portion of our economy applied to both industries has increased dramatically, yet we don't hear news reports and congressional hearings focused on reducing spending on computers and computing services. What is the difference?
- Is health care a *right* or a *privilege*?

References

Centers for Disease Control and Prevention. (1999, September 20). *Table 89. Discharges, days of care, and average length of stay in non-federal short stay hospitals* [On-line]. Available: www.cdc.gov/nchs/products/pubs/pubd/hus/tables (Accessed May 9, 2000).

Cunningham, R. M., Jr. (1983, 16 January). More than a business: Are hospitals forgetting their basic mission? *Hospitals*, pp. 88–90.

Edwards, M., Garland, M., Bonazzola, M., & Crawshaw, R. (1999, Fall). "Care" that cares: Medicine's essential patient-centered ethic. *Pharos*, pp. 20–23.

Engel, C. (1999, March). Health services industry: Still a job machine? *Monthly Labor Review*, pp. 3–14.

Health Care Financing Administration. (2000, January 10). The nation's health dollar: 1998. In *National health expenditures, 1998* [On-line]. Available: www.hcfa.gov/stats/nhe-act/tables/chart.htm (Accessed May 8, 2000).

Moskowitz, D. *1999 Health care almanac & yearbook*. New York: Faulkner & Gray.

Relman, A., & Reinhardt, U. (1986). Debating for-profit health care. *Health Affairs, 5*(2), pp. 5–31.

U.S. Bureau of the Census. (1996, February). *Current population reports* [On-line]. Available: www.census.gov.

CHAPTER

3

Paying for Health Care Services

Chapter Objectives

After completing this chapter, the reader should have an understanding of:

- The origin and development of health insurance in the United States.
- The variety of health insurance plans available.
- The government programs of Medicare and Medicaid.
- How health care providers are paid.
- Problems inherent in each of the health insurance plans and payment mechanisms.

INTRODUCTION

Estimates vary concerning how many people in the United States are protected against the costs of health care. Some say that insurance and government programs cover about 85 percent of the U.S. resident population, leaving over 43 million Americans without any protection at all ("Uninsured Grab Federal Policy Spotlight Again," 1999). Although the exact figures may change depending on the source of data, the fact remains that many people are still unprotected from health care costs and must rely on whatever out-of-

pocket funds they might have available to them or on charity to pay for care. For some of the unprotected, securing access to care can be difficult. Even among those who are insured or enrolled in a government program, we find those who are underinsured and do not have adequate protection against hospital, physician, nursing-home, dental, and drug charges. There are shortcomings in both private insurance and government programs, and these should be a cause for social concern.

THE INSURED POPULATION

The United States has what is primarily an employment-based health insurance system. The majority of people who have health insurance obtain it through their place of employment (*group policies*). Some policies, however, are taken out on a nongroup basis (*individual policies*) by the self-employed and others who are not eligible for group enrollment. The principal differences between group and individual coverage are that group insurance generally costs less and has a broader range of benefits.

Most insured people (an estimated 166 million in 1997) have what is referred to as private insurance—policies with Blue Cross and Blue Shield or one of the large commercial insurance companies (Aetna, Prudential, Cigna, etc.). Some 35.8 million people were protected against health care costs in 1998 under the Medicare program, a government entitlement program principally for those over the age of sixty-five, which also protects a small number of younger people (approximately 3 million) who fall into certain disability categories. Another 278.8 million people received benefits in 1998 under Medicaid, a federal/state government program designed to pay for health care for certain categories of the very poor. Many of these people (some 3.1 million) were Medicare enrollees who became eligible for Medicaid because of their low income (U.S. Census Bureau, 1999).

Protection against health care costs is also available through various other government programs: for military personnel; for their dependents in the military system and through a program known as the Civilian Health and Medical Program of the Uniformed Services (CHAMPUS); for Native Americans and Alaskan Natives through the Indian Health Service; for veterans who are totally dependent on the Veterans Administration system for care; and for long-term residents of federal, state, and local psychiatric hospitals and prisons.

We must emphasize that the figures cited about the number insured and otherwise protected are estimates, and the estimates vary depending on the rate of unemployment in the country, business conditions, and the changing eligibility standards for Medicaid and other government programs. Those not protected by health insurance or by government programs are not only the unemployed. They also include part-time employees, people between jobs, employed persons whose incomes are too high to qualify for Medicaid but not high enough to afford health insurance, those working in some small businesses that do not offer health insurance, and some who choose not to have health insurance. In fact, most of those without insurance in 1998 were in paid employment (see Figure 3–1).

People who have the protection of health insurance often feel a sense of satisfaction, but inadequate coverage against the costs of medical care can be a cause for great social concern. Some health insurance policies exclude coverage for conditions that existed at the time of enrollment (preexisting conditions). Other policies insist that the insured must wait a cer-

tain period of time (typically one year) before a pre-existing condition is covered. Most policies place a limit on how much is paid for hospital care, physician care, nursing-home care, and the like through annual limits, lifetime limits, and/or fee schedules. In an effort to make consumers more aware of health care costs and therefore more responsible health care consumers, many policies require portions of the costs to be paid by the insured, including the following:

- **Deductibles:** money the patient must pay before the insurance policy provides benefits
- **Coinsurance:** a percentage of the costs of each service that must be paid by the insured along with the insurance policy payment (e.g., a payment of 80 percent of the cost by the insurance and 20 percent of the cost by the consumer)
- **Copay:** a flat fee paid for each type of service (e.g., the patient pays $10 for each physician visit or $5 for each prescription filled)

Why do we have such a variety of policies with so many limitations that ultimately force the patient or patient's family to meet a significant portion of the costs of care? Why can't we have a comprehensive benefit structure for all people? What good is all the insurance if it does not *protect?*

The answers to these questions are rooted in at least two factors: social choice and historical developments that shaped the health insurance industry. Victor Fuchs, in his book *Who Shall Live?* (1974), offers this explanation as it relates to social choice:

> The most basic level of choice is between health and other goals. While social reformers tell us that "health is a right," the realization of that "right" is always less than complete because some of the resources that could be used for health are allocated to other purposes. This is true in all countries regardless of economic system, regardless of the way medical care is organized, and regardless of the level of affluence. It is true in the communist Soviet Union and in welfare-state Sweden, as well as in our own capitalist society. No country is as healthy as it could be; no country does as much for the sick as it is technically capable of doing.
>
> The constraints imposed by resource limitations are manifest not only in the absence of amenities,

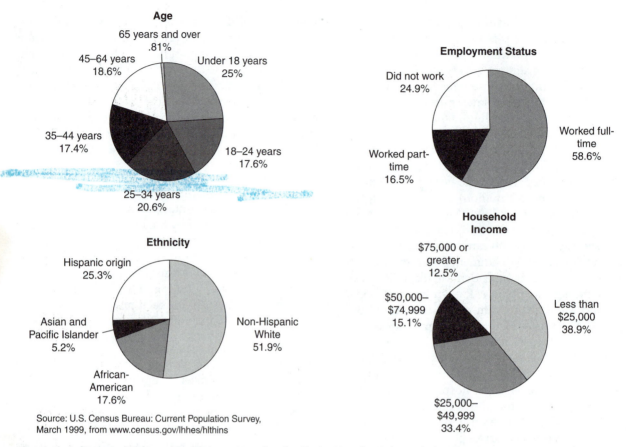

Figure 3–1 Persons Without Health Insurance for the Entire Year, by Selected Characteristics, 1998

delays in receipt of care, and minor inconveniences; they also result in loss of life. The grim fact is that no nation is wealthy enough to avoid all avoidable deaths. . . .

Within limits set by genetic factors, climate, and other natural forces, every nation chooses its own death rate by its evaluation of health compared with other goals. . . . If better health is our goal, we can achieve it, but only at some cost. (pp. 17–19)

Although most Americans express concern over the numbers of uninsured, we have been unwilling to provide comprehensive coverage even for a limited population group—the elderly. As each year passes, benefits are cut and the elderly are forced to pay more. In theory, universal health care coverage is desirable. However, fear of increased taxes, government control, and loss of some benefits by those with extensive health insurance, prevents us from moving toward implementing the theory.

A second answer to the questions posed earlier lies in the history of health insurance in the United States, and in the principles of health insurance rate structuring.

HISTORY OF HEALTH INSURANCE

The year 1929 is generally credited as marking the birth of modern health insurance. It was in that year that Justin Ford Kimball established a hospital insurance plan at the Baylor University Hospital for the schoolteachers of Dallas, Texas. As a one-time superintendent of the Dallas public schools, he was sensitive to the plight of schoolteachers, particularly so when he found many of them had unpaid bills at the hospital. Working from hospital records, he calculated that the schoolteachers as a group "incurred an average of 15 cents a month in hospital bills. To assure a safe margin, he established a rate of 50 cents a month" (Anderson, 1975, p. 19). In return, the schoolteachers were assured twenty-one days of hospitalization in a semiprivate room.

Kimball's success spread, and over the years his approach was the model for what became the Blue Cross plans around the country: the concept of assuring the benefit not of cash but of *service,* the emphasis on semiprivate accommodations, and even the time frame of twenty-one days of benefits.

Though 1929 is cited as the beginning, there were antecedents. Anderson (1975) notes, for example:

> Between 1916 and 1918, attempts were made by 16 state legislatures from New York to California to establish some form of compulsory health insurance, essentially a mechanism to help families pay for health services, which were already being felt as costly and unpredictable episodes. The necessary mass political support in the states was not present, however, and the solid opposition of the American Medical Association, insurance companies, and the pharmaceutical industry, not to mention business and industry opposed to unaccustomed payroll taxes, stopped the movement. (p. 17)

The Health Insurance Institute (1978) also cites antecedents:

> When health insurance began some 130 years ago, it met a far simpler need—coverage against rail and steamboat accidents. The nation's first health insurance company came into being in 1847. Three years later another company was organized specifically to write accident insurance. By 1864, coverages were available for virtually every type of accident. At the turn of the century, 47 companies were issuing accident insurance.
>
> In addition, the mutual aid society concept, which originated in Europe, was adopted in the United States in the latter half of the 1800s. Small contributions were collected from members of workers' groups in return for the promise to pay

cash benefits for disability through accident or sickness. Fraternal benefit societies also were important early providers of health insurance in the U.S.

Mutual benefit associations, or "establishment funds," began in 1875 in the United States. These funds—sometimes financed partially by employers—provided small payments for death or disability of workers in a single organization.

Both accident insurance companies and life insurance companies entered the health insurance field in the early 1900s. At the beginning, the insurance largely covered the policyholders' loss of earned income due to a limited number of diseases, among them typhus, typhoid, scarlet fever, smallpox, diphtheria, and diabetes. . . .

This was the birth of modern health insurance. The demand for the new product grew as the Depression of the 1930s deepened. Out of this emerged the Blue Cross service concept, which foreshadowed insurance company reimbursement policies for hospital and surgical care. Also during the 1930s, insurance companies began to emphasize the availability of cash benefit plans for hospital, surgical, and medical expenses. The first Blue Shield type of plan for surgical and medical expenses was formed in 1939. (p. 7)

In addition, there was the single hospital benefit plan organized in 1912 at Rockford, Illinois; the Grinnell, Iowa, hospital plan in 1921; and the Brattleboro, Vermont, plan in 1927. Each offered payment for limited hospital services. But the idea as developed at Baylor by Kimball was the model that spread. The American Hospital Association (AHA) asked Kimball to describe the Baylor plan at its annual meeting in 1931. Other hospital people also developed interest, and by 1935 there were fifteen hospital insurance plans in eleven states, and six additional plans developed during 1936. "Concurrently, there was a move to create a coordinating agency of some sort to give the now rapidly growing movement a national focus and a broad base" (Anderson, 1975 p. 36). This was done within the framework of the AHA, evolving over the years to a semiautonomous body and eventually to a completely independent Blue Cross Commission and, later, Blue Cross Association.

Anderson notes that the early leadership came not from hospitals but from early pioneers, farsighted individuals, some of whom were hospital account-ants. The hospitals, says Anderson, were "timid in their backing of prepayment." It was, after all, a new idea, an experiment. "Originally, the plans covered only employees and not their dependents; the de-pendents were an unknown and feared quantity ac-tuarially. But common sense and equity would shortly have it that dependents should be covered too, and so they were" (Anderson, 1975, p. 43).

The Blue Cross movement surged ahead in the 1940s, with a nationwide enrollment of 6 million sub-scribers in 1940 spread through 56 independent Blue Cross plans. "By 1945, the enrollment was up to 19 million in 80 plans, and by the early 1950s, it was 40 million. By that time, private insurance companies were also coming up from behind after an early lack of interest in insuring against hospital costs" (Ander-son, 1975, p. 45).

The Health Insurance Institute (1978) states:

> During World War II, as a result of the freezing of wages, group health insurance became an important component of collective bargaining. Even greater impetus came in the postwar era when the U.S. Supreme Court ruled that employee benefits, including health insurance, were a legitimate part of the labor-management bargaining process.
>
> After that, health insurance protection expanded rapidly. For instance, in 1950 some 77 million people had hospital expense insurance. By 1976, some 177 million Americans were protected, or more than eight out of ten of the civilian non-institutional population.
>
> Traditionally, the greatest emphasis has been on hospital coverage because health services revolve around the hospital as the center of medical technology. The dramatic progress of surgery and its increasing cost also spurred the demand for insurance for these expenses. In 1950, 54 million people had surgical expense insurance. By 1976, this coverage had tripled, with 167 million having such protection. In 1950, more than 21 million people had coverage for physicians' fees other than surgery. In 1976, 163 million persons were covered. (p. 8)

As Blue Cross began to demonstrate the feasibility of covering hospital expenses through the insurance mechanism, pressures to do likewise for physician services also developed. The pressures accelerated following the 1932 report of the Committee on Costs of Medical Care, with its challenge to organized med-icine. In 1939 the California Medical Association es-tablished the California Physicians Service, which was the first of what became known as the Blue Shield plans for payment of doctors' bills. Like Blue Cross, Blue Shield operated on a *service benefits* principle: The California plan provided complete physician services at a rate of $1.70 per month (Hawley, 1949):

> Enrollment was limited to employed persons earning less than $3,000 per year. Physicians were reimbursed on a "unit" basis, the unit having a par value of $2.50 (the fee for an office visit), with other services being valued at multiples of this unit (unit value scale). Experience in the early years, however, was unfavor-able, as demand of services far exceeded expectations, and the effect was to devalue the unit. So, beginning in 1941, all contracts were modified. (p. 36)

We might digress for a moment to note two things. First, California developed the unit-value scale. (A similar concept known as the relative-value scale was developed for Medicare in the 1990s and will be de-scribed later in this chapter, in the "Paying Physi-cians" section.) Most Blue Shield plans did not, how-ever, use this method for establishing their schedules of payments. Second, the need to devalue the unit was acceptable to the medical profession because the plan was medical society sponsored: The physicians were obligated to deliver the service regardless of what the plan could pay. Such an arrangement is ac-ceptable if one has a say in the management, as the physicians did. Throughout the Blue Shield move-ment, physicians had dominated the boards of direc-tors not only because they underwrote the plan but also because the plans were truly *their* response to the challenge for national health insurance and because the plans met the AMA principles of keeping medical matters in the hands of physicians.

A similar situation existed with Blue Cross. The participating hospitals agreed to accept the Blue Cross payment as full payment for care in a semipri-vate room. If the Blue Cross plan could not pay the agreed-upon cost, then the hospital would accept whatever Blue Cross could pay and *not* bill the patient for any additional monies. Thus, Blue Cross offered its subscribers *service benefits* rather than lump-sum or *indemnity benefits*. In the early days of Blue Cross, quite a few plans had to pay hospitals less than 100 cents on the dollar, and hospitals tended to dominate Blue Cross boards. Both Blue Cross and Blue Shield have changed or are in the process of changing their board structures because the underwriting of the plan by the providers of service is now less a fact of life. We might note here that even when Blue Cross paid a hospital full cost, it was frequently discounted. Since the hospital was assured payment, the discounted amount was acceptable.

Medical society sponsorship of the Blue Shield plans had its origins as early as 1917 in the state of Washington. There, county medical societies established "county medical service bureaus" that contracted with employers to provide medical care for employees. According to Hawley (1949), these bureaus developed as a result of competitive abuses that arose among some of the medical care plans in the state.

Both Blue Cross and Blue Shield were service-benefit plans, relying mainly on type of accommodation (semiprivate room) as the determinant of service-benefit eligibility. Blue Shield relied on income of the patient or patient's family. Blue Cross provided benefits for subscribers who used private rooms, and Blue Shield provided benefits for patients who were above income by having the patient pay the additional charges, if any.

Blue Cross worked quite well. The Blue Shield service-benefit principle did not work well. The reasons for this failure were historical and developmental. When Blue Shield first began, physicians commonly charged patients on a sliding fee scale: charging the wealthy more to pay for care of the poor, and so on. The early Blue Shield payments for various services were designed for the going rate in the ser-vice-benefit income category. As the economy developed, and along with it inflation, the Blue Shield schedule of payments provided service-benefit payments for fewer and fewer subscribers because they were increasingly above the maximum income. Blue Shield made the same dollar payment for services rendered, but because the patient was above the

service-benefit income level, the patient frequently had to pay an additional amount to the physician.

This situation led some Blue Shield plans to develop different types of contracts with different service-benefit income levels, allowance schedules geared to each level, and, of course, premiums geared to the allowances. But still the Blue Shield service benefits, when geared to subscriber income, did not work well because of inflation and the difficulties in determining subscriber income. It was left to the patient to discuss his or her income level with the physician, and both parties were reluctant to talk about money when the patient was sick. Resulting misunderstandings were common. In time, many Blue Shield plans (as well as commercial insurance and eventually Medicare) developed contracts with *usual, customary,* and *reasonable* (UCR) allowances (this will be described further in the "Methods of Paying for Health Care Services" section later in this chapter).

Another problem faced by Blue Shield with regard to service benefits developed as a result of the changing health system. Initially, radiology, pathology, and anesthesiology were hospital services covered by Blue Cross. During the 1950s and 1960s, many of the hospital-based physicians in these specialties moved out from under the hospital umbrella to do their own billing while still housed in the hospital, and many also established their own offices. Blue Cross generally was not allowed by law to pay for physician services as such, but only for hospital services. Blue Shield rate structures were not geared to pay these professional services because they had never been calculated or anticipated in structuring of the rates. For a while, the subscribers were caught in a bind and had to pay the bills until Blue Shield was able to adjust its rates to incorporate these benefits. But then Blue Shield had to get the groups, mainly the employers, to go along with the increased rates. As one can imagine, not all were willing to do so unless they had to, and those who worked with unions would not do so until the next round of collective-bargaining sessions began, when these new benefits could become a management concession.

Both Blue Cross and Blue Shield also faced similar situations in later years as new, often expensive, technology developed. If they paid for equipment under existing rates because payments were close to or at cost, hospitals would be encouraged to expand and pass the increased costs on to Blue Cross. The new equipment would be averaged with all other costs and be built into what all admissions would cost. If Blue Cross covered such items, a rate increase would eventually be necessary, and a rate increase would give competitors an advantage. The pressures on both Blue Cross and Blue Shield became even more acute as they acted as fiscal intermediaries (the agency handling the payments) for Medicare. The federal government sought to pressure the Blues (a term frequently used for the Blue Cross/Blue Shield movement) and others to stem rising costs. Pressure also came from state governments, which were affected by the rising costs of Medicaid. If the Blues held the line, the federal/state Medicaid program would benefit.

Generally, the Blue Cross plans provided great support and assistance to the developing Blue Shield plans. Typically, they used the same salaried sales forces, the same personnel systems, the same offices, and sometimes the same executive staffs. Although the governing boards were generally different and the corporations generally separate from a legal standpoint, in nearly all states special enabling legislation for both plans made them legally different from ordinary insurance companies. In some states, there were bitter conflicts between the Blue Cross plan and local medical societies that sponsored Blue Shield. These conflicts even reached the national level in 1948, for example, when the AMA opposed a proposed merger of Blue Cross and Blue Shield at the national level for purposes of enrolling national accounts.

Why the conflict? The AMA's position was based on fear that it would be accused of restraint of trade, and well it might have been. It also feared that Blue Cross, representing the hospitals, would dominate the national joint venture, and the views of medicine would not be adequately represented (Anderson, 1975). Like the conflicts within the states, this reflected an age-old fear on the part of physicians that nonmedical people would tell doctors how to practice medicine. Hospitals, by the same token, were wary of physicians telling them how to run the hospital. Such conflicts become more pronounced as one moves up the hierarchies. In small towns, the physicians and

hospital people may get along fine (but not always) in their small hospital. As organizations become larger, the need for a bureaucracy develops and, with it, the insensitivities, misunderstandings, and resulting fears that pervade all large social institutions and organizational arrangements.

Though a mechanism for enrolling national accounts was eventually successful, not until 1978 was there a successful merger of the national Blue Shield and Blue Cross organizations. Part of the reason for the successful merger was that by 1978, under pressures from state insurance departments and the federal government, the Blue Cross and Blue Shield plans were less than surrogates for the providers; they were becoming true third-party payers.

HEALTH INSURANCE RATE STRUCTURING (PREMIUM CALCULATION)

Premium errors in the early days of Blue Cross came about because the plans did not have a reliable statistical base available for predicting what their utilization would be. No one else had the data either. Thus, for a given premium, should Blue Cross provide fourteen days of in-hospital care or twenty-one days or thirty days? Should it cover maternity? What about medical conditions that exist at the time a person joins Blue Cross? If a preexisting condition exists when a person joins? Should that person have to wait a period of time before the condition is covered, or can it be covered immediately? A great deal of information had to be weighed into the equation for calculating what the premium should be.

To illustrate this dilemma in simple form, let us suppose that a community of 100 people is debating whether or not to join Blue Cross and be covered for only one kind of hospitalization: removal of the gallbladder. Let us further assume that the cost of care in the hospital is $200 a day and that, on the average, a person who has undergone gallbladder removal stays in the hospital for five days. Let us further assume that, on the average, one can predict five cases a year for every 100 people.

Given these assumptions, Blue Cross could anticipate for that community a cost of $200/day × 5 days × 5 cases, or $5,000. But the laws governing Blue

Cross as a nonprofit company generally require Blue Cross to set aside an additional sum of money for the unforeseen. This would be a *contingency fund,* or *reserves.* In this instance, the law might require Blue Cross to provide for a possible sixth case, thus another $1,000. In addition, the people at Blue Cross have to live; they need income and therefore must be paid for their services, which include selling the policy, negotiating with the hospital, and administering the claims. They also need an office in which to work, and that means rent, electricity, fuel bills, and so on. Typically, for Blue Cross these costs amount to about 6 percent of its income. Thus, in this case we must add about $360 for administration. The total cost to Blue Cross would thus come to $6,360.

Blue Cross can thus say to the community: We calculated a rate; it is a *community rate* to cover all of you for gallbladder removal. Since there are 100 people, it will cost each of you $63.60 a year for coverage, about 17 cents a day. That will cover you only for hospital care relating to gallbladder removal. It will not cover the doctor's bill or other conditions or admissions for gallbladder when surgery is not performed. You get what you pay for, and all you are paying for is gallbladder surgery. If all of you join *now,* you will be covered immediately—no waiting periods—and all of you are covered even if you have gallbladder problems before joining. We can do this because you represent the average, and we have calculated our premium rate on that basis.

It is this kind of exercise that Blue Cross went through originally in deciding how much to charge and for what. In real life, however, it was much more complicated because Blue Cross covered most acute conditions. Moreover, because Blue Cross worked with the community rate idea, in the beginning it enrolled not communities but representative bodies or groups of the community—typically, groups of employees.

Let us carry our hypothetical model a step further. Let us suppose that not everyone in the community or group of 100 wants to join. Let us suppose that only 20 people choose to do so. Blue Cross would probably refuse to let only 20 people join, because the group of 20 is not a community average and thus does not meet requirements of a community rate. In all probability, more than one gallbladder case would occur in the 20

people. Blue Cross would probably not allow a group such as this to be organized even at a higher rate. But let us suppose that instead of only 20, 60 people want to join. Now Blue Cross has a problem. Is an average of 60 people enough? Probably not. But can't the rate be tinkered with to make the group financially acceptable? Though each Blue Cross plan has its own enrollment requirements, in this hypothetical case Blue Cross might well say that it could enroll the group of 60 but that the rate would have to be adapted. Blue Cross could change the rate or impose an eleven-month waiting period for preexisting conditions—in this case, for any gallbladder surgery— if the subscriber had any reason to believe he or she had abdominal problems.

Let us assume now that in the next isolated community or employee group, there are four people. They hear about the Blue Cross coverage and seek to join. But here Blue Cross would probably say that a community or group of four is not typical for its rate. However, Blue Cross might say that if any member of that group of four wants to join, it will write an individual contract or policy, but it will not cover any gallbladder operation if the subscriber has reason to believe something is amiss. Moreover, Blue Cross will charge more for the policy because of higher risks and higher administrative costs (contracting, billing, and so on for four individual policies rather than one group). Thus, Blue Cross and Blue Shield typically offer *nongroup* enrollment for those who are not eligible for *group* enrollment. But what about that group of 20 people? They cannot get nongroup enrollment because Blue Cross must rely on group enrollment if it is to succeed in its mission of covering everyone at a community rate. By denying the 20, Blue Cross will encourage them to become a pressure group within the larger group, agitating for more people to seek Blue Cross enrollment.

We can appreciate the need for minimum enrollment if we make another assumption. Let us suppose that two more groups of 100 people each want to join, and let us assume that all 100 join in each group. The two groups contribute $2,000 to the contingency fund. The first group (60 subscribers) also probably contributes to that fund. We do not know for sure, but the waiting period (the Blue Cross equalizer) has probably assured us that instead of five cases, there will be only three. Proportionally, $600 from the 60-person group would go into the contingency fund. Thus, there would be $2,600 in the fund.

Let us further suppose that a fourth group, also of 100, joins. As the year progresses, Blue Cross may find that this group has many more than five gallbladder operations. Let us say it has eight. The group's premiums cover five of those operations; the group's contingency fund contribution covers a sixth. That would leave Blue Cross $2,000 short if it did not have the contributions from the other groups to cover the high-utilization group. If there were no other groups, but only this group with eight operations, Blue Cross would have to seek a rate increase, and it might have to ask the hospital this year to underwrite the Blue Cross policy by accepting $6,000 as though $8,000 were paid. If Blue Cross had not adhered to its enrollment minimum, it would have fewer reserves and would have less money to pay the hospital. One can say, in fact, that enrollment minimums not only protect the hospital but also protect the subscribers against rate increases. This is how Blue Cross and Blue Shield developed. They gambled, they made mistakes, but they won more than they lost.

Enter now another complication. Let us suppose that one of our groups of 100 is a community of young people in their twenties working for the same company. The employer provides them with Blue Cross coverage, as well as a life insurance policy and a good retirement plan. The complication is that another large insurance company would love to get the insurance policy and the retirement plan away from a competitor. It has a handle on this business by way of health insurance. It could offer a health insurance policy with about the same benefits as Blue Cross at a lower cost because the group is low risk. It would base its rate on the group's experience (or performance). Alternatively, the insurance company could charge the same as Blue Cross but provide greater benefits. The commercial company does not need the unused premium money from the low-risk group to carry the losses incurred with a high-risk group, as does Blue Cross. If the commercial company enrolled a high-risk group, its rate would bear a relationship to its experience or anticipated claims performance.

With an experience-rated policy, the commercial insurance company is thus not likely to lose, even if it does not get the life policy and retirement plan business. At worst, it takes a loss for one year only and then adjusts its premiums accordingly the next year. But what is the effect on Blue Cross? Blue Cross does not have as much money in the contingency fund. If, moreover, the competition takes away too many low-risk groups, Blue Cross is forced to seek a rate increase that, in turn, might make it noncompetitive.

Blue Cross has thus had to engage in experience rating also, simply to remain competitive and to keep a contingency fund. But the process has undermined the concept of the community rate and has driven up health insurance costs. The result is higher premiums for those who are sicker.

In practice, the group commercial insurance companies did not provide quite as high a ratio of benefits on the income dollar as Blue Cross and Blue Shield. Their indemnity benefit packages were, however, typically very good. In many cases, the competition stimulated Blue Cross and Blue Shield to do better, but it also had adverse cost effects on some groups because the community rate concept was undermined.

In recent years, the underwriting by hospitals and physicians has been inconsequential because the economic pressures that exist today prevent any subsidization. Hospitals and doctors do not subsidize the inability of Blue Cross or Blue Shield to pay 100 cents on the dollar. Instead, rates rise, and subsidization by hospitals can be considered a luxury. As noted earlier, even in the best of times, in many areas the Blue Cross plan never paid hospitals 100 cents on the dollar but negotiated a discounted rate because Blue Cross was assuring payment.

HEALTH INSURANCE TODAY

At one time, we could describe four basic groups that provided protection against the costs of health care services: commercial insurance companies, the non-profit Blue Cross and Blue Shield plans, health maintenance organizations (HMOs), and government plans. However, changes have occurred among third-party payers just as they have occurred among health care delivery organizations. Many new forms and many hybrid forms of health plans are now available. We have already discussed the development of Blue Cross and Blue shield at length, but let us continue now with a description of the early forms of health plans and then move on to more contemporary forms.

Commercial Insurance

Most private health insurance companies (commercial insurance companies) restrict their business to group coverage, generally through place of employment; Aetna, Prudential, and Cigna are examples of such companies. Other companies focus primarily on individual policies, and the benefits of these nongroup plans tend to be most limited in terms of the amounts paid for care, the types of care covered, and who can get coverage.

The group commercial companies, because they emphasize group enrollment, are able to be less restrictive. If a large group is enrolled, then all members of the group can be enrolled and no person will normally be excluded because of poor health. Some group commercial companies selectively exclude people with health problems from enrolling in small employee groups or charge higher rates than for the rest of the small group members. This practice, known as *selective medical underwriting*, was designed to hold down the cost of the insurance for other employees. This practice of excluding individuals out of small groups undermines the very purpose of insurance as a way to spread the risk. Concern over selective underwriting has led many states to prohibit the practice.

The benefits provided by the group insurance companies tend to be more liberal than those provided by nongroup companies, but what is covered and what is not vary depending on what the group wants and is willing to pay for. As with Blue Cross and Blue Shield, the benefits may vary in terms of the number of days covered in hospital, the dollar amounts paid for surgical and medical care, whether home and office medical care is included, and whether nursing-home care, visiting-nurse services, dental, vision, and major medical expenses are covered.

Nearly all people enrolled in commercial insurance plans and the nonprofit Blue Cross and Blue Shield plans are covered for hospital and physician care; lesser numbers are covered for dental and eye care, though such coverage is growing. *Major medical expense insurance*, sometimes called *catastrophic insurance*, was first introduced in 1951 by the commercial companies and also became available through Blue Cross and Blue Shield plans. Typically, major medical insurance covers 80 percent of all residual medical expenses (i.e., it covers 80 percent of all expenses not covered by the regular hospital, medical, and surgical policies) after the insured pays the deductible. The deductible may vary from $100 to $200 or more, depending on what the group wants and is willing to pay for. For catastrophic illness, the bills can mount, so these policies tend to pay 80 percent up to a maximum of perhaps $250,000 or more.

Both deductibles and coinsurance are mechanisms designed to limit costs and to give greater responsibility for the use of services to the insured. The assumption is that the insured will not likely incur unnecessary expense for overuse of medical care. To the extent that these mechanisms are successful, we can appreciate them; but for the person who really needs the added services, the costs can be significant, and deterrence may not be in the best interest of the patient. In recognition of this problem, many policies now set a limit of $2,000 to $3,000, which the patient has to pay, after which the policies pay all costs. When the payment of costs is shared between an insurance company and the patient, or between two companies, it is said that the policy is *coinsured.*

Insurance companies are regulated by the states. Each state sets standards for fiduciary responsibilities, minimum coverage, reporting responsibilities, disclosure responsibilities to policyholders, and so on. Within this framework, large interstate businesses have difficulty complying with multistate regulations when providing health insurance benefits to employees in diverse locations (e.g., large companies like AT&T or General Electric have plants and offices in many states). In 1974, Congress passed the Employee Retirement Income Security Act (ERISA). Although a major thrust of the legislation was to set standards for securing retirement plan funds, the act also set regulations by which employers could establish self-insured health benefits plans. In other words, employers could set aside funds to pay for employees' medical expenses and pay them directly from the fund rather than purchasing a group plan from an insurance company. Self-insured plans were defined as *employee health benefits plans* and differentiated from *health insurance*. As such, health benefits plans were exempt from state regulations. Interstate employers could thus set up plans that were the same for all of their employees without regard to their geographic location.

ERISA also provided other benefits to employers who self-insured. Not only did it remove state regulation from the benefits plans, but the federal regulations covering these plans were very liberal. Federal regulations addressed the process rather than the content of employee benefits plans—reporting requirements, disclosure, and fiduciary conduct. Unlike state regulations, the federal regulations did little to set standards for minimum coverage or reduction or termination of benefits. Employers had more latitude in deciding just what procedures and/or treatments would be covered by the benefits plans.

Employer self-insured plans are often difficult to differentiate from health insurance for employees because employers often contract with well-known insurance companies to administer their plans. But the difference is significant operationally. Although the issue is outside the scope of discussion in this text, ERISA has become problematic when states attempt to establish statewide universal health insurance for all residents because ERISA exempts employee benefits plans from any state regulations.

Government Plans

Government plans fall into another category of third-party payers for health care. In this category are a number of programs that have already been cited, such as those for military personnel and their dependents; for veterans for service-connected disabilities and for non-service-connected disabilities if they are unable to afford private care; and for Native Americans and Alaskan Natives. But the principal programs with which we are concerned are *Medicare*

and *Medicaid*. These programs were established when Congress amended the Social Security Act in 1965, adding to it Title XVIII (Medicare legislation) and Title XIX (Medicaid legislation).

Medicare

Medicare is a health insurance program for persons age sixty-five and above, regardless of income or wealth. In 1972, provisions were added to cover people under sixty-five who are entitled to Social Security or Railroad Retirement disability benefits for at least two consecutive years, and those who suffer from end-stage renal (kidney) disease (ESRD) that requires a kidney transplant or routine dialysis treatment.

Medicare consists of two parts: Part A primarily for inpatient care, and Part B for ambulatory care. Part A provides coverage for in-hospital care, skilled nursing care, hospice, and home health care. Part A benefits are financed by Social Security taxes, require no premium payment by the beneficiary, and are automatic for those sixty-five and over. Although Medicare provides health care coverage without a premium cost to the beneficiary, it is not by any means free health care. Benefits include deductibles and coinsurance provisions. Some of the benefits (for the year 2000) are as follows (Health Care Financing Administration, 1999a):

- **Up to 90 days of inpatient care for each benefit period.** A new benefit period begins after the patient has been out of hospital and/or skilled nursing facility for 60 consecutive days. The inpatient hospital deductible is $776 for each benefit period. There is also a $194-a-day coinsurance for the sixty-first through ninetieth days, and a $388-a-day coinsurance for each "nonrenewable, lifetime reserve day (60 extra days of hospitalization)."
- **Up to 100 days in a skilled nursing facility,** with Medicare paying the full cost for the first 20 days and the patient paying $97 a day for each day thereafter. To be eligible for this benefit, the patient must have been in the hospital for three consecutive days prior to being transferred to skilled nursing care.
- **Unlimited home health visits by a participating home health agency** for *part-time* skilled nursing care, physical therapy, or speech therapy for patients

confined to their home and certified as needed by a physician. The deductible does not apply to home health visits.

- **Hospice care in a home or homelike environment for the terminally ill.** A wide range of medical and social services is available, including medical, nursing, and social work services, respite care, and short-term inpatient care, as well as homemaker services. All services are available without charge to the patient except for some sharing of the cost for outpatient drugs and inpatient respite care.

Many of the elderly have additional insurance to cover the Medicare deductibles and copayments (referred to as Medigap, or Medicare supplemental insurance). A small number of people over sixty-five who are not automatically eligible for Medicare because they had insufficient work experience to accumulate the necessary Social Security credits may get Medicare coverage by paying a monthly premium ($301 in 2000).

There is one additional factor that Medicare beneficiaries must bear in mind: Hospital care must be needed and must be a type of care that can be provided only by a hospital. If the hospital's utilization review committee or another peer review organization (PRO) does not approve the hospital stay (determines that inpatient care was not needed) after the patient's admission, then there can be a retroactive denial of benefits, and the patient may have to pay all costs or the hospital may have to bear the loss.

Part B of Medicare is supplementary medical insurance; it is optional, and Part A beneficiaries must pay for it if they agree to enroll; most people do subscribe to it (see Table 3–1). In fact, Part B enrollment is automatic unless the person informs Social Security that he or she does not want coverage and that deductions to pay for it should not be made from his or her Social Security checks. Part B provides some important insurance benefits:

- Payment of *reasonable* physician charges is covered in Part B (after the patient pays the initial $100 annual deductible).
- As in Part A, the payment is not full payment. Medicare pays only 80 percent of what it deter-

Table 3–1 Medicare Aged and Disabled Enrollees by Type of Coverage for Selected Years, 1966–1998

Year	Medicare Part A: Hospital Insurance	Medicare Part B: Supplemental Insurance
1966	19,082,454	17,735,966
1970	20,361,152	19,584,387
1975	24,640,497	23,904,551
1980	28,066,894	27,399,658
1985	30,589,468	29,988,763
1990	33,719,118	32,629,109
1995	37,134,949	35,684,584
1996	37,661,881	36,139,608
1997	38,052,242	36,460,143
1998	38,432,477	36,780,731

Source: Health Care Financing Administration, 1999b.

mines to be reasonable. If the physician accepts *assignment* (i.e., agrees to accept the Medicare fee), the physician is allowed (in fact is *required*) to bill the patient for the remaining 20 percent. If the physician is unhappy with the amount Medicare determines as "reasonable," he or she may decline to accept assignment for some of the fee and may elect to have the 80 percent paid to the patient and thus be free to bill the patient for whatever amount the physician feels is appropriate. There are limits, however, on the amount a physician may charge for nonassigned cases. Regulations now impose a maximum charge to the patient of 115 percent of the amount Medicare has established as reasonable. A number of states have passed legislation making assignment mandatory for all Medicare cases in their states.

- Hospital outpatient, ambulance, and emergency department services are paid under Part B and are subject to the same $100 deductible. Medicare pays 80 percent of the approved amount; the patient is responsible for the remaining 20 percent.
- A number of other services and supplies, such as outpatient physical and speech therapy, diagnostic x-ray examinations, wheelchairs, artificial limbs, limited chiropractic services, and so on, also fall under Part B.

Part B (Supplemental Medical Insurance) cost Medicare beneficiaries $45.50 per month in the year 2000. Additional costs come out of federal general revenue. As health care costs go up, so do the premium charges, but the law requires that the premium increase be limited to the percentage rise in Social Security income.

The Health Care Financing Administration (HCFA) under the Department of Health and Human Services oversees the Medicare program. It handles some payments directly, but most payments for care are made by *fiscal intermediaries* for Part A and *carriers* for Part B, with whom HCFA contracts. The contractors are mainly Blue Cross, Blue Shield, and commercial insurance companies. Contractors must rebid for the position approximately every three years.

Medicare has clearly helped the aged and other eligibles pay for needed health services. Many of the beneficiaries are on fixed incomes and may still have to pay considerable sums when hospitalization and skilled nursing facility care are necessary. There are also some expensive items not covered by Medicare, such as prescription drugs, hearing exams and hearing aids, and eyeglasses.

Although Medicare payments represent a sizable portion of most physicians' incomes, getting physicians to accept assignment has not been easy. Some physicians accept assignment in all cases, but many more accept assignment on a selective or case-by-case basis, presumably basing the decision on whether they think the patient can afford to pay more than the fee Medicare has established as being reasonable. Some physicians never accept assignment. Massachusetts dealt with this issue by requiring that all physicians accept assignment in all cases if they wish to retain their license to practice there. A number of states have since adopted similar legislation.

Congress began to deal with this problem first by instituting a Medicare participating physician (MPP) program, whereby physicians who agreed to participate would accept all cases on assignment. Those who did not agree to accept all cases on assignment would have to bill all transactions to Medicare, but would not receive direct payments. Payment would go to the patient, and the physician would have to bill the patient. There would be no case-by-case decision whether to accept assignment. Congress also directed that the names of all participating physicians be published so that Medicare patients could determine beforehand whether a physician was an MPP. Other incentives to participate include shorter turnaround time for payments, rollover of Medicare payment information to Medigap insurers to reduce paperwork for participants, and access to toll-free telephone numbers for support services. The number of physicians accepting assignment has thus increased significantly because of actions by various federal and state government.

Although the direct costs of care borne by Medicare recipients are still considerable, the cost of benefits paid by the government has been frighteningly high, far exceeding the early calculations when the legislation was being considered. Expenditures by Medicare continue to rise despite various cost containment efforts, posing a political dilemma. If Medicare is to continue to meet its obligations, raising taxes to meet the rising demand and rising costs as we have in the past is not popular with wage earners and businesses. Some of the increased costs are being shifted to the patient through higher deductibles and higher Part B premiums. Denying access to care is tempting, and many countries do this, but it does violate our values, our sense of what is right. Rationing care may mean denying access to care, and we are a society accustomed to having all the medical care we desire.

While Congress struggles with ways to deal with the cost of the Medicare problem, it also recognizes the shortcomings of the benefits. During the 1999–2000 legislative session, Congress debated "Medicare Part C" prescription benefits. As of this writing, no legislation has been passed, but proposals focused on paying prescription costs above a threshold amount that would first be the patient's responsibility. Congress recognizes that many seniors, although living longer active lives, are dependent on prescription drugs to help control chronic conditions such as heart disease, arthritis, diabetes, and the like. In a time of concern over cost containment, developing a plan to ease the cost of prescriptions for the elderly has not been easy. Democrats and Republicans do not agree on how to finance any additional Medicare benefits, especially with the advent of the aging of the Baby Boom generation into the Medicare population in the next ten years.

Medicaid

Medicaid, authorized by Title XIX of the Social Security Act, is a federal- and state-financed program to provide health insurance for low-income Americans: the *categorically needy* and the *medically needy*. Originally the eligibility for benefits was determined through eligibility for cash assistance (welfare) through the Aid to Families with Dependent Children (AFDC) program (for single parents and children) and the Supplementary Security Income (SSI) program (aged, blind, or disabled). All states must cover these persons as "categorically needy." States also covered the "medically needy": persons who have enough money to live on, but not enough to pay for significant specific medical costs they incur. Medicare beneficiaries who have low income and limited resources may receive help paying for their out-of-pocket medical expenses from their state Medicaid program. Those who are eligible for both Medicare and Medicaid are referred to as *dual eligibles;* in essence, Medicaid becomes their supplemental, or Medigap, insurance. It is up to each state to define income eligibility; determine the type, amount, duration, and scope of services; set the rate of payment for services; and administer its own Medicaid program (Health Care Financing Administration, 1999c). It should be noted that Medicaid standards for low income differ from state to state, most based on some percentage of the federal poverty level. These amounts are very low, excluding many persons with what we would consider low incomes, but not low enough to qualify for Medicaid benefits.

Each state's Medicaid program must at least provide for inpatient and outpatient hospital services; physician services; medical and surgical dental services; nursing-facility services; home health care; family planning services; rural health clinic services; laboratory and x-ray services; pediatric and family nurse practitioner services; federally qualified health center services; nurse-midwife services; and early and periodic screening, diagnosis, and treatment (EPSDT) of children under twenty-one. A state, at its option, may elect to pay for dental services, prescribed drugs, eyeglasses, intermediate-care facility services, and other services.

Medicaid is financed from general tax revenues. The federal government share currently ranges from 50 percent in the most wealthy states to 80 percent in those states with the lowest per capita personal income. Medicaid was originated as a fee-for-service, vendor payment program with payments made directly to the provider. Providers participating in Medicaid must accept the Medicaid payment as payment in full and cannot bill additional amounts to the patient. Because those eligible for benefits have very low incomes, cost sharing through deductibles, coinsurance, or copayments is not very logical.

Like Medicare costs, Medicaid costs have risen rapidly (see Table 3–2). In 1992, Medicaid expenditures exceeded $75 billion, and by 1997 they were more than $123 billion (Parnuk, Makuc, Heck, Reuben, & Lochner, 1998). Outlays for 1999 were $190 billion, with $108 billion paid by the federal government and the balance paid by the states (Health Care Financing Administration, 2000a). These costs have been of growing concern to both state and federal governments. In most states, increases in Medicaid expenditures are outpacing increases in state revenues. Because payments have not grown with inflation, more and more physicians are limiting the number of Medicaid patients they treat; some have withdrawn from the program totally. The refusal to participate is not just financially driven. Physicians experience difficulties with excessive paperwork, changing enrollment status of beneficiaries, long delays in payment, and other program deficiencies.

But the states are not sitting by idly. In the past, many were forced to reduce the number and scope of optional services and to be more restrictive about eligibility of the medically needy. Other options were to impose limits, such as limitations on the number of days for in-hospital care, and limitations on the amounts paid to physicians, hospitals, and nursing homes.

Rather than simply reduce the number of persons eligible for Medicaid, state governments have tried many innovative approaches to stabilize their Medicaid programs. The state of Oregon extended Medicaid benefits to *all* residents who were below poverty level. This action added many more people to the Medicaid roles. To pay for the cost of care for these new Medicaid enrollees, the state mandated managed care for all Medicaid patients and developed a list of medical services in priority order based on the effectiveness of the services. The program does not pay for

Table 3–2 Medicaid Recipients and Payments for Selected Years, 1975–1997

	1975	1980	1985	1990	1995	1996	1997
	Numbers in Millions						
All recipients	22.0	21.6	21.8	25.3	36.3	36.1	33.6
	Percent of Recipients						
Aged (65 and over)	16.4	15.9	14.0	12.7	11.4	11.9	11.8
Blind and disabled	11.2	13.5	13.8	14.7	16.1	17.2	18.3
Adults in families with dependent children	20.6	22.6	25.3	23.8	21.0	19.7	20.2
Children under age 21	43.6	43.2	44.7	44.4	47.3	46.3	45.5
Under Title XIX	8.2	6.9	5.6	3.9	1.7	1.8	4.3
Amount in billions							
All payments	$12.2	$23.3	$37.5	$64.9	$120.1	$121.7	$123.6

Source: Parnuk, Makuc, Heck, Reuben, & Lochner, 1998.

those procedures that have little or no beneficial effect, even though they were on the federal government's regular Medicaid list. The plan offers a basic benefit package that stresses prevention and covers most, but not all, of the usual Medicaid treatments. It goes beyond the customary Medicaid benefits by providing coverage for dental and hospice care, prescription drugs, routine physicals, and most transplants. A broadly representative commission of health professionals and community leaders developed the list of medical treatments and their prioritization. The federal government had to approve the plan but rejected it in mid-1992 because the prioritized list might have violated the federal Americans with Disabilities Act. The plan, according to Oregon's governor, enjoyed the support of leading disability groups in Oregon because they believed it would help more than harm those who had disabilities. The Oregon commission reorganized the list, deleted references to "quality of life," and extended coverage to some controversial treatments (Office for Oregon Health Plan Policy and Research, 1998). The Clinton administration approved the revised plan in March 1993 for a five-year demonstration period.

This acceptance of the Oregon plan signals that the Clinton administration recognized the need for drastic action and would give the states flexibility in dealing with the problems associated with health care re-

form. Between 1993 and 1996 the HCFA approved waivers for eighteen states to expand Medicaid coverage to an additional 2 million people (Health Care Financing Administration, 2000a). In many states the waivers consisted of adopting managed care programs in an attempt to control costs and provide more comprehensive care to their enrollees. This approach shifts the risk from the state to the managed care providers. When the managed care plans have been given realistic budgets, they have been successful. However, in areas where payments to managed care programs are too low to provide care, the same problems have occurred as those found in fee-for-service Medicaid plans (see the next section for more about managed care).

Waivers are necessary in order for states to move to managed care Medicaid plans because of the original concept of the Medicaid program. The 1965 legislation emphasized that Medicaid recipients should receive care through "mainstream" American medicine. That meant care provided by private physicians in their offices, and choice of providers of care. Managed care, with its limited "panel" of providers and restrictions regarding in-network facilities, technically violates the original concept of the Medicaid structure—thus the need to obtain a waiver from the federal government. With any innovative delivery plan, states must prove that recipients will receive benefits that are the same, or better, than those mandated by the federal government.

Medicaid programs were drastically affected by the Personal Responsibility and Work Opportunity Reconciliation Act of 1996 (welfare reform). It replaced AFDC with the state-run Temporary Assistance for Needy Families (TANF) program that separates eligibility for cash assistance from eligibility for Medicaid. The law made it easier for states to expand Medicaid to more working families and to offer families at least six months of Medicaid after they leave welfare for work. The federal government provided some $500 million in matching funds to support these changes (Health Care Financing Administration, 2000a).

In 1997, Congress also created the State Children's Health Insurance Program (SCHIP) to reach more children whose parents earn too much to qualify for Medicaid but too little to purchase health insurance. SCHIP gives the states three options for covering children: (1) design a new children's health insurance program, (2) expand current Medicaid programs, or (3) provide a combination of both. As of September 1998, 2 million children were enrolled in SCHIP plans in all fifty states. However, still more incentives are being proposed to find and enroll children who are eligible and have not been enrolled and to simplify the Medicaid enrollment process (Health Care Financing Administration, 2000a).

Managed Care

At one time the terms *managed care* and *health maintenance organization* (HMO) were synonymous. However, *managed care* now describes a wider range of services and practices that have come to revolutionize the practice of medicine and the delivery of health care. In its broadest sense, managed care is a health care delivery system that in some way places the provider in the position of managing the utilization of health care by the consumer (patient). Managed care has five very important characteristics:

1. A select panel of providers
2. Comprehensive health services
3. Quality tracking
4. Utilization review
5. Cost containment

There are various types of managed care, but perhaps the three broadest categories are HMOs, preferred provider organizations (PPOs), and point-of-services (POS) plans. These are described in the sections that follow, although with a reminder that they are not the only managed care plans available and that in many instances it is very difficult to draw distinctions among various managed care plans.

Health Maintenance Organizations

HMOs are perhaps the most restrictive of managed care plans. The term *HMO* may refer to a specific organization (such as Kaiser Permanente) or a health insurance plan (Aetna U.S. Health care, United Health care, etc.), which adds to the confusion and makes descriptions even more difficult. The basic characteristics, however, are the same for the organization or the health plan. The main characteristic is the gatekeeper concept. A primary care physician (PCP) or other health care professional is the case manager. All care for the patients is directed (in conjunction with the patient) through the PCP, including referrals to specialists, orders for diagnostic tests, and any surgical or other treatment procedures. As the case manager, the PCP receives payment on a capitated basis—a fixed payment per patient per month. By providing as much needed care as possible in-house, the PCP controls costs (for the HMO) often connected with specialty care. The PCP determines the appropriate setting for care by providing referrals when necessary. Services provided outside the realm of the PCP must be provided by other HMO network providers (contracted with the HMO for discounted fees). If a patient chooses health services with a provider outside the network or seeks services without a referral from the PCP, the HMO will not pay for the service and the patient is responsible for any costs incurred; that is one way of shifting risk. But the real shift of risk is to the PCP. The capitated fee is fixed. The PCP receives the same fee regardless of the number of times the patient is seen and regardless of the range of services provided by the PCP. In some cases, the PCP may also be at risk for some of the costs associated with referring a patient for additional treatment—at risk either for admonishment by the HMO's administration (through utilization review) or through loss of income if there is a pool of money withheld from the PCP to pay for specialty care.

Another very important feature of the HMO is the emphasis on preventive care. One very effective way of reducing overall health care costs is to keep the population healthy. Traditionally, health insurance has really been "sick care insurance," paying for services only when they are medically necessary. Therefore, traditional health insurances do not pay for routine exams or care that "rules out" illness. HMOs not only pay for routine exams, they encourage them and monitor that patients receive preventive care such as immunizations and screenings. Some even provide services such as smoke-enders programs and discounts on health club memberships.

Although the phrase *health maintenance organization* seemed new to most consumers and health care providers in the 1980s, the idea of paying for services on a fixed fee or capitated basis appears throughout U.S. medical history. It became most prominent, however, during the 1940s with the development on the East Coast of the Health Insurance Plan (HIP) of Greater New York, and on the West Coast of Kaiser Permanente. Expansion of the HMO approach was modest—some would say slow—until the 1970s, when the costs of health care began to soar and when these costs became a concern both to government and to the business community. The federal government took the initiative in 1973 with passage of the Health Maintenance Organization Act. The act provided financial incentives for the development of what then became known as HMOs by providing start-up money and instituting regulations requiring firms of twenty-five or more employees who offered health insurance to employees to include an HMO option if it was available in the firm's area. The act also preempted state legislation prohibiting HMOs and granted Federally Qualified Status (certification that the HMO met a minimum package of benefits) to encourage Medicare and Medicaid populations to enroll in HMOs. The government saw in the HMO approach a way to control rising costs of health care, a sizable portion of which it paid for through Medicare and Medicaid. The HMO approach thus shifted the risk arising from increased costs caused by heavy utilization from the government to the provider of services.

Despite subsidies, HMO growth was slow, but by the 1980s HMO enrollment had increased (see Table 3–3), in part because of the continued rising cost of health care. Even as federal subsidies ended, HMOs began to develop all over the country, spurred on by the prevailing idea that through competition and utilization control, costs could be controlled. Businesses, like the government earlier, found HMOs appealing because they seemed like a good way to hold down rising costs; no longer would the employer pay without limit. If the costs rose above the limit, the HMO would be responsible for absorbing the costs. Declining hospital bed occupancy (explained in the section "Paying Hospitals" later in this chapter) and a large supply of physicians (some said an oversupply) gave the HMOs the necessary leverage to compete for business, offering employers lower costs and offering hospitals and doctors an assured flow of patients in return for greatly reduced fees.

HMOs promised lower health care costs based on the efficiency of delivering services in a coordinated and comprehensive fashion. Initial cost reductions came mainly from a reduction in inpatient and specialty care, not from a reduced quality of care. As the HMOs competed with one another for their share of the market, some critics feared HMOs would begin to curtail services in order to keep their costs low. They would not openly ration care but would more subtly ration by making patients wait for appointments, ordering fewer diagnostic tests, reducing the amount of nonemergency surgery, and signing up only those employee groups that appeared to be young and healthy.

More than 28 percent of the population belonged to HMOs in 1998. The highest concentrations of enrollees are in the West and Northeast, and in large metropolitan areas. The number of HMOs grew so rapidly during the 1980s that many did not have the management skills or the number of enrollees necessary to survive. Many of the HMOs merged or disappeared during the late 1980s, resulting in fewer HMOs with a steady but slower growth in the number of persons enrolled (see Table 3–3). HMOs caused

Table 3–3 HMOs and Enrollment, According to Model Type and Geographic Region, United States, for Selected Years, 1980–1998.

	1980	1985	1990	1996	1998
Plans	**Number**				
All plans	235	478	572	562	651
IPA[a]	97	244	360	332	317
Staff, group, and network	138	234	212	108	116
Mixed	—	—	—	122	212
Enrollment	**Number of Persons (in Millions)**				
Total	9.1	21.0	33.0	50.9	76.6
Model	**Percent of HMO Enrollees**				
IPA[a]	1.7	6.4	13.7	20.1	32.6
Staff, group, and network	81.3	69.6	58.4	26.0	18.0
Mixed	—	—	—	34.5	39.2
	Percent of Population Enrolled in HMOs				
Total	4.0	8.9	13.4	19.4	28.6
Geographic region					
Northeast	3.1	7.9	14.6	24.4	37.8
Midwest	2.8	9.7	12.6	16.4	22.7
South	0.8	3.8	7.1	12.4	21.0
West	12.2	17.3	23.2	28.6	39.1

Source: Parnuk et al., 1998.
[a]Individual practice association.

a restructuring of the way health care is marketed, delivered, and financed in almost every metropolitan area of the country.

There are many varieties of HMOs, but they can be categorized into four types:

1. **Staff model** HMOs employ physicians directly, provide care through central offices, and pay physicians by salary (the insurer and the health care provider are one).
2. **Group model** HMOs contract with one independent, multispecialty group practice to provide physician services. The HMO pays the group practice a negotiated per capita rate, and the group practice determines what each physician will be paid—typically a salary plus incentive payments.

The HMO sends all of its patients to that group, and the group sees only the HMO's patients.

3. **Network model** HMOs resemble the group model. The only difference is that the HMO contracts with more than one independent multispecialty group practice.
4. **Individual practice association** (IPA) HMOs contract with an association of individual physicians in solo practice or with group practices to ensure the provision of services to HMO members. Payment schemes vary from capitation to fee for service, as well as variations on these types of payment. Unlike the other HMO models, IPA physicians usually provide services in their own offices and see other patients in addition to their HMO patients. In 1998, about 49 percent of HMOs were IPAs.

No study has shown one model to be superior to the others, but the IPA model seems to be the most predominant in number of plans, number of persons enrolled, and percent of HMO enrollees. The group and staff models, although once the icons of HMOs, have been declining in strength over the years. The structure of HMOs is changing and becoming more diversified, as indicated by the number of mixed HMO plans and number of enrollees in those plans. HMOs are a continually changing mix of nonprofit and for-profit organizations.

The initial reduction in health care expenditures for HMO members was due mainly to a reduction in hospital admissions and a greater reliance on outpatient services, not a reduction in physician services. However, many of those initial reductions have since stabilized, and employers are not saving as much money as they had hoped. Employers continue to press to keep costs down without sacrificing quality. Even though HMO premiums continue to increase more than employers expected, and in some cases more than the premiums for traditional fee-for-service plans, employers are still turning to HMOs, often by passing more of the premium cost to employees if the employees opt for fee-for-service plans.

Membership in HMOs typically offers some advantages for enrollees, such as a predictable cost for health care, broader coverage for more routine care (e.g., physical examinations), and no claim forms to fill out and submit. Disadvantages often cited are the requirement of choosing a physician affiliated with the HMO, the need to get approval before hospitalization or specialty care, and the difficulty of securing payment for care that the insured receives when outside of the home geographic area.

Physicians may find HMOs advantageous because they offer a guaranteed income if in a staff, group, or network model; those in an IPA model may appreciate the possibility of expanding their patient base. Disadvantages for physicians that are often cited include some loss of autonomy, minimal input into quality assurance and utilization review criteria (except in the IPA model), possible alteration of referral patterns, increased outside influence on treatment decisions, and possible reduced earnings.

Although studies have shown lower hospital utilization rates for HMOs, the results are not altogether persuasive on two accounts. First, some critics believe that many HMOs have enrolled groups that are not representative of the population, that they have sought younger groups of enrollees, who would tend to be healthier, and have avoided those groups from which high utilization could be expected—principally the poor and the elderly. Second, many believe that some of the reduced utilization may stem from rationing—for example, not doing elective surgery that would serve only to improve the quality of life. HMOs are increasing their enrollments; however, they are facing increasing competition from another type of managed care: preferred provider organizations.

Preferred Provider Organizations

PPOs are primarily a phenomenon of the 1980s and have grown dramatically. A PPO is an arrangement in which a limited number of health providers—physicians, hospitals, and others—agree to provide services to a defined group of people at a negotiated fee-for-service rate, which is usually discounted from the normal rate. There are incentives for enrolled people to use the preferred providers because the costs of provider services are fixed, and except for routine office visits, they are typically paid for in full (or at least at 80 percent of the fee). If the enrolled person goes to a provider outside the network (a nonpreferred provider), a lesser payment is paid (typically only 70 percent) and the patient must pay the balance.

PPOs have attracted enormous interest as a way to contain costs while retaining the patient's choice of physician and retaining the fee-for-service type of payment. PPOs may be sponsored by insurance companies (including Blue Cross and Blue Shield plans), employers, hospitals, or physicians. Some hospitals and physicians have joined together to form physician-hospital organizations (PHOs) in response to economic competition and as a mechanism for capturing and securing a share of the market, lest they lose patients. PHOs form their own preferred provider networks to contract with insurance companies or directly with employers to provide care to groups of consumers (patients) at a discounted rate rather than waiting for insurance companies to come to them to contract for a PPO. The PHO is usually an affiliation for contracting purposes rather than a complete merger of organizations.

The success of PPOs depends on the recruitment of cost-effective physicians and hospitals. The competition must be strong enough for these providers to be willing to negotiate discounted rates for PPO members. PPOs, like HMOs, also depend upon management activities to keep costs down. These activities may include prior authorization for hospital admission (precertification), concurrent and retrospective utilization reviews, and mandatory second opinions for surgery.

Physicians like the PPOs' feature of maintaining fee-for-service, office-based medical practice. Many physicians see PPOs as a way to compete with HMOs. As suggested earlier, they see an opportunity to enlarge their patient base or to preserve their current patient base. PPOs do not restrict physicians to a single plan. Most physicians have participation agreements with more than one PPO and with other types of plans in addition to the PPO.

In the PPO, physicians lose some of their autonomy as in an HMO, but they must accept some controls. External utilization review may leave the physician with less opportunity to influence the design and operation of reviews. Fee schedules are usually discounted, so the physician must see more patients to maintain the same level of income; however, many physicians view the PPO as a better option than participation in an HMO.

PPOs appeal to patients because they allow freedom of choice of physician or hospital for care. If the patient prefers to use a provider outside the network, he or she bears some share of the costs. Admittedly, the additional cost may effectively deter them from exercising that option, but that is the purpose of the PPO concept.

Point-of-Service Plans

POS plans, sometimes called open-ended HMOs, are the most recent model of managed care and are somewhat of a hybrid of the HMO and PPO concepts. This model requires the insured to choose a primary care physician (PCP), who manages the overall care of the insured. The PCP provides as much care as possible and appropriate, makes referrals to specialists, and provides preventive services. The insured pays only a copay for the PCP's services and referred services. However, the insured has the option of seeking the care of a specialist without a referral or choosing doctors and hospitals outside of the network of providers if he or she is willing to pay a portion of the costs. POS plans differ from PPOs in the low cost to the insured for staying with care provided and referred by the PCP. Over 11 million people were in POS plans in 1998 (the number are included in total HMO enrollment in Table 3–3). This model of managed care is most attractive to consumers because of its greater range of choice of providers, whereas an HMO will not pay any of the costs of providers outside the network. However, the cost for a POS plan is greater than that for the other managed care models, reflecting the fact that greater flexibility comes at a greater cost (Parnuk et al., 1998).

Managed Care Trends

Managed care plans are expected to continue to grow at the expense of traditional forms of health insurance. All insurance forms are in intense competition and are altering the plans they offer to respond to the demands of health care purchasers. The future for managed health care delivery systems will probably be a combination of the positive features of both PPOs and HMOs (as seen in the point-of-service plans). The traditional, unrestricted, fee-for-service system of payment is really unheard of today. Even the most flexible of health plans contains some discounted payments to providers, some utilization review, and some restrictions to beneficiaries as to what services will be covered.

The future holds contention and possibly frequent litigation because vital professional and public interests are at stake. Antitrust issues will be raised with increased frequency as physicians are excluded from participation in some HMOs and PPOs, and as complaints arise over what are claimed to be anticompetitive practices and price fixing. Patients will question the managed care organization's refusal to provide access to certain treatments or denial of care. In 2001, Congress will debate a patient protection act for the fifth time and question whether managed care has gone too far in its control over decisions that should be left to the patient and his or her physician. Consumers have asked for the right to sue their health plans when denial of services results in adverse health conditions. Physicians have asked for the return of medical decision making into the hands of the practitioner and out of the realm of administrators. All of this is a focus on quality of care, which has become questionable under the aura of cost containment in health care delivery.

METHODS OF PAYING FOR HEALTH CARE SERVICES

Just as the types of health insurance have changed over time, the methods by which insurance plans pay for services has also changed, although no insurance company has one plan or one method of payment. Paying for health care will be discussed in the sections that follow, without a specific type of insurance in mind, although the reader will be able to recognize how certain types of payments are attached to certain insurance plans, or at least historically began that way.

Paying Hospitals

In the early years of hospital insurance, hospitals were paid at cost. The hospital simply kept an account of the costs involved in caring for the patient; added a small amount for uncompensated care, medical education, and new construction; and billed the insurance plan. The insurance plan in turn paid the hospital's full charges. The problems are obvious. Hospitals had no incentive to operate efficiently. In fact, the more services provided and the longer the patient stayed, the more the hospital got paid. Health care expenditures rose rapidly.

In an effort to stem the rise in cost of hospital care, many approaches were taken. Some insurance companies reimbursed hospitals on the basis of average costs—based on area providers. Hospitals were compared to one another and paid an average of their combined costs, often based on a daily rate. These

rates were eventually negotiated in an attempt to lower the daily rate. However, this approach did little to contain costs because hospitals still had the incentive simply to keep the patient longer (even after well enough to be discharged) in order to recoup some costs.

Because the federal government is responsible for a large portion of hospital costs under Medicare and Medicaid, it is the driving force in attempts to contain increasing hospital costs. Dissatisfied with retrospective cost-based reimbursement, the government, beginning in 1972, conducted several demonstration projects to evaluate a wide variety of alternative payment systems. After ten years of research, a prospective payment system (PPS) was chosen as a viable alternative to the retrospective cost-based reimbursement for Medicare patients. In 1983, Congress amended the Social Security Act to provide Medicare payment for inpatient hospital services under a prospective payment system in which payment is made at a predetermined, specific rate for each discharge according to the patient's treatment classification in one of almost 500 diagnosis-related groups (DRGs). The DRG takes into account the patient's principal diagnosis, principal surgical procedure (if there is one), any complicating conditions (comorbidities), and type of discharge. Each DRG is assigned a weight relative to the standard (1.00), and each hospital is assigned a fee for the standard. Payment becomes a simple formula:

$$\text{Weight} \times \text{Standard} = \text{Payment}$$

The legislation still provided for capital-related costs and adjustments, such as urban/rural location, teaching hospitals, low-income case mix, and outlier cases.

The transition to this PPS was made in a four-year phase-in period until 1988, when prospective payment went into full effect. The results were dramatic. DRG payment means a single payment to the hospital for the care of the patient regardless of the costs incurred. If the hospital incurs greater cost for the care of the patient than provided by the DRG, the hospital must bear the cost. If the hospital provides care to the patient at less than the DRG payment, the hospital still retained the full payment. DRGs were truly an incentive for hospitals to operate more efficiently.

It is important to note that other conditions changed somewhat in accord with the implementation of DRGs. Technology facilitated the move of many previously considered inpatient procedures to the outpatient setting. New medications made the medical management of many conditions preclude or delay surgical intervention. Coupled with DRGs, these broader environmental conditions changed the face of hospital care. Beginning in the mid-1980s, hospitals saw dramatic decreases in patient length of stay and in occupancy rates. Many hospitals responded by developing more outpatient services, converting inpatient beds to short-stay units, and developing market plans to stay financially viable. Many of these efforts resulted in the type of vertical integration and horizontal integration seen in the case study of the Baptist Memorial Health Care Corporation presented in Chapter 1. DRGs were a significant cause of these dramatic changes, along with the competition introduced by managed care structures.

Medicare introduced DRGs into hospital compensation methods. However, it did not take long for other third-party payers to adopt this method. It made sense—force hospitals to run more efficiently by shifting the cost risk to them. It also made sense for other third-party payers to protect themselves. On a cost basis, hospitals might simply have shifted any losses incurred from serving Medicare patients to the payers who were still paying at cost.

Payment by diagnostic category has become the norm for hospitals. Managed care organizations negotiate similar flat-rate payments. Prospective payment is also spreading to other service areas that previously remained under cost plus reimbursement or daily rates. The Balanced Budget Act of 1997 brought prospective payment systems to hospital outpatient services, certain community mental health services, certain home health care services, and certain rehabilitation services. Hospitals branched out to provide some of these services in order to protect themselves from losses of inpatient revenues, but now even that avenue seems to be closing (Health Care Financing Administration, 2000b).

The outpatient prospective payment system (OPPS) consists of groups of services known as ambulatory payment classification (APC) groups, based on services that are similar clinically and require similar resources. Actual procedures are isolated from ancillary procedures; for example, laboratory tests or imaging might be paid for separately from surgery. However, actual surgical procedures include such things as anesthesia, supplies, and recovery rooms. The outpatient prospective payment system went into effect on July 1, 2000 (Health Care Financing Administration, 2000b).

With the early introductions of prospective payments, there were many questions about quality of care. Terms like *quicker and sicker* defined the fear that patients were going to be discharged from hospitals before they were well enough to go home and would simply end up returning to the hospital in a short time, even sicker than the first time around. This did not prove true. However, it was obvious that costs were simply being diverted to home health agencies, which were now seeing more patients than ever because patients did require some additional care after hospital discharge. Nursing homes saw an increase in shorter-stay patients, who spent their rehabilitation periods in this less expensive setting than the hospital prior to going home. Costs for home health care and skilled nursing home care rose—resulting in the introduction of DRG payments for these services several years later.

The Balanced Budget Refinement Act of 1999 included provisions to adjust payments and protect against certain losses (budget-neutral provisions).

Paying Physicians

Physician and hospitals are paid separately (Blue Cross pays hospitals, Blue Shield pays physicians). This is true even when physicians perform services within the hospital. When a patient is admitted to a hospital, the hospital receives a facility fee and the physician receives separate payment for his or her services (surgical fee, consult, etc.). When we think of physician payments, however, we ordinarily think about payment for office-based care. Early forms of health insurance paid physicians on a fee-for-service basis. Physicians had their own fee schedules for various office visits and procedures and simply charged the patient or the insurance plan the amount of the fee. The more patients the physician saw, and the more procedures the physician performed, the greater the physician's income.

In time, many of the Blue Shield plans (as well as commercial insurance and eventually Medicare) developed contracts with *usual, customary,* and *reasonable* (UCR) allowances. These were schedules for payment for physician services based on the physician's history of charges (usual), the prevailing charges for physicians in the same specialty in the same locality (customary), and reasonable charges (the maximum the insurer was willing to pay). For each type of service, the insurer would pay the *least* of the usual, customary, or reasonable charges for that particular physician.

Enrollees covered under UCR payment schedules would not incur the cost of the physician's service if the patient used a physician who agreed to accept the insurance plan's UCR payments as full payment (such a physician is called a participating physician, referring to the physician's contract to participate in the insurance plan). If the physician is not a plan participant, then the payment is an indemnity payment (cash payment to the patient), and the physician may charge whatever he or she thinks is appropriate. The patient is responsible for any payment to the physician beyond what the insurance plan has provided. While UCR held down the amount of payment per visit or procedure, it did very little to reduce the number of visits or procedures performed. Just as in full fee-for-service payment, the incentive to overserve remained.

Until the early 1990s, Medicare paid physicians through the UCR system. Increasing costs, however, led Medicare to investigate alternative payment methods, just as it had with hospital costs in the 1980s. Medicare's answer to physician payment was the Resource Based Relative Value Scale (RBRVS), which was based on three main factors:

1. Total work performed by the physician for each service
2. Practice costs, including the cost of malpractice insurance
3. Cost of specialty training to perform the service

The relative-value scale is based on a model developed by a Harvard research group and relates the value of each medical procedure to others, a dollar conversion factor, and a geographic factor. RBRVS redistributes money among physicians by increasing the amount paid for cognitive services (listening, diagnosing, explaining, and advising patients) and decreasing the amount paid for invasive procedures (e.g., surgery) and diagnostic tests distributed through the Medicare fee schedule used to pay for physician services. Thus, primary care physicians had their income from Medicare patients increase while surgeons' fees decreased. The decrease for surgical and other specialized care is not a statement that these services are any less important because of RBRVS, but historically the services had been overvalued in relation to other medical procedures. Payment according to RBRVS began in 1992 and was phased in over a five-year period. Some insurance companies are following Medicare's lead and are also using the RBRVS to revise their payments to physicians.

RBRVS, when first introduced, was quite controversial. Specialists feared a drastic reduction in income, which did happen in selected specialties. Primary care practitioners never quite saw increases in their income as they were projected, but they did see some improvements. Perhaps the most difficult aspect of RBRVS was the concept of "evaluation and management" (E&M) codes—the method used to bill Medicare for office visits and consultations with patients. The evaluation and management codes take into account whether the patient is new to the physician or is an established patient, the extent of medical history taken during the visit, the extent of the examination done, and the amount of medical decision making on the part of the physician necessary in order to come up with a diagnosis and treatment plan for the patient. Obviously, these are very subjective criteria, and folding them all into an appropriate billing code is a difficult task, to say the least. How to document all of this information to substantiate the chosen billing level is another difficulty. The use of evaluation and management coding is still being discussed and clear regulations governing their use were not found until 2000. It is also important to note that while RBRVS attempted to balance the discrepancy between primary care practitioners' and specialists' payments, it did nothing to limit the incentive to overtreat. The more procedures a physician performed, the more the physician got paid.

Another type of physician payment is the discounted fee for service (mentioned in the discussion of PPO plans earlier in this chapter). Discounted fee for service is simply a negotiated fee scheduled between the physician and the insurance plan. The physician agrees to a reduced fee schedule in return for the potential increase in patients covered by the insurance plan (or in some cases, an assurance that the physician will not lose patients because of his or her enrollment in the insurance plan).

A physician payment plan introduced by managed care is *capitation.* As mentioned before, capitation is a fixed payment per patient per month. In return for the capitated payment, the physician agrees to provide a negotiated range of services. The monthly payment remains the same whether or not the patient requires any care that month. In other words, if a physician agrees to a panel of 100 patients at $10 per month per patient, the physician receives $1,000 per month. That $1,000 remains the same whether the physician sees none of the patients that month or sees all 100 patients every day that month! The physician is at financial risk for the range of services to which he or she agreed. Under capitation, it is in the physician's best interest to keep the panel of patients as healthy as possible. This is the built-in incentive in managed care for preventive services. It is also, unfortunately, an incentive to undertreat, in direct opposition to the incentive to overtreat that is built into fee-for-service medicine.

SUMMARY

Paying for health care services has had a long and complicated history. Hospitals, nursing homes, physicians, and other health care providers have all been paid differently. Third-party payers have had a significant presence since the first half of the twentieth century, and yet the term *third-party payer* means something significantly different from what it meant then. Containing costs has been the major focus in health care delivery for a very long time, particularly with the growth of the Medicare and Medicaid programs and the government's involvement as a third-party payer. Cost became a significant issue because the government's resources are limited, mainly by the taxes it imposes. Raising taxes to pay increased costs is never a popular option. Without raising taxes, however, the government faces reduced spending in other areas in order to keep pace with rising health care costs. And so it becomes a matter of allocating resources: Defense, education, transportation, other social services, or health care—which is more important in any given budget year?

Government is not the only entity concerned with costs. Employers and insurance companies also face dilemmas caused by increased health care costs. Insurers must absorb these costs and face decreased profits or pass on these costs through higher premiums for their insurance products. Employers must incorporate the cost of rising health insurance premiums into their own costs, consider raising prices of their products or services to cover that cost, or pass the increased cost on to employees through shared premium payments.

Managed care has had a significant impact on the delivery and cost of health care. However, managed care has brought with it new considerations and conflicts, mainly regarding choice and access to care. But the overriding struggle in health care today is the pressure to contain costs while providing quality care, and it remains to be seen if both goals can be met.

ACTIVITY-BASED LEARNING

Insurance Project

As a new employee, you have been given the following information regarding three insurance plans offered by your employer. Option 1 is a form of PPO (preferred provider organization) plan that gives you the option of seeking services from participating providers for little or no cost or seeking services from nonparticipating providers for additional out-of-pocket expense to you. The two HMO plans, Option 2 and Option 3, provide coverage for services from participating providers and *no* coverage for services outside the network of providers. You must choose your health insurance plan for an extended time period. You will not be able to change plans until the next enrollment period (on January 1 of the next calendar year).

Scenario 1

Choose a health plan assuming the role of a person in his or her mid-twenties, newly married and planning on having your first child in the near future. You and your spouse seem to be relatively healthy at the present time (the male has a family history of heart disease, the female a family history of breast cancer). You each have your own family physician, and the female spouse has heard about a wonderful obstetrician/gynecologist she would like to see, should she become pregnant.

Scenario 2

Choose a health plan assuming the role of a person in his or her late forties with a spouse and three children. One child is about to enter college away from home, the second is in high school, and the third is twelve years old. The college-age child is very active in sports, you are concerned that the high school student may be anorexic, and the twelve-year-old has a long history of allergies. You and your spouse are relatively healthy; the occasional flu, sprains, and screening exams for your age group are expected.

Questions

- Which health insurance plan would you choose under each scenario?
- Why did you make each choice?

Your choice of health plans need not be the same for both situations, but you must give specific reasons why you chose the same, or different, health insurance plans for each of the scenarios.

Since these are theoretical situations, you do not have some of the basic information you would otherwise have, such as a list of participating providers. Such information might influence whether or not you would have the access to providers with whom you are familiar and whether or not you would incur additional expenses to get some services you felt were important to you. You will therefore need to make some basic assumptions about those options. It would be helpful to report those basic assumptions in your response as it relates to how you made your insurance plan choice. Perhaps an interesting way to approach this is to think in terms of the worst-case scenario.

Option 1

Benefits	In Network	Out of Network
Office visit	$10 visit	Basic medical ($250 deductible; 80%/20% to maximum of $2,500)
Specialty office visit	$10 visit	Basic medical
Diagnostic/therapeutic services:		
X-rays	$10 outpatient $25 inpatient	Basic medical
Lab tests	$10 outpatient $25 inpatient	Basic medical
EKG/EEC	$10 outpatient $25 inpatient	Basic medical
Radiation/chemotherapy	No cost	Basic medical
Women's health/OB-GYN:		
Pap tests	$10 outpatient $25 inpatient	Basic medical
Mammograms	$10 outpatient $25 inpatient	Basic medical
Pre- and Postnatal visits	No cost	Basic medical

(continues)

Option 1–*continued*

Benefits	In Network	Out of Network
Other services:		
Emergency room	$25 copay	Basic medical
Ambulance	$35 copay	$35 copay
Inpatient mental health	No cost	$2,000 deductible
	Unlimited time	50% allowance
		30 days max
Outpatient mental health	$15 visit	$500 deductible
	Unlimited	50% allowance
		30 days max
Inpatient drug rehab	No cost	$2,000 deductible
	Lifetime max: 3 stays	50% allowance
		1 stay per year
		Lifetime max: 3 stays
Inpatient alcohol rehab	Same as above	Same as above
Outpatient drug/alcohol rehab	$10 copay	$500 deductible
	Unlimited visits	50% of allowance
		30 visits max
Durable medical equipment	No cost	Basic medical
Prosthetics	N/A	Basic medical
Orthotics	N/A	Basic medical
Rehabilitative care	No cost after	$250 deductible
	hospital%	50% of allowance
	$10 copay outpatient	$1,500 max
Diabetic supplies	No cost	Basic medical
Hospice	No cost	Basic medical
	No limit	
Skilled nursing facility	No cost	Basic medical
	365-day limit	
Prescription drugs	No coverage	No coverage
Chiropractic care	$10 copay	$250 deductible
		50% of allowance
		$1,500 max
Dental (preventive)	No coverage	No coverage
Vision	No coverage	No coverage
Hearing aids	$600 max every 4 years	Same
Podiatry	$10 copay	Basic medical
	No routine	
Family planning services	$10 copay	Basic medical
Your cost through payroll deductions:	$100 per month for family coverage	

Options 2 and 3

Benefits	Option 2 (In-Network Coverage Only)	Option 3 (In-Network Coverage Only)
Office visit	$5 visit	$5 visit
Specialty office visit	$5 visit	$10 visit
Diagnostic/therapeutic services:		
X-rays	$5 visit	$10 visit
Lab tests	$5 visit	No cost
EKG/EEC	$5 visit	No cost
Radiation/chemotherapy	$5 visit	No cost
Women's health/OB-GYN:		
Pap tests	$5 visit	No cost
Mammograms	No cost	No cost
Pre- and postnatal visits	$5 first visit, then no cost	No cost
Other services:		
Emergency room	$35 copay	$50 copay
Ambulance	No cost	No cost
Inpatient mental health	No cost 30 days max	No cost 30 days max
Outpatient mental health	Lesser of $25 or 50% 20 visits max	Lesser of $25 or 50% 20 visits max
Inpatient drug rehab	No cost 30 days max	No cost 30 days max
Inpatient alcohol rehab	Same as above	Same as above
Outpatient drug/alcohol rehab	$5 copay 60 visits max	$10 copay 60 visits max
Durable medical equipment	No cost	No cost
Prosthetics	No cost	No cost
Orthotics	No cost	No cost
Rehabilitative care	Inpatient 60 days max at no cost Outpatient 60 visits max at $5 copay	Inpatient 90 days max at no cost Outpatient 45 visits max at $10 copay
Diabetic supplies	$5 per item	No cost
Hospice	No cost No limit	No cost Lifetime max: 210 days
Skilled nursing facility	No cost No limit	No cost 360-day limit
Prescription drugs	$5 copay No contraceptives	$5 copay for generic $10 copay for brand
Chiropractic care	$5 copay	$10 copay
Dental (preventive)	$5 copay Children under 12 only	No coverage

(continues)

Options 2 and 3–*continued*

Benefits	Option 2 (In-Network Coverage Only)	Option 3 (In-Network Coverage Only)
Vision	$5 copay Discount eyeglasses	$10 copay Limit to every 2 years Discount eyeglasses
Hearing aids	No coverage	$600 every 3 years Children under 19 only
Podiatry	$5 copay No routine	$10 copay No routine
Family planning services	$5 copay	$5 copay for PCP $10 copay for specialists
Your cost through Payroll deductions	$60 per month for family coverage	$40 per month for family coverage

A QUESTION OF ETHICS

- In the discussion of payment to physicians, we see that fee-for-service structures can be an incentive for overtreatment (the provision of unnecessary services). Conversely, we see that capitation payments can be an incentive to underserve (withhold necessary services). From an ethical standpoint, which method of payment is more appropriate, in your opinion?
- Despite various government programs, over 40 million people remain without health insurance. Is it society's responsibility to provide health care services to all?
- Should there be limits to the amount of medical care provided, and should those limits be applied only to those who cannot pay? In other words, is a two-tiered system of health care appropriate— basic health care for the poor and full-coverage health care for those who can pay?

References

Anderson, O. (1975). *Blue Cross since 1929: Accountability and the public trust.* Cambridge, MA: Ballinger.

Fuchs, V. (1974). *Who shall live? Health, economics, and social choice.* New York: Basic Books.

Hawley, P. R. (1949). *Non-profit health service plans.* Chicago: Blue Cross Commission and Blue Shield Commission.

Health Care Financing Administration. (1999a, October 25). *Medicare deductible, coinsurance and premium amounts* [On-line]. Available: www.hcfa.gov/stats/mdedco00.htm (Accessed May 12, 2000).

Health Care Financing Administration. (1999b, June 30). *Medicare enrollment trends 1966–1998.* Available: www.hcfa.gov/stats/enrltrnd.htm.

Health Care Financing Administration. (1999c, August 2). *Overview of the Medicaid program.* [On-line] Available: www.hcfa.gov/medicaid/mover.htm (Accessed March 14, 2000).

Health Care Financing Administration. (2000a, April 12). *Fact sheet: Ensuring Medicaid coverage to support work* [On-line]. Available: www.hcfa.gov/facts (Accessed September 24, 2000).

Health Care Financing Administration. (2000b). *Outpatient prospective payment system quick reference guide* [On-line]. Available: www.hcfa.gov/medlearn/refopps.htm (Accessed September 26, 2000).

Health Insurance Institute. (1978). *Source book of health insurance data 1977–78.* Washington, DC: Author.

Office for Oregon Health Plan Policy and Research. (1998). *A brief history of the Oregon Health Plan*

and its features. [On-line]. Available: www.
ohpr.state.or.us/ohp/welcome_historyohp.htm

Parnuk, E., Makuc, D., Heck, K., Reuben, C., &
Lochner, K. (1998). *Health, United States, 1998:
With socioeconomic status and health chartbook.*
Huntsville, MD: National Center for Health
Statistics.

Uninsured grab federal policy spotlight again. (1999,
March 15). *American Medical News,* pp. 5–6.

U.S. Census Bureau. (1999, March). Health insurance
coverage: 1998. In *Current population survey*
[On-line]. Available: www.census.gov/hhes/
hlthins/hlthin98.

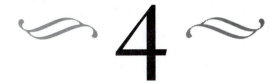

CHAPTER
4

Medical Education

Chapter Objectives

After completing this chapter, the reader should have an understanding of:

- The history of medical education.
- The difference between undergraduate and graduate medical education.
- How medical education is financed.
- The determination of physician competency through licensing and certification.
- Current trends in medical education.

INTRODUCTION

The physician today is a person vastly different from the practitioner in seventeenth- and eighteenth-century America. Today's physician pursues a rigorous course of study and clinical practice under the close supervision of faculty who are typically at the forefront of the health professions. Not only must today's physician pass courses in a premedical curriculum at a college or university and courses offered by the medical school, but he or she must also complete a year of general residency and pass the licensing exam. Nearly all physicians, moreover, now undertake at least three years of additional supervised specialty training in a nationally accredited residency training program on completion of their basic medical education. In most states, physicians must also participate in approved continuing medical education programs in order to maintain licensure.

While state law does not require certification in the physician's area of expertise, most hospitals, managed care organizations, and insurers do require certification, as well as licensure and continuing education. The end result is a person licensed by the state government, certified by a specialty board, and competent to diagnose and treat most illnesses while knowing when to refer the patient for specialty care.

Licensure and certification do not guarantee that every physician is excellent, that all are competent, that all provide the best possible medical care, or that diagnostic and treatment errors are not made. However, they do say that most physicians are competent and that the patient has some grounds for assessing competency. Licensure and/or accreditation have been the benchmarks in the past, while new methods for assuring quality of care have been elusive.

MEDICAL TRAINING AND KNOWLEDGE IN COLONIAL AMERICA

In colonial times, women in the family treated most of the sick at home. They used medicinal herbs, relied on family and friends for advice, and later used medical guides that were specifically published for laypeople. During that period, people with little or no training could also treat the sick and be regarded as physicians. Most "physicians" were trained under an apprenticeship system, and there was no organized method for testing the competence of those practitioners or their students. No effective organizations or formats existed to attest, by the granting of a license, to the physician's competence (Packard, 1963).

In the traditional British categorization of practitioners, physicians typically held university medical degrees and practiced what we would call internal medicine. The apothecary was not a physician nor university trained. He was trained as an apprentice and was concerned with the dispensing of drugs. People frequently sought medical advice from the apothecary as they do from today's pharmacist, but the apothecary became, in Britain, the equivalent of a general practitioner. The surgeon (know as the chirurgeon) was also apprentice trained.

These distinctions became blurred in colonial America, for very few physicians came to the New World. There were, according to William Smith's 1758 *History of New York,* no medical schools in America to train them (Packard, 1963). Furthermore, there was only one hospital in all the colonies, the Philadelphia Hospital, and it had been open for only a few years. The first medical school was established in 1756 at the College of Philadelphia (later, University of Pennsylvania). The second school was at King's College (later, Columbia University), founded in 1768. By the time of the Revolutionary War, neither school had made significant medical manpower contributions to the total number of medical practitioners in the colonies. Accurate figures are hard to obtain, but it appears that the Philadelphia school graduated fewer than ten students a year from 1768 to 1773. The first class at King's College, in 1769, consisted of two students.

Shryock (1960) notes that on the eve of the Revolutionary War, there were approximately 3,500 established practitioners in the colonies, of whom fewer than 5 percent held degrees. Most of those who held degrees in medicine were from European, mainly British, medical schools.

Some of the early non-medical-degree practitioners were simply learned men[1]—ministers, planters, lawyers, teachers—who could gather a smattering of knowledge from books they read and could apply that knowledge. Those who aspired to medical practice apprenticed with established physicians for a number of years. Upon completion of the training period, during which time the apprentice would watch and assist his preceptor and read his books, the physician would give the apprentice a signed testimonial that constituted the certificate of proficiency. The real competence of the "graduate" from apprentice training was as good or as bad as the preceptor, as the books available, and as the conscientiousness of the apprentice. Some physicians in colonial times, however, may not have had any qualifications other than "an interest in the sick and assurance enough to hang out a shingle" (Corner, 1965).

Apprenticeship to a single physician was common because there was, until 1752 in Philadelphia and 1791 in New York, no institution that could rightly be called a hospital.[2] With the opening of the Pennsylvania Hospital (described in Chapter 7), however, a significant new pattern of training began to develop. Physicians not only began to take their ap-

---

[1]At this point, the use of the word *men* is appropriate, for medicine was a male domain. Female involvement in "medical" matters was confined to midwifery, and to the extent that some of them received formal training, it was frequently provided by medical practitioners. The first female medical school graduate was from the Geneva Medical College around 1850. See "Women in American Medicine," by R. H. Shryock, 1950, *Journal of the American Medical Womens Association,* 5(9) (reprinted in Shryock, 1966).

[2]The New York Hospital apparently served briefly during the Revolutionary War as an American military hospital, until the British occupied New York, at which time it became for seven years a barracks, and possibly also a military hospital, for British and Hessian soldiers. It was not until 1791 that the hospital admitted its first civilian patient. See *Commission on Hospital Care,* 1947, p. 439.

prentices with them to the hospital to assist, but they also began to allow other students to follow them as they examined and treated their hospital patients. So many students sought this privilege that the hospital resolved in 1763, "It is the unanimous opinion of the Board that such of them at least who are not apprentices to the Physicians of the House, should pay a proper Gratuity for the Benefit of the Hospital for their privilege" (Packard, 1963, p. 323).

By 1773 the hospital had decided to regulate this system so that an aspiring physician could pay a fee to the hospital and be formally apprenticed to the institution for five years. Upon completion of the apprenticeship, the institution granted a certificate. In 1765 the University of Pennsylvania established a medical department, and the hospital apprentices attended lectures there. This practice continued until 1824, when the hospital required future residents to be regular graduates from the medical college before taking up their hospital appointments (Packard, 1963).

NINETEENTH-CENTURY MEDICAL EDUCATION

Only four medical schools—Harvard University (1783), Dartmouth College (1797), the College of Philadelphia, and King's College—had been established by 1800. These schools were not like medical schools of today. Three or four faculty members were sometimes all that were available, but not always even that many. Corner (1965) tells us that Dartmouth "appointed the formidable Harvard graduate Nathan Smith to be a one-man medical faculty. For ten or 12 years he alone ably taught all the courses" (p. 57). The science and art of medicine were extremely limited in what they could offer in the way of cure, and one can appreciate, therefore, the great appeal in the nineteenth century of cultists and quacks. However weak the first schools were, they marked an important forward step. Stevens (1971) notes that "the foundation of the medical school in Philadelphia . . . was a part of the movement by university trained physicians to organize and rationalize medicine on a European model and to institute recognizable educational standards" (p. 17). Men with European medical training dominated the early medical faculties at Philadelphia, Harvard, and Columbia, and even at Dartmouth. As

the number of medical schools grew, and as more and more U.S. medical graduates went abroad to Edinburgh, London, Paris, and other cities of Europe, many returned and gravitated to the medical school faculties, and they championed reform.

Three local physicians in Castleton, Vermont, established the first proprietary medical school in 1818 (Stevens, 1971). Whether it was an improvement over apprenticeship to a single physician we can only guess, but the school did survive until 1862. For some time the school was, in form, the medical department of Middlebury College, and some of its faculty were people of considerable ability (Norwood, 1944). In Boston, the Tremont Street School, established in 1838 by four physicians, including Oliver Wendell Holmes, and the Boylston Medical School were among the better private schools (Packard, 1963). The Tremont Street School flourished and offered lectures in embryology and anatomy, surgical pathology, chemistry, auscultation and percussion, and microscopic anatomy. The faculty consisted mostly of moonlighting Harvard faculty, something at which we should not be surprised, since rarely did a faculty member in those days rely solely on medical school income. The school thus had a close relationship with Harvard and eventually became Harvard's summer program.

The Boylston Medical School opened in 1849. Despite opposition from Harvard, it received authority to grant degrees in 1854. It had a good faculty, illustrated by the fact that soon after receiving degree-granting authority, Harvard recruited the best of them, and the school "faded out of existence" (Packard, 1963).

In medicine, as in most other endeavors, those who are most expert initiate the effort to raise standards and elevate the level of practice (Stevens, 1989). The effort was evident in medicine as medical professionals were involved in the founding of university medical schools, the early establishment of medical societies, and the initiation of medical journals. All of these steps were designed to share knowledge, to communicate, to improve the quality of practice, and to establish a profession in which standards and esteem were comparable to those of European colleagues.

Medical licensure was rarely effective in the colonial and postcolonial periods, mainly because there were insufficient numbers of well-trained practitioners. Georgia was the first state to restrict medical licenses to graduates of medical schools (1821). However, opposition to licensure was strong from the apprentice-trained physicians, to whom licensure loomed as a threat; from other kinds of quasi health practitioners, whose practices were threatened; and from many segments of the lay population that resented medical elitism. By the middle of the nineteenth century, many licensure acts were either repealed or so drastically altered that they were rendered ineffective (Stevens, 1971). However, the trend toward formalized medical education was firmly established.

As the decades advanced in the nineteenth century, more and more medical practitioners were educated in medical schools. A decreasing percentage came from the apprenticeship system. In the absence of a strong licensing mechanism, the measure of a physician's competence came to rest on the standard of whether or not the physician had graduated from a medical school with a Doctor of Medicine (MD) degree.

This new standard encouraged development of a large number of new medical schools—some at universities that were ill equipped to support and nourish them, and a great many freestanding schools with no university ties. Sometimes a school consisted of two rooms, one for lectures and one for dissections. There were few, if any, laboratories, and very limited libraries. Many schools were located in rural areas with no hospital or other clinical facilities.

The notion of university-based medical education came to the United States primarily from Scotland. University of Edinburgh–trained physicians strongly influenced the structuring of the schools at Philadelphia and Columbia. University-based medical education was also dictated by the absence of strong hospitals in colonial America that could provide the milieu for excellence. In England, however, a number of medical schools grew up around such long-established hospitals as St. Thomas' and Guy's, from which came the acceptable model of freestanding and hospital-based schools in the nineteenth-century United States. By then, hospitals were more common in the United States than they had been in the latter part of the eighteenth century, though not all of the new medical schools could claim meaningful hospital affiliation.

Some of the new nonuniversity schools were good and had reputable faculties. Some of the schools were weak and were allegedly set up to make money because the professors in most of the schools (good and bad) were paid directly by each student for attendance at lectures. Even the quality of education at the "better" schools left much to be desired, as depicted by Burrow (1963):

> When Charles Eliot became president of Harvard in 1869 (the year that the institution provided its first microscope for medical students), his early effort to institute written examinations for medical degrees met opposition from the director of the medical school who asserted, with little exaggeration, that a majority of the students could hardly write (p. 9).

Under such conditions, one can sympathize with those in the population who relied on quacks of various sorts or who cherished their apprentice-trained doctors as being as good as any coming out of a university medical school. Medical science was rather primitive, with a very limited understanding of the causes or options in the treatment of disease.

During the 1870s, Harvard increased its length of training from two to three years, instituted written exams, and then required a college degree or the passing of a qualifying exam for admission. In 1892 the training was lengthened to four years. In 1893, Johns Hopkins University launched its pioneering effort in medical education with a four-year curriculum. This curriculum became, as we shall see, the model used to reform all medical education.

The American Medical Association and Its Influence on Medical Education

The American Medical Association (AMA) was founded in 1847 with a primary goal of improving medical education. At the organizational meeting in Philadelphia, the Committee on Medical Education was established. The first pronouncement of the committee was to criticize "medical instruction which does not rest on the basis of practical demonstration and clinical teaching (Johnson, 1947, p. 888).

Although its primary goal was reform of medical education, the AMA's efforts were diluted for many years because so many of its members had an interest of one sort or another in continuation of the weaker schools. The vested interest not only was financial investment and return but also included a desire to buy time so that the improvements could be made. Some practitioners did not want to see their schools put out of business. Some were skeptical about what reform would accomplish. In its 1872 report, the Committee on Medical Education observed that it was easier to find defects in the system than to propose remedies because of the influence of medical school professors in the AMA (Johnson, 1947).

In 1876, twenty-two medical schools organized the Association of American Medical Colleges (AAMC) as part of the effort to improve the quality of medical education. This new organization also struggled over issues to establish higher standards, and higher graduation requirements in particular (Coggeshall, 1965). Both the AMA and the AAMC thus encountered the problem that besets all representative bodies: To continue to exist, the organization, like the elected politician, must retain the support of its constituency. Get too far ahead and the effort flounders because it does not enjoy support from the majority of the membership. Standards thus tend to be minimal, so that most of the present members can meet them. Progress is still made, as it was by the AMA and the AAMC, but with incremental steps so as not to lose the constituency.

Even though Harvard lengthened its curriculum to three years in the early 1870s, it and other institutions could not move the AAMC on this matter in 1876. Not until 1891 did the AAMC support a three-year training period, only to have Harvard a year later again go its own way and lengthen its curriculum to four years. John Hopkins, as we have noted, introduced its four-year curriculum after Harvard, in 1893. The AAMC was persuaded in 1894 also to support a four-year curriculum. The organization played an important role, increasingly so from the 1890s on, but clearly it did not have enough clout to bring about the necessary reform by itself. It was at this point that the AMA began to play a significant role.

In 1901 the AMA was restructured to become a more representative body by lessening the influence of medical educators in its governing House of Delegates. In 1904 the House of Delegates acted on a report of the Committee on Medical Education and created a new Council on Medical Education. The council's functions were to report annually on the existing conditions of medical education, suggest means and methods by which the AMA could favorably influence medical education, and act as the AMA's agent in its efforts to elevate medical education (Johnson, 1947). The council still exists, and its annual report, published in the *Journal of the American Medical Association* (Barzansky, Jonas, & Etzel, 1999), offers a definitive account of the current state of medical education.

But even before the council's work began, leadership in the AMA was making progress. Beginning in 1902, the *Journal of the American Medical Association (JAMA)* published medical school failure statistics on state board licensing examinations, a form of exposure that could not help but embarrass and lead to institutional reform. In 1907 the assessment grouped schools into four classes determined by percent of failure. The council subsequently decided to rate each school on the basis of not only the state board exam performance but also such factors as entrance requirements, medical curriculum, laboratory facilities, hospital facilities, faculty quality, library, and research. The resulting scores would place each school in one of three categories: Class A (acceptable), Class B (doubtful), and Class C (unacceptable). Each school was visited, and the findings were reported.

The council chairman noted that "the Council was very lenient in its markings," and of the 160 schools, 82 were in Class A, 46 in Class B, and 32 in Class C. The classifications were not published; however, each school was notified of its standing. The result of the report was a great wave of improvement in medical education, from changes in curriculum to mergers of schools (Johnson, 1947).

The improved situation was evident. The AMA's work was clearly facilitated by effective leadership in the organization, as well as by medical educators from some of the better schools, who were also working within the AAMC. The AAMC began to inspect the schools and put pressure on the poorer schools to improve or get out of the association. There was, however, a clear political constraint on the AMA classification of schools. The ratings were made leniently, perhaps in recognition of the fact that it had to take one step at a time if it was to be effective and that to be successful in this, it had to rate a clear majority of schools as acceptable. This was perhaps as far as the AMA could go by itself. Some council members felt that any additional improvements would come only through the assistance of the Carnegie Foundation for the Advancement of Teaching (Johnson, 1947).

The Flexner Report and Reform

In 1905 the Carnegie Foundation had set out to investigate all of the professions (law, medicine, theology). When contacted by the Council on Medical Education, the Carnegie Foundation, impressed by the efforts being made to improve medical education and by the large amount of data available, agreed to conduct an independent investigation. Abraham Flexner of the foundation began the study of medical education in 1909. Flexner was not a physician, but an educator, and his study was mainly an educational survey. He identified five factors that would provide him with conclusive data as to the quality of a school:

1. Entrance requirements
2. The size and training of the faculty
3. The financial resources and expenditures of the institution
4. The quality and adequacy of the laboratories provided for instruction in the first two years.
5. The relations between the medical school and hospitals

He secured the data through interviews with the dean and the faculty and through observation of the facilities, particularly laboratories and equipment (Flexner, 1940).

The Carnegie Foundation published Flexner's formal report, *Medical Education in the United States and Canada,* in 1910. Though controlled in language, the report provided a candid, searing critique of medical education in both the United States and Canada. It named schools, their assets, and their liabilities, and it offered a prescription for each school, for each state and region, and for the country as a whole. Where schools were no more than business ventures, Flexner said so. Some medical schools, such as Dartmouth, were recognized for excellent preclinical training but criticized for a lack of opportunities in clinical training. Still others received high praise (for more details, see Flexner, 1910).

The Flexner report caused some schools to close and some to consolidate. Some allegedly closed before the report's publication in order to escape the criticism (Flexner, 1940). In all, Flexner recommended that the number of schools be reduced from 155 to 31. By 1920, the number of schools was down to 85. By that time, however, the need for more than 31 was apparent because of population increases and new knowledge that permitted more to be done for patients.

The report, coming from an independent body, strengthened the hand of medical reformers in the AMA, AAMC, state medical societies, and, importantly, state licensing boards. Licensing legislation in the states mandated more rigorous control. The AMA's Council on Medical Education, moreover, leaned on people in the state societies, even before the Flexner study, to see to it that reform-minded people were appointed to state licensing boards. Many boards began to set new requirements, which included increasing the length of medical training and providing students with modern laboratories, libraries, and clinical facilities (Stevens, 1971).

The increased leverage provided by the work of the AMA and the AAMC was evident in their increased coordinated efforts, leading, in 1942, to the establishment of the Liaison Committee on Medical Education (LCME), which developed educational program guidelines, inspected schools, and became the official accredited body for medical schools. The joint efforts of the AMA and AAMC were supported by the growing number of medical graduates from the better schools, who, in their own ways, were persuasive within their state societies, before legislative bodies, and with the public.

But the final leverage for reform came from foundations and individuals whom the foundations could persuade. Flexner's influence here was a critical factor. Shortly after his report, he joined the General Education Board, a Rockefeller charity, which poured enormous sums into medical education. Flexner estimated that the General Education Board's $50 million for medical education had been successful in getting other contributors to come up with half a billion dollars or more from 1919 to 1928, a period when the dollar bought much more than it does today (Flexner, 1940). The monies went to the better schools and to those that showed promise of moving in the direction laid out in Flexner's report. University medical schools usually had a better academic reputation and a more solid financial base than proprietary schools, and therefore they acquired the new money that became available for medical education. Because of this influx of money, universities gained control of medical education (Ludmerer, 1985).

MODERN MEDICAL EDUCATION

Today, medical education typically begins with premedical education consisting of four years of study that end with a baccalaureate degree from a college or university. Most premedical students major in the sciences, although they can, in fact, major in almost any academic program, as long as they take the specified

science and other courses required by the medical school to which they apply for admission. Almost 10 percent of students who entered medical school in 1998 had advanced degrees (Barzansky et al., 1999).

Many students are attracted to medicine because it is a prestigious, well-paying profession. Competition for entrance to medical school is very intense. In 1999 there were 125 U.S. and 16 Canadian medical schools fully accredited to award the MD degree. About 41,000 persons applied to medical schools in 1998. Of these, 42 percent were accepted (Barzansky et al., 1999). Once accepted, students are seldom dismissed for poor academic standing. Usually they are allowed to repeat all or part of the academic year if they are in academic difficulty. The AMA's Council on Medical Education reports data on medical school application and admissions, as Table 4–1 shows.

The number of medical school students increased during the 1970s and decreased somewhat during the 1980s. There was a sharp increase in applicants in the early 1990s; however, that took a downturn in 1997. Applicants in 1997 were down by 8.4 percent from 1996, and 1998 applicants were down 4.7 percent from 1997. The decrease in the number of applicants is reflected among female applicants, male applicants, and groups considered to be

Table 4-1 Medical School Applications and Admissions during a Twenty-Year Period, 1978–1998

Academic Year	No. of Applicants	Number of Accepted Applicants	First Year Enrollment (No.)
1978–79	36,636	16,527	16,620
1988–89	26,721	17,108	16,781
1989–90	26,915	16,975	16,749
1990–91	29,243	17,206	16,803
1991–92	33,301	17,436	17,027
1992–93	37,410	17,464	17,001
1993–94	42,808	17,362	17,090
1994–95	45,365	17,317	17,048
1995–96	46,951	17,357	17,024
1996–97	46,968	17,385	16,904
1997–98	43,020	17,313	16,844
1998–99	41,004	17,379	16,790

Source: Data from the Association of the American Medical Colleges Data Warehouse, May 26, 1999. Reprinted with permission from *JAMA* (Barzansky, Jonas, & Etzel, 1998, 1999).

under-represented. Since 1994, the number of applications submitted per person has continued to stay around twelve, reflecting a continuing recognition on the part of applicants of the difficulty of being admitted (Barzansky et al., 1999).

Women made up 44.4 percent of the 1998 total first-year medical school enrollment and 43.2 percent of all medical school students. The percentage of female medical school students has consistently been rising, notably since the 1970s (see Table 4–2). Minority group members made up 34.6 percent of the 1998 total first-year enrollment and 33.8 percent of all 1998 medical school students (see Table 4–3) (Barzansky et al., 1999).

Table 4–2 Women in U.S. Medical Schools during a Twenty-Year Period, 1978–1998

Academic Year	Women in Entering Class (%)	Total Women Enrolled (%)	Graduates (%)
1978–79	4,184 (25.2)	15,293 (24.4)	3,445 (23.0)
1988–89	6,205 (37.0)	22,902 (35.1)	5,225 (33.5)
1991–92	6,777 (39.8)	24,911 (38.0)	5,483 (35.7)
1994–95	7,191 (42.2)	27,497 (41.0)	6,216 (39.1)
1996–97	7,268 (43.0)	28,217 (42.3)	6,609 (41.6)
1997–98	7,325 (43.5)	28,447 (42.6)	6,622 (41.5)
1998–99	7,450 (44.4)	28,705 (43.2)	6,872 (42.6)[a]

[a]Estimated in April 1999.

Source: Data from the Association of the American Medical Colleges Data Warehouse, May 26, 1999. Reprinted with permission from *JAMA* (Barzansky et al., 1998, 1999).

Table 4–3 Race and Ethnic Background of Medical Students, 1998–99

	First-Year Enrollment[a]			Total Enrollment		
	Men	Women	Total No. (%)	Men	Women	Total No. (%)
African-American	516	838	1,354 (8.1)	2,033	3,133	5,166 (7.8)
Native American/ Alaskan Native	84	68	152 (0.9)	302	253	555 (0.8)
Mexican American	262	191	453 (2.7)	1,051	775	1,826 (2.7)
Puerto Rican	113	101	214 (1.3)	432	404	836 (1.3)
Puerto Rican (mainland)	60	56	116 (0.7)	239	220	459 (0.7)
Other Hispanic	169	150	319 (1.9)	745	533	1,278 (1.9)
Asian/Pacific Islander	1,795	1,400	3,195 (19.0)	7,055	5,296	12,351 (18.6)
All other students[b]	6,341	4,646	10,987 (65.4)	25,927	18,091	44,018 (66.2)
Total	9,340 (55.6)	7,540 (44.4)	16,790 (100)	37,784 (56.8)	28,705 (43.2)	66,489 (100)

[a]Includes students repeating the year.

[b]Includes whites (not of Hispanic origin) and non-U.S.-citizen foreign students of various races and ethnic backgrounds.

Source: Reprinted with permission from *JAMA* (Barzansky et al., 1998, 1999).

The premedical grade point averages of those matriculating continue to fall in the A to B range. Medical school admission is based, however, on a number of factors in addition to grade point average. These include performance on the Medical College Admission Test (MCAT), which nearly all accepted applicants take, as well as recommendations and interviews. The MCAT is an objective test that measures knowledge of science (biology, chemistry, and physics), ability to solve science problems, analysis and reading skills, and quantitative skills. In 1991 the MCAT was modified to strengthen the evaluation of skills such as critical thinking, verbal reasoning, and communicating, which have become more important because the vast expansion and change in medical knowledge requires physicians to rely less on rote memory. The new MCAT includes two nonscientific essays to help assess these skills (Association of American Medical Colleges [AAMC], 1999b).

Another weighted factor in medical school admission is the report from the student's premedical advisers. In many schools, this confidential report is a committee report, which serves to minimize risks of bias. Interviews of applicants are also considered important in asserting personality factors that tests and recommendations may not reveal. Not all schools or medical educators are satisfied with the interview because it is fraught with the risk of interviewer bias, and the search continues for other methods of assessing the personal qualities necessary for the best practice of medicine.

Nearly all leaders in medical education endorse the desirability of a broad liberal education in the arts, humanities, and social sciences, in addition to study in the biological and physical sciences during the premedical years. They recognize that such an education can enhance patient communication, improve understanding of the influence of social and economic problems on disease and convalescence, and enable physicians to acquire an understanding of the past that will help them contribute constructively to changes in society. However, because of the keen competition for admission to medical school, premedical students have tended to "play it safe" by emphasizing the biological and physical science courses at the expense of studies in other subject areas. Although medical schools are beginning to articulate more clearly and implement admission policies that give broadly educated applicants the same chance of admission as those with an intensive scientific education, this changing emphasis needs to be recognized more clearly by premedical counselors and by students preparing for medical school

The *premedical student* is an undergraduate working toward graduation and a baccalaureate degree. Baccalaureate graduates who go on to graduate school in, say, nutrition or philosophy and who study for a master's degree or Doctor of Philosophy degree (PhD) are, during this period of study, called graduate students. This is not the case for medical students. Although they typically hold a baccalaureate degree, in medical school they are considered undergraduates; hence, *undergraduate medical education* refers to medical schools and the training of physicians who will, on graduation, be awarded a Doctor of Medicine (MD) or Doctor of Osteopathy (DO) degree.

Graduate medical education refers to formalized post-MD or post-DO training in an approved internship or residency. *Postgraduate or continuing medical education* refers to formalized training on a short-course or short-term basis for physicians who have completed a period of graduate medical education; it generally includes refresher courses or intensive courses to develop new skills.

Undergraduate Medical Education

The typical medical school program lasts four years. A few universities today integrate their premedical and medical school programs and require less time to earn the MD degree. The Liaison Committee on Medical Education (LCME) accredits the programs, which award MD degrees. The U.S. Secretary of Education and the Council on Postsecondary Education recognize accreditation by the LCME, adding to its legitimacy (LCME, 1999). The American Osteopathic Association (AOA) accredits osteopathic medical schools. The U.S. Secretary of Education and the Council on Postsecondary Education also acknowledge the AOA's legitimacy in this role.

Medical School Curriculum

Although the structure of medical education has not changed significantly for almost fifty years, new ways of teaching are being introduced to cope with the vast amount of information and the changing way in which medicine is practiced. The first two years of medical school have changed little; they are devoted largely to the basic medical sciences (anatomy, physiology, biochemistry, histology, pharmacology, microbiology, etc.), with lectures crammed full of facts. The amount of scientific material to be learned has increased dramatically, and most schools have responded by adding the latest scientific findings in still more lectures. Many schools have incorporated electives and some patient contact during the first few years in response to student pressures. During the final two years, students rotate through clinical clerkships in which they acquire clinical skills and give general medical care. Students are assigned patients on whom they conduct histories, physical examinations, and some laboratory tests. The students are actively involved in the diagnosis and treatment of these patients under the supervision of the resident and faculty.

The clinical experience ranges from primary to tertiary care in a variety of inpatient and outpatient settings. Usually students do clerkships in internal medicine, obstetrics and gynecology, pediatrics, psychiatry, and surgery. Most schools allow students some elective courses or other clerkships during the final year. The number and duration of these vary from school to school. Society, government, and expanding knowledge continually pressure medical schools to add to the content of their curricula. However, the undergraduate years of medical education should emphasize a broad perspective of medicine. Medical school graduates are not expected to become experts in all subjects and are not prepared for immediate independent, unsupervised practice; instead, they are prepared to enter a program of graduate medical education.

Most medical schools now require courses to facilitate a humanistic approach—courses designed to improve doctor-patient relationships, to enhance communication skills, and to grapple with social and ethical issues (Robinson, 1999). The AAMC has stressed the need to address the humanistic aspect of medicine, as well as the need for medical students to become competent in the computer area to manage the staggering amount of available information and to enhance independent learning (AAMC, 1984). Where medical informatics was once the domain of medical researchers and information managers, it is now embedded in all aspects of medical training, including clinical care.

Although medical schools have considerable freedom to design and implement educational programs within the general criteria stated by the LCME, all schools provide an extensive knowledge of the basic biomedical sciences and exposure to the major clinical disciplines. Studies calling for curricular reform appear to be having some effect, as most medical schools are decreasing the number of didactic lectures while increasing problem-based and computer-assisted learning, and placing greater emphasis on social and ethical issues (LCME, 1999).

Whatever the curriculum, most medical schools require that students take Steps 1 and 2 of the United States Medical Licensing Examination (USMLE). The USMLE was established by the National Board of Medical Examiners (NBME) and the Federation of State Medical Boards of the United States (FSMB). The examination has three parts, the third of which assesses the knowledge and understanding of biomedical and clinical science necessary for the unsupervised practice of medicine. It consists of computer-based case simulation and is the basis for state licensing and insurance.

Osteopathic Medicine

About 5 percent of medical practitioners (approximately 38,000) have become fully qualified to practice medicine by earning the Doctor of Osteopathy (DO) degree (American Association of Colleges of Osteopathic Medicine, 1998a). Osteopathic medicine represents an approach to medical practice employing all the methods traditionally associated with physicians (diagnostic testing, medication prescriptions, surgery), but it also advocates the value of osteopathic manipulative treatment "to relieve pain, restore range of motion, and enhance the body's capacity to heal" (American Association of Colleges of Osteopathic Medicine, 1998b). The osteopath is a physician, licensed in all fifty states to practice medicine and surgery.

The osteopath is trained in essentially the same way as the allopathic physician (the physician trained in the MD schools) and in most of the same specialties. An individual must graduate from an osteopathic medical school (there are currently eighteen in the United States). Applicants typically have a four-year undergraduate degree, take the MCATs, and go through a personal interview to assess their interpersonal communications skills. The curriculum emphasizes preventive medicine and holistic patient care. After completion of the osteopathic medical school curriculum, DOs serve a one-year rotating internship. Many DOs then choose residency training if they wish to practice a medical specialty (American Osteopathic Association, 1999).

As a school of medicine, osteopathy developed following the Civil War under the leadership of a former army physician, Andrew Taylor Still. On the basis of the role that the musculoskeletal system plays in the body's effort to resist and overcome illness and disease, Still believed that manual manipulation was useful in stimulating the body's ability to fight disease (American Association of Colleges of Osteopathic Medicine, 1998a). Because his theories received little support from the established schools, Still branched off and opened the first osteopathic school in 1892. Others followed. Flexner included osteopathic schools in his 1909 study, and his report resulted in reform also in osteopathic medical education.

Osteopathy was strong in the Midwest, where most of the osteopathic schools were, and still are, located. Because it was a competing approach to medical practice, and because the AMA had long sought a unified voice for medicine, considerable antagonism developed between the two groups. For many years osteopaths were unable to secure licenses in some states and were given limited licenses in others. Today, however, they are licensed in all states, with the same rights and responsibilities as MDs. In eight states they are licensed by an MD medical board, probably because there are not enough DOs in those states to justify a separate or a joint board. In twenty-five states there is a joint MD-DO board. In the remaining states, the osteopaths have their own licensing boards.

The tension between MDs and DOs has subsided in recent years. Each group has now inspected each other's schools and satisfied themselves of one another's worth. Members of each group serve on one another's faculties and have privileges in the same hospitals. Before that, osteopaths had to develop their own hospital system. Occasionally, we hear of an allopathic hospital that will not give privileges to the osteopathic physician, but this is increasingly rare.

Although the AMA apparently wanted to absorb the osteopathic movement, the osteopaths felt it better to stay apart, believing that they could work more effectively for objectives they valued if they were outside the AMA framework. DOs were thus prohibited by the American Osteopathic Association (AOA) from joining MD medical societies, but enforcement of this prohibition was apparently ignored in states where there were relatively few osteopaths. Professional association is important for physicians, and if there were not enough DOs to support a local DO organization, the medical societies would do! The AOA prohibition against DO membership in the AMA and other allopathic societies was dropped in the summer of 1979. In 1983 the AMA granted observer status in its House of Delegates to the AOA.

Is there any real difference between what an osteopath does and what an allopath does? Osteopathic philosophy speaks of understanding the whole person and treating the patient as a total unit. But many allopaths, particularly those in primary care specialties, speak in the same terms. Manipulative therapy is considered unique, but some manipulative therapy seems to be part of physical medicine and rehabilitation (a specialty within allopathic medicine) and is used to some extent when the MD refers a patient for physical therapy. The average MD is not trained to use manipulative therapy at this time, but some osteopaths assert that they really do not use it anyway.

What is clear, however, is that the osteopathic school, while encompassing all of the traditional medical specialties, stresses family practice more than does the allopathic approach. Approximately 57 percent of osteopaths are in primary care fields (American Association of Colleges of Osteopathic Medicine, 1998b), whereas the percentage of allopaths in primary care fields is only about 40 percent (Moskowitz, 1999). This difference, however, may be a passing one, because some osteopaths do select non-primary care specialties, and there is growing pressure for and interest in the primary care specialties within allopathy. Many osteopathic physicians complete their graduate training in allopathic residency programs. Most of the MD specialties examine DOs for certification after the DOs have met their respective requirements. Comparison of the specialties between the two groups of physicians indicates remarkable similarities.

The osteopathic physician is very different from the chiropractor. The osteopath is a licensed physician; the chiropractor, although licensed, is not a physician. Chiropractors use manipulative procedures and physiotherapy, and are permitted to take x-ray films for diagnostic purposes. However, their range and scope of treatment options are more limited than a physician's.

Cost of Medical Education

The cost of training a physician is high, and tuition in most schools covers only a small portion. Nationally, tuition and fees constitute only 4% of revenue for school and university activities. The greatest source of revenue for medical schools comes from practice plans (revenue from patient care), which amounted to nearly 34 percent of total revenue for 1997–98 (Krakower, Williams, & Jones, 1999). Grants and hospital support also provide significant portions of medical school income (see Table 4–4). Revenue proportions differ for public and private organizations, as well as for nonprofit and for-profit organizations. Because of the varied sources of funds and differing

Table 4–4 Revenue (in Millions) Supporting Programs and Activities at All Accredited U.S. Public and Private Medical Schools: 1995–96, 1996–97, 1997–98

Revenue Source	Public Schools (n = 74)			Private Schools (n = 51)		
	1995–96	1996–97	1997–198	1995–96	1996–97	1997–98
Federal appropriations	93	106	107	24	18	21
State and local government appropriations	2,793	2,819	2,968	140	148	152
Tuition and fees	469	494	517	833	881	926
Endowment[a]	126	141	170	389	394	455
Gifts	291	318	347	434	532	548
Parent university support	156	160	183	84	88	94
Practice plans[b]	5,600	5,851	6,189	5,118	6,093	6,370
Hospitals/medical school programs	2,227	2,596	2,731	2,536	2,877	3,010
Miscellaneous sources	587	609	607	593	626	684
Total grants and contract	4,249	4,557	4,916	5,227	5,551	6,000
Total revenue	16,591	17,650	18,736	15,377	17,209	18,261

[a]Includes unrestricted and restricted endowment.
[b]Includes practice plan, network affiliation, and other medical service organization funds.

Source: Prepared by the Association of American Medical Colleges from data from the Annual Medical School Questionnaire, Part 1-A, of the Liaison Committee on Medical Education. Totals may not sum because of rounding. Reprinted with permission of *JAMA*.

accounting practices, it is difficult to determine exactly what it costs to train a single physician.

For a great many years after World War II, federal monies, in the form of research contracts and grants, fueled expansion in medical education. The monies came not to the deans of the medical schools but to the individual researchers. The most adept could get the grants and thereby hire more faculty, travel to meetings, and attract more residents, who were also paid out of grants. Highly specialized areas became more attractive. Reinforcing this way of obtaining funds was the reward system. Medical schools reflected the universities of which they were a part; the rewards of promotion and salary increases went to those who brought in the most grant money and who published. Relatively small amounts of the grant money went directly for support of medical education; most was for research.

Change occurred during the early 1960s. There was a widely perceived doctor shortage, and Congress responded by passing the Health Professions Education Assistance Act of 1963. The primary purpose of the act was to increase the supply of professional health care personnel. The legislation provided direct federal assistance to medical schools in the form of construction grants, student loans, and financial distress grants. In 1965 the law was amended to provide direct institutional support for operating expenses on the condition that schools expand their enrollments to eliminate the doctor shortage. The Comprehensive Health Manpower Training Act of 1971 greatly increased support for operating costs, and it established a "capitation grant" of $2,500 per student for the first three years and $4,000 per student for the last year of medical schools. However, schools that received capitation grants were required to increase their enrollment. As a result, the financial condition of medical schools greatly improved, and their enrollments increased from 31,491 in 1962–63 to 47,546 in 1972–73 (50 percent). When the legislation expired in 1974, the doctor shortage was perceived to have disappeared, but the legislation was nonetheless renewed in 1976.

The 1971 Comprehensive Health Manpower Training Act required for the first time that institutions carry out certain programmatic activities in addition to increasing student enrollment as a condition for receiving capitation grants. To qualify for the grants, institutions had to present a plan to implement projects in at least three of nine categories described in the legislation. Categories included promoting interdisciplinary training, establishing a team approach for providing health services, and establishing programs in drug use and abuse and nutrition, among others. This was the first time the federal government had intervened in the internal program decisions of medical schools. The legislation also expanded student loan and scholarship opportunities, and provided grants to initiate, expand, or improve professional training programs in family medicine.

As in all other areas of health care delivery, medical education programs struggled to cope with the cost containment efforts of the 1980s and 1990s. Graduating medical students carry heavy educational debt. Loans accounted for approximately 80 percent of available financial aid (Beran & Lawson, 1998). About half of all graduating medical students carry debt of over $75,000, and nearly one-third carry debt of over $100,000 (Yom, 1998). Yet estimated future earnings for physicians are uncertain as the health care delivery system continues to undergo change.

THE DEVELOPMENT OF MEDICAL SPECIALTIES

Most physicians in the colonial and postcolonial periods were general practitioners. The state of medical science was rather primitive, hardly justifying a specialist. Surgical practice was limited, until 1846, by the absence of anesthesia. Physicians who did develop special skills or interests and became known for them remained primarily general physicians, practicing their specialties (such as obstetrics or surgery) only on occasion. Shryock (1966) reminds us that this was the age of bleeding and purging (the former carried on as late as the 1870s), when illness was attributed to a generalized problem such as "impurities of the blood or the existence of excessive tension or laxity in the nervous and vascular systems." Under such a philosophy, there was little need for specialists. Surgery was limited largely to trauma cases.

During the first half of the nineteenth century, a growing number of U.S. physicians went to France for advanced study. During this period, French investigators were effectively proving the errors of bleeding and purging, as well as the ineffectiveness of many drugs then in common use. Their investigations pointed to specific pathology in different locations and systems of the body, there being no single or simple explanation for disease. These findings made the notion of specialization appealing to those physicians whose interest was excited by special health problems.

It was not until the 1860s that specialties began to make headway. Resistance to specialties was at times vigorous, and the issues were complex. Fishbein (1947), in his history of the AMA, summarized issues pertaining to specialization in a report at the association's 1866 meeting. Many of those same issues persist to this day:

- Should a patient go first to the general practitioner or directly to the specialist?
- Will the specialist treat the whole patient?
- Will the surgeon operate because that is what a surgeon is taught to do?
- Does specialty practice lead to unnecessary procedures?
- Will people study specialty medicine for the sake of the higher fees paid to specialists?
- Don't we want the best medical care, and isn't the specialist the best?

In 1859, scientific sections of the AMA began to form. Initially they focused on what were then well-defined areas of scientific interest as the AMA delegates saw them: anatomy, physiology, chemistry, practical medicine, obstetrics, and surgery. Obstetrics became part of the new Section on Obstetrics and Diseases of Women and Children in 1873. Children were separated to become a Section on Diseases of Children in 1879. Ophthalmology, laryngology, and otology sections were formed in 1878, and so on. The AMA responses to specialty interests were often slow because of the occasional reluctance of AMA membership to recognize the validity of the specialty. Though it is true that the specialist may tend to draw paying patients away from the general practitioner, there is also considerable evidence that a specialist practicing in

too isolated an environment runs grave risks of providing bad medical care because of the tendency to magnify concerns of the specialty and to be insensitive to the contributions and skills of other specialties. The resistance to some specialty development was thus genuinely concerned with quality of patient care, as well as the economics of medical practice.

General practitioners' concerns on the economic score were also well founded. By the mid-twentieth century, in some larger cities specialists were able to squeeze general practitioners out of many hospitals. The argument advanced by the specialists was, if you're sick enough to be in the hospital, you're sick enough to need a specialist. The general practitioners fought back. In 1947, general practitioners formed the American Academy of General Practice, with state and local chapters applying pressure for hospitals to add general practice departments. To prove their worth, members of the academy were required to have 150 hours of approved continuing education credits every three years. Family practice replaced general practice and became a recognized specialty in 1969. The American Academy of General Practice is now the American Academy of Family Physicians (AAFP).

Because of the slow response by the AMA to specialty interests, the specialists began to form their own societies and associations. These groups, by and large, did not fight the AMA but simply went their own way. Often, some members held leadership positions both in the AMA and in their specialty group. The specialty organization could focus more quickly than the more generally oriented AMA on the problems and concerns of the specialty. Some of the early specialty groups were the American Ophthalmological Society (1864), the American Otological Society (1868), the American Gynecological Society (1876), the American Association of Obstetricians and Gynecologists (1888), and the American Pediatric Society (1888). There were also state and local specialty societies—some established before the national body, some later. Specialty journals followed. In many cities the specialty was advanced by the presence of specialty hospitals and clinics. In most large cities today, one can find specialty hospitals still thriving or only recently merged with other hospitals. Eye and ear hospitals are perhaps the most common example.

These special hospitals and clinics became, in the late nineteenth and early twentieth centuries, the foci for training in those specialties because, generally speaking, the most outstanding practitioners were affiliated with those institutions. This is not to suggest, however, that some outstanding specialists did not practice and train others in the more generally oriented hospitals.

The Development of Standards in Graduate Medical Education

There was no standard at the turn of the twentieth century for what constituted adequate training in a specialty. Courses were offered by medical societies, hospitals, specially founded schools, and universities. The programs of study lasted anywhere from a few weeks to three years. Flexner (1910) described the postgraduate school as "established to do what the medical school failed to accomplish. . . . The postgraduate school was thus originally an undergraduate repair shop. . . . Urgency required that in the shortest possible time the young physician already involved in responsibility would acquire the practice technique which the medical school had failed to impart" (pp. 174–177).

The "repair shop" to which Flexner referred was also the rationale in the later part of the nineteenth century for the internship. Over time, the internship became standard practice, requiring an additional year of supervised training to give the medical graduate (still, in a sense, a student) that extra bit of on-the-job training necessitated by the medical schools' adoption of the Harvard practice of not requiring an apprenticeship before medical school. This need for additional training was also what motivated many physicians to go abroad. As Stevens (1971) notes, the internship tended to emphasize either medicine or surgery and thus became an introductory phase of specialization.

Early specialty training was thus erratic, and in the absence of accepted standards, the quality of specialty care ran from excellence to complete incompetence. Anyone who wanted to become a specialist did

so. There was no mandated course of study or training, nor was a license granted for specialty practice. State licensure acts focused on the basic qualifications for medical practice. A physician, once licensed, had no legal constraints placed on him or her but could legally do all that fell within the definition of medicine and surgery.

To be sure, many, perhaps even most (we have no way of really knowing), of the specialists were conscientious. They sought to learn by taking special courses, by going abroad, and by reading books and journals. They sought further information and fostered research through local, state, and national specialty societies. When one of their members secured a reputation for special skills, others went to work with that person. With the advent of anesthesia, antiseptic techniques, new instrumentation, and new technology learned from the Civil War battle casualties, as well as from European research, a new era began to open. Hospitals grew in number because now people could go to them for general and special surgery with less fear of pain and more assurance that they would survive the encounter and improve as a result of it.

This new era posed new problems. The new opportunities unlocked the specialties, but the advances in most of the specialties entailed surgery. Prior to the onset of this new technology, surgery included sewing a laceration, setting a bone, or amputating and was the domain of the general practitioner (GP). Now, however, surgery became more complicated, and the better surgeons wanted to restrain not only the GPs but the less qualified surgeons as well.

As noted earlier, this could only mean cutting the volume of paying patients for the GP. It meant that the GP's image to the public might be lowered, that the GP might come to be viewed as a less-than-complete physician. In fact, by 1947 the AMA's Council on Medical Education had to issue a special report on the prestige of general practitioners (Stevens, 1971). The better surgeons, on the other hand, argued that GPs had no business inside the abdomen. This view led, as noted earlier, to the attempt to keep the GP out of urban hospitals and, in many areas of the country, to restricting the practice of the GP in the hospital to non-surgical cases.

The American College of Surgeons (ACS), which was established in 1912, set specific requirements in an effort to improve the skills of physicians it accepted into fellowship. Stevens (1971) notes that "prerequisites included a one-year internship, three years as an assistant, fifty case abstracts, visits to surgical clinics, and for graduates of 1920 and after, two years of college before medical school" (p. 92). This suggested a pattern for certifying specialists. Clearly, the ACS requirements raised standards to improve surgical practice. Though the college could not license surgeons, it could pass professional judgment by approving of accomplishments and behavior of surgeons. As a voluntary group, however, it could judge only those who appeared voluntarily before it. Once a practitioner was accepted into fellowship, the ACS could do little to monitor continued excellence; such monitoring came much later. All these developments by the ACS were important, but not enough. The next step was to inspect the places in which internships were provided—that is, the general and specialty hospitals around the nation. Both the AMA and the ACS moved on this front.

The AMA began to pay attention to the internship at the time it established its Council on Medical Education. The council surveyed hospitals that were offering internships and in 1914 published its first list of approved internship hospitals. At about the same time, the ACS began to think about establishing hospital standards for surgical practice. In 1916 it received a Carnegie grant for this purpose. The first list of hospitals that the ACS felt met its standards was ready in 1919, but the conditions encountered in its survey were so bad that the college suppressed the list. In 1924 the Council on Medical Education began to approve hospitals for residency (specialty) training programs. A key requirement at that time was that the hospital must first have approval for internship programs.

Residency training in one of the recognized specialty fields also posed some problems as it developed. Originally, the residency represented an extra period of clinical training following the internship for a few elite young physicians who wished to become teachers or leaders in medicine. By the mid-1960s, however, nearly all medical school graduates were taking three or more years of residency (specialty) training after an internship. The growth of the specialties was a direct result of new knowledge and new technology, enabling physicians to do more than ever before to help people in need. As with internships, residency programs proliferated into hospitals of all types and sizes. In some teaching hospitals there was little, if any, full-time staff, few of the attending physicians were interested in teaching, and the resident's educational experiences and practice were poorly supervised and coordinated. Some hospitals did not have an adequate number or variety of patients, and in some, where there were senior staff, the staff were so involved in research that they often neglected to teach the residents. In addition, many residency programs were planned, monitored, and appraised only by members of one individual medical service (medicine, surgery, pathology, etc.)—sometimes only by a single person, the chief of the service.

The need for reform was evident to many medical educators and to leaders of the AMA. The AMA once again assumed a leadership role and commissioned the Citizens Committee on Graduate Medical Education, chaired by John S. Mills, who was then president of Western Reserve University. The Mills Commission (as it became known) consisted of eleven members, only three of whom were physicians.

For the second time in its history, the AMA requested an outside examination of the medical education process. The mandate this time was to examine graduate medical education—the internship and the residency—and to make recommendations to improve this part of a physician's formal training. The Mills Commission's report, *The Graduate Education of Physicians,* was issued in 1966 (Citizens Commission on Graduate Medical Education, 1966). Among key recommendations was a call for the elimination of the independent internship, meaning that no internship be approved unless it is linked with and part of an approved residency training program. The first year of each residency program, however, should be one that gives the resident a broad clinical experience. The commission further recommended that this change in the nature of the internship should not mean an additional year of residency training.

Another key recommendation related to the role of the hospital. The commission felt that the existing autonomy of individual hospital departments and the programs they developed was not appropriate, but that the hospital as a whole had to play some role in residency programs in terms of providing resources and facilitating the cooperation of other hospital departments and services. The commission went so far as to recommend that accreditation of residency training programs be given to the institution rather than to the individual services involved. There were many other recommendations, but these are the ones of most concern in this discussion.

The Mills report is an excellent example of a health policy plan. Although not completely implemented, it led to considerable discussion within the medical profession and to positive reforms in line with the spirit of the report. In late 1970, the AMA's House of Delegates endorsed the concept that the first year of graduate medical education be in a program approved by the appropriate residency review committee (which each specialty board had) rather than by the AMA's Council on Medical Education. Thus, in effect the AMA said that it would no longer review and approve internships, that internships would have to be integrated with residency training programs. In fact, since 1975 the AMA has stopped approving internships and has ceased the use of the term *internship* in its *Directory of Residency Training Programs*. The AMA's position was reaffirmed and strengthened in 1982 when its House of Delegates adopted a recommendation from its Council on Medical Education that the first year of postdoctoral medical education for all graduates consist of a broad year of general training.

Modern Graduate Medical Education

Graduate medical education today consists of a period of supervised training in a medical specialty in an approved clinical setting following graduation from medical school. Hospitals provide the large majority of graduate medical education opportunities, but ambulatory settings are beginning to play a more important role. Historically, the larger general hospitals, particularly those affiliated with medical schools

or those that had approved residency training programs for specialty training, attracted U.S. and Canadian medical graduates. Positions in smaller unaffiliated hospitals were filled mainly, if at all, by international medical graduates. In the larger general hospitals, there was usually a salaried, full-time director of medical education who saw to it that the educational experiences of both interns and residents were appropriate. In the latter hospitals, the director of medical education typically filled that role on a voluntary or part-time basis. In both instances there was concern that the educational aspects of the program were being neglected while the services provided by the residents were being emphasized.

Today, graduate medical education includes training in specialties and subspecialties (the residency) and training preliminary to the residency program (a one-year general residency, or the transitional year). Accreditation of graduate medical education programs is granted by the Accreditation Council for Graduate Medical Education (ACGME), which is jointly sponsored by the American Medical Association, the Association of American Medical Colleges, the American Board of Medical Specialties, the Council of Medical Specialty Societies, and the American Hospital Association. Accreditation is based on an evaluation of both the institution and the program it provides (ACGME, 2000). Recent studies of medical education have called for more resident training to take place outside of the hospital with ambulatory patients in a primary care setting because much of the preliminary work and treatment formerly done in hospitals is now done in ambulatory settings (Ebert & Ginsberg, 1988; New York Academy of Medicine, 1988).

In 1998 there were over 7,500 active residency training programs in the United States. The largest number of programs was in internal medicine, followed by family practice, and then pediatrics (Miller, Dunn, & Richter, 1999). From 1993 to 1997, the total number of residents remained fairly constant. In 1998, however, the number of residents decreased slightly. The number of residency programs continues to rise, a trend attributable to the rise in the number of subspecialty slots. As a result, some residency programs have no residents, and subspecialty residencies average fewer than three on duty (Miller et al.).

Securing a Residency and Becoming a Specialist

The National Resident Matching Program (NRMP) is a computerized service that matches resident applicants with approved hospital training programs. The aim is to meet the desires of the hospitals and the would-be residents to the greatest extent possible. Additional aims are to eliminate, if possible, pressures and special inducements that tend to skew the distribution of interns and residents, leaving some hospitals with many unfilled slots and other hospitals oversubscribed (National Resident Matching Program, 1999).

The NRMP was introduced when there were twice as many positions available each year as there were graduating seniors. By the 1980s that ratio had changed because of the increased number of U.S. and international medical school graduates applying for residencies. The decrease in options in residency programs is beginning to concern some medical school graduates, who are anxious to be accepted in top-quality programs, in a specific specialty, and in a desired geographic location. Acceptance into the "right" residency is considered as important as being accepted into the "right" medical school. Concerns regarding residency placement will become even more acute as medical education systems review policies that will help to bring balance to the physician-patient ratio and the specialist-generalist ratio. This topic is covered more extensively in the discussion on financing graduate medical education.

In 1998 a total of 35,823 applicants participated in the NRMP, competing for 22,541 positions offered by 3,814 programs (National Resident Matching Program, 1999). For the 1999–2000 training year, first-year residents received an average annual stipend of $34,985, which represents an increase of approximately 3 percent over the previous year. For the second year of graduate medical training, the average base salary was $44,523, indicating an increase of about 2.3 percent over the previous year (AAMC, 1999a).

Traditionally, resident physicians have worked long hours while gaining the clinical experience necessary to practice medicine. However, the number of hours residents should be on duty is controversial and was questioned in 1987 when the state of New York investigated the number of hours residents

worked following mishandling of an emergency case. The residents involved had been on duty for an extended period of time. New York set rules to govern the working hours of residents in order to minimize the risk of future misadventures that might be attributable to residents being too tired to think clearly. The rules require an average eighty-hour work week and shifts limited to twenty-four hours followed by sixteen hours off (*AMA Member Communications, 2001*). Some program faculty objected because the rules could interfere with continuity of care. Additional controversy revolves around increased costs of training with limitations on work hours.

Prior to the 1990s, resident training focused largely on acute care in the tertiary care setting, reinforcing the physician's decision-making skills, the use of large regimens of diagnostic tests over a short period of time, and wide variations in treatment planning based on the customs and training of the faculty involved. The setting of the inpatient acute care facility also fostered specialty training rather than primary and preventive care (family practice, pediatrics, internal medicine, etc.). Since the mid-1980s, much of the delivery of health care has been moving from the inpatient to the ambulatory setting. Prospective payment and new technology have reduced lengths of stay, promoted less-invasive techniques, and encouraged prevention over intervention. The 1997 budget reconciliation agreement provided incentives to train physicians in ambulatory sites by making direct medical education and indirect medical education payments available to such sites (Young & Coffman, 1998).

Specialty Boards

To become a specialist today in a particular medical area, a physician must pass a qualifying examination administered by a specialty board (following medical school, the general residency, and the specialty residency). The physician is then certified as a diplomate (diploma holder) of that specialty by the appropriate specialty board. The various boards are legitimized by their sponsors: the specialty society (or societies) in that area and the appropriate specialty section of the AMA. The first specialty board, the American Board for Ophthalmic Examinations (renamed the American Board of Ophthalmology in 1933), was developed in 1917 by the AMA's Section on Ophthalmology, the American Ophthalmological Society, and the American Academy of Ophthalmology and Otolaryngology. The second specialty board, developed in 1924, was the American Board of Otolaryngology. Other boards followed in the 1930s and later.

The American Board of Ophthalmology set the pattern for specialty recognition in the nation. The logic for legitimacy was simple: Any specialist worthy of recognition belonged to one or more of the sponsoring groups. This did not mean that a physician could not be a competent specialist without belonging. It did say that if that self-styled specialist wanted outside professional recognition of competence, he or she had to belong to one of the societies or to the AMA scientific section. If the specialists belonged, then the society or AMA section, as a representative body, could legitimately sponsor a specialty board. Over a span of time, each of the specialty societies modified its requirements for membership. One common element, however, became certification by the appropriate specialty board.

The number of specialty boards in 1995 stood at twenty-four (American Board of Medical Specialties, 1995). Application for the development of a specialty board is submitted to the Liaison Committee for Specialty Boards (LCSB), a joint creation of the AMA's Council on Medical Education and the American Board of Medical Specialties (ABMS). The ABMS is a coordinative body representing the twenty-four existing approved specialty boards, with five cooperating or associate members who are there for liaison purposes: the American Hospital Association, the Association of American Medical Colleges, the Council of Medical Specialty Societies, the Federation of State Medical Boards of the United States, and the National Board of Medical Examiners. The ABMS was established in 1933 as the Advisory Board for Medical Specialties when there were only four existing certifying boards, but the trend toward establishment of specialty certifying boards was clearly established. The board was reorganized, and its name was changed to the American Board of Medical Specialties in 1970. The major purposes of the ABMS are to act as a spokesperson for approved specialty boards, resolve problems that arise among specialty boards, deal with the approval of new specialty boards and types of certification, and prevent duplication of effort among boards.

Specialty certification in the United States is voluntary. Certification in a medical specialty is separate and distinct from the license to practice medicine in a state. The trend is toward certification as "virtually all United States graduates . . . undertake residency training and seek specialty certification" (American Board of Medical Specialties, 1982). There are no legal requirements for a licensed physician to seek specialty board certification in order to offer specialty services. Even though certification is not a form of licensure, it is often required for certain appointments, such as hospital medical staff privileges, participation in health care insurance programs, and participation in managed care plans.

Establishment of many specialty boards inevitably led to conflicts over definition of the specialty. So long as the specialty, however defined, did not pursue a formal legitimizing process, the need for precise definitions was not imperative. Once the boards were established, however, definitional, or domain, or "turf," problems arose.

Organizational conflicts also arose. The AMA, for example, at many points sought to bring things under its umbrella, believing that the stronger the AMA was in terms of being *the* voice of American medicine, the more persuasive it could be in bringing about lasting improvements. Others, on the other hand, saw organizational development outside the AMA, but not in opposition to the AMA, as a more effective mechanism. Sometimes the disagreement over strategies was in part a conflict of long-term versus short-term objectives. Clearly the AMA was not altogether happy that the specialties developed outside its structure, for it wanted a unified medical profession. The AMA viewed the specialty sections as focal points for the dissemination of knowledge to all physicians, and not just to serve the needs of the highly trained specialists (Fishbein, 1947). A major step was taken by the AMA in late 1977 to bring the specialty societies into its policy-making framework (*American Medical News*, 1977a). Despite some competitiveness and disagreements, the AMA and most of the specialty organizations sought ways to work together for the good of their profession and of the public.

The development of specialty organizations also brought about issues of terminology. A physician who completed all specialty requirements except the final board examination was, until recently, said to be *board eligible* in that specialty. Some specialties, such as orthopedic surgery, require the person to be a board-eligible practitioner in the specialty area before being permitted to take the examination. In other cases, the board-eligible person practices in the specialty area until the examination is scheduled and results are reported. In some cases, the board-eligible person never bothers to take the examinations. Since "board eligible" can cover a multitude of competencies as well as sins (including those who fail the board examinations), there is a move by specialty boards to drop the use of this phrase and, on inquiry, to state precisely what a person's status is in the certifying process. When the physician passes the specialty exam and is awarded a diploma, he or she is then said to be a diplomate (holder of a diploma) or board certified.

In 1973 the ABMS adopted a policy urging voluntary, periodic recertification of medical specialists by all member boards. In 1980 the ABMS issued guidelines to assist member boards with the recertification process. Most boards require recertification within a ten-year period, although family practice and pediatrics require recertification in seven years. Most boards require a written examination. A smaller number require oral exams or other forms of assessment. The ABMS also calls for publication of members' certification status in the ABMS directory (American Board of Medical Specialties, 1995).

The time required for training in a specialty varies with the specialty (see Table 4–5). The training program is known as the *residency* in a particular clinical area. The person being trained is a graduate of a med-

Table 4–5 Length of Some Residency Programs and Their Recertification Requirements

Residency Program	GY-1: General Residency	Includes GY-1	Years of Training	Subspecialty Training	Years to Recertification
Family practice		X	3		7
Emergency medicine		X	3		10
Pediatrics		X	3	2 years	7
Internal medicine		X	3	2 years	10
Obstetrics/gynecology		X	4		10
Pathology		X	4		N/A
General surgery	X		3	1–3 years	10
Neurological surgery	X		4		N/A
Orthopaedic surgery	X		4		10
Otolaryngology surgery	X		4		N/A
Urology	X		4		10
Anesthesiology	X		3		10
Dermatology	X		3		10
Neurology	X		3		10
Nuclear medicine	X		3		10
Ophthalmology	X		3		10
Physical medicine	X		3		10
Psychiatry	X		3		10
Radiology, diagnostic	X		3		N/A
Radiation Oncology	X		3		10

Source: Data from the American Board of Medical Specialties (1995), the American Association of Medical Colleges, and the National Resident Matching Program (1999).

ical school and while in the residency is known as a *resident.* The AMA's annually published *Essentials of Accredited Resident Training Programs* (available at www.acgme.org/acgme/intro.htm) spells out the general requirements for approval and accreditation of residency programs. It also describes the specific requirements that apply to the respective specialties. Each accredited residency program is responsible for providing the training as specified in the *Essentials.*

Graduate Medical Education Financing

The cost of graduate medical education (GME) involves resident salaries, the administration of the programs, the cost of having more complicated cases, and the increased cost of patient care (increased use of diagnostic services and length of stay) associated with the hospital's teaching function. As a result, the cost per case at teaching hospitals is higher than at comparable nonteaching hospitals (Bajaj, 1999b).

Until recently, financing GME was not a major problem. About 80 percent of residents' training costs were supported by patient care revenues, but now costs are rising rapidly and are paid for largely by government programs. Private insurance companies do not directly support medical education, and decreased payments for patient care have ended the type of cost shifting that once allowed for indirect support of GME built into higher patient charges. Federal and state governments, which were willing to subsidize GME when there was a shortage of physicians and when funds were more plentiful, are now searching for ways to reduce their support. Medicare is now the major source of funds for GME. It subsidizes GME indirectly with adjustments to the diagnosis-related group (DRG) payments to teaching hospitals. Direct GME payments to hospitals under Medicare were once based on the hospital's cost of training. Since 1985, direct GME payments have been capitated and are linked to a "per resident" amount (Bajaj, 1999a). Reimbursement to hospitals from Medicaid is hardly adequate to cover essential patient care, and yet government is looking for ways to contain costs in that area also.

GME funding is also coming under scrutiny because of a perceived imbalance in the physician-population ratio and an oversupply of specialists and undersupply of generalists. Medicare has changed its funding policies to take the first step toward curtailing an overabundance of doctors. The new rules cap the number of residency slots Medicare will fund, permits payments to nonhospital providers, and provides incentives for facilities to reduce the number of residents they train (Martin, 1998). Prior to 1997, Medicare payments to HMOs included an adjustment for medical education but contained no requirements for the HMO to provide medical education. The new legislation decouples GME payments from HMO payments (Young & Coffman, 1998).

MEDICAL LICENSING

In the second half of the nineteenth century, many states established or reestablished licensing boards. But not all states at the turn of the twentieth century required passing a state board licensing examination to practice medicine in that state. Texas, in 1873, was the first state to establish a state board of medical examiners. By the turn of the twentieth century, thirty-seven states required credentials of some sort for licensure, and twenty-three of these states required more than a diploma. Some states also began to recognize the credentials and licenses of certain other states on a reciprocal basis; hence the practice of reciprocity came into being (Womack, 1965).

Practices for governing the qualifications for medical practice differed widely. Some states scrutinized candidates with care, while others did not; some required examinations, while others did not. The need for some kind of national standard was apparent to many, but to bring this about was not easy. As with so many efforts at change, resistance is often encountered. For example, the National Confederation of State Medical Examining and Licensing Boards (founded in 1891) considered the question of a national examining board but disapproved the idea. In 1902, four states established the American Confederation of Reciprocating Examining and Licensing Boards (Derbyshire, 1969). The organization increased in membership as it focused on "improving educational standards and promoting uniform legislation for medical licensing." In 1912 the two organizations merged to form the Federation of State Medical Boards of the United States. Despite initial disagreements over aims of the federation, by 1978 all medical (MD) boards were members, as well as nine osteopathic examining boards and the medical boards of some Canadian provinces.

During the early part of the twentieth century, some in the AMA were interested in national licensure, but this never became a strong movement because of constitutional concerns over the question of states' rights. This is a nice way of stating two related points of view: concern over federal bureaucratic control of the right to practice and concern by state boards about their rights (self-preservation). Many persons involved believed that the state boards were better able to assess competence to practice medicine. It is important to note that any national system would have to have standards low enough that most states could qualify. Otherwise, a national system would not be acceptable. Why, then, should a state board with very high standards opt for a system that would lower that state's standards? This is, in part, why the federation's early successes were limited.

However, reformers wanted to see standards raised throughout the nation, as well as increased reciprocity. In addition, they wanted a mechanism in the federal services to ensure high-quality physicians. The idea, then, of some kind of national examining system as a means for comparing medical graduates from the different schools gained acceptance, and this led, by 1915, to the formation of the National Board of Medical Examiners (NBME).

The AMA's endorsement of the NBME came in 1916, and with that endorsement the NBME was fully legitimized. The NBME quickly began work, administering the first examination in late 1916. Thirty-two applicants asked to take the examination, but only sixteen were considered sufficiently qualified. Womack (1965) reports that only ten took it, and only five passed. Initially, eight states indicated that they would accept NBME test results for licensure. Over the years, as testing procedures improved, and as state boards were reassured that the NBME would not usurp their prerogatives and become the licensing agency, more and more states accepted the results. But there were many variations, and some states in-

sisted on creating their own examinations, constructed from the NBME pool of questions, graded by the NBME, but administered by the states under their own names. Some states, moreover, insisted on special basic science examinations, which often became a barrier to licensure (Derbyshire, 1969). The original intent of licensure and examination was to deal not so much with physician deficiencies, but with chiropractors, cultists, and the like.

Despite the significant advances brought about through the NBME examinations, state structuring of some examinations by boards whose personnel were always changing and who generally had no expertise in testing procedures, coupled with state determination of pass levels, prompted concern. Some states rarely failed applicants, while others had high failure rates. These variations posed very real problems in terms of facilitating reciprocity of licenses among the states. In addition, the NBME examinations were not given to graduates of foreign medical schools. (See the section on international medical graduates later in this chapter.)

The problems that arose from variations among the states concerned enough of the state boards that a move began toward improving the situation by creating one national test. The Federation of State Medical Boards (FSMB) developed the Federation Licensing Examination (FLEX) from NBME questions. FLEX was accepted by all state boards for medical licensure until 1994. Each state administered the exam, which was graded by the NBME, and recorded by the federation for reference purposes. The grade was then reported to the appropriate state boards. All states had set the pass level at the FLEX weighted average of 75, although individual states differed about the number of times FLEX could be taken.

FLEX was taken by graduates who wished to practice in the few states where the NBME was not accepted, by a few medical school graduates who did not have an NBME certificate, and by international medical graduates. The great majority of medical school graduates took the NBME examinations (the "National Boards") to receive licensure.

Finally in 1992, after nearly a century of debate about a national licensing system, the FSMB and the NBME together introduced a single, uniform examination for the medical licensure called the United States Medical Licensing Examination (USMLE). The USMLE replaced the NBME examinations and FLEX. No other national examination was available after 1994.

The USLME is a three-step examination. Steps 1 and 2 can be taken during undergraduate medical school and are often folded into the curriculum as a measure of performance or criteria for advancement. Step 3 is taken after completion of medical school in conjunction with the applicant to practice in a particular state. Most states require completion of the one-year general residency in addition to undergraduate medical school in order to obtain licensure (USMLE, 1999a).

Since spring 1999 the USMLE has been administered on computer, reflecting the introduction of technology into more areas of education and evaluation (USMLE, 1999b). For additional information on the USMLE, see the Web site at www.usmle.org.

CONTINUING MEDICAL EDUCATION

Lifelong learning is essential for members of the medical profession (as for many other professions). Many physicians pursue their continuing medical education informally by reading journals, having conversations with colleagues, and attending presentations or discussions at medical staff or medical society meetings. Some physicians might participate voluntarily; since the 1970s, however, participation has largely become a requirement. Many states require participation in continuing medical education for relicensure, state medical societies require it for membership, and specialty societies require it for membership and recertification. This requirement has come into question by some because there is no convincing correlation between continuing medical education and improved patient care. In an age of quality assurance, continuing medical education is only one of the tools used to measure the physician's abilities. As previously mentioned, more emphasis has been placed on reexamination for recertification in specialties. Competitive forces have brought about new evaluation methods such as outcomes measurement and adherence to practice guidelines. A more in-

formed patient-consumer gathers information from multiple sources in determining quality of care.

INTERNATIONAL MEDICAL GRADUATES

The United States has always attracted graduates of foreign medical schools, who come for a variety of reasons: to escape wars, religious persecutions, and other repressions, as well as to seek new opportunities for adventure, economic well-being, and so on. In the eighteenth and nineteenth centuries, these physicians often provided a level of expertise very much needed in this land. Following World War II we began to experience a new wave of physician immigration: graduates of European schools who sought to establish a new life in the United States, in large measure because of the dislocations resulting from the war or of the economic chaos that reigned in the postwar period. As Europe was reconstructed, the flow of physicians waned.

A new group of physicians began to come to the United States to establish new lives and to get advanced training; some came under the guise of obtaining advanced training, but hoped to stay. They came from Asia. During the 1950s and 1960s, the flow from Asia did not contribute much to the permanent physician supply in the United States because our immigration laws were weighted heavily against Asians and Africans. Changes in 1968 and 1970, however, opened the gates to immigration from all countries. Physicians came in large numbers from a former U.S. colony (the Philippines), from newfound military allies (South Korea, Thailand, Iran, Taiwan), and from India. We welcomed them because they helped fill the physician shortage that we were beginning to experience as a result of a rapidly growing population, hospital expansions, and expansions due to research and technological advances that enabled physicians to help people in ways that were not previously feasible.

The international medical graduates (IMGs), formerly called foreign medical graduates (FMGs), provided medical services in three important areas: residencies providing patient care in teaching hospitals that were unable to fill their residency positions with U.S. medical graduates; patient care for the medically underserved areas of the inner city; and specialties such as pathology and institutional psychiatry that have not tended to attract U.S. medical graduates. Many of these physicians came from medical schools that were relatively unknown to us, and many had language difficulties (though not the Indians, who, as a result of British imperialism, had received excellent English-language training). The unknown quality of the foreign schools raised legitimate questions about the adequacy of their student training and their graduates' competence. The language barriers caused communication problems between doctor and patient, as well as between the IMG and his or her American colleagues.

It should be emphasized here that Canadian physicians are not considered foreign trained. Because of the similarities between the U.S. and Canadian educational systems and the medical school accreditation process, graduates of approved Canadian schools are considered eligible to be examined by all state boards on the same basis as U.S. graduates, and about half the states grant reciprocity.

For a long time it was relatively easy for IMGs to come to the United States for graduate medical training and to remain in this country for an indefinite period of time. Many foreign medical graduates took the medical knowledge and language reading ability test developed in the 1950s by the Educational Commission for Foreign Medical Graduates (ECFMG). The test was administered in many overseas locations, but it was advisory only and not legally binding. The failure rates were disturbingly high. IMGs could also enter the United States with or without ECFMG certification and take positions in places that did not attract enough U.S. medical graduates (e.g., state mental hospitals and inner-city indigent hospitals). Then, in 1974 the Coordinating Council on Medical Education reported an increasing concern that the United States had become overly dependent on IMGs to provide medical services, especially in hospitals. The report also stated that the IMGs coming from so many different countries, cultures, and educational institutions were not screened vigorously enough and might jeopardize the health and safety of the patients they treated. Testimony before a congressional committee in 1974 described the variety of practices that

were occurring and the serious questions about the quality of care being provided by many of the IMGs. Some states, because of the physician shortage in certain areas, issued temporary licenses (*American Medical News*, 1977b).

The data and the official reports that focused on the IMG problem, along with the emerging realization by others that there could be an excess supply of physicians by the 1980s, resulted in amendments to the Health Professions Educational Assistance Act of 1976. The amendments placed restrictions on the number of IMGs entering and remaining in the United States. In addition, the legislation mandated that IMGs who wished to enter the United States as immigrants on the basis of their medical skills and qualifications would have to pass Parts 1 and 2 of the NBME examination, or their equivalent, and be competent in written and oral English. The Visa Qualifying Exam (VQE) was subsequently developed and certified as equivalent. Failure rates were high—80 percent for 1977 and 1980. IMGs performed better on the clinical portion than on the part testing basic medical science knowledge.

In 1984 a new test, the Foreign Medical Graduates Examination in Medical Sciences (FMGEMS), replaced the VQE for ECFMG certification. ECFMG certification is necessary for graduates of foreign medical schools who want to be licensed and practice in the United States. At the present time, IMGs who are not U.S. citizens are required to pass either the FMGEMS or the new USMLE (basic science and clinical components), as well as an English-language proficiency test, to become certified.

To be eligible to take the basic science portion of the FMGEMS, applicants must have completed at least two years at a medical school listed in the *World Directory of Medical Schools*. To take the clinical portion, the applicant must have graduated from such a school.

About half of the IMGs today are U.S. citizens who were unable to gain admission to a U.S. or Canadian medical school and so took their training in foreign countries. Virtually all of these IMGs plan to practice in the United States. The exact number of those studying abroad is not known, but fewer are now accepted in residency programs. In 1984 there were 1,831 U.S.

citizen IMGs (USIMGs) accepted in residency programs in the United States, but in 1990 only 929 were accepted—a 61 percent decrease. This decrease is due in large part to the efforts of U.S. medical organizations and the government to limit the numbers of both USIMGs and IMGs because there is still uncertainty about the adequacy of their training.

Most of the U.S. nationals studying in foreign medical schools are concentrated in schools located in Mexico and the Caribbean. The accrediting bodies in those countries do not assess schools by the same criteria as are used for U.S. and Canadian medical schools, and all but a few of these schools are proprietary. It is generally believed that they lack the resources and teaching facilities, particularly the clinical teaching facilities, to provide an adequate undergraduate medical education. Because of the weak clinical teaching facilities, some students transfer to U.S. schools to complete their undergraduate training. Other countries also attract U.S. students, especially Italy, Hungary, and Spain. Students there also frequently seek to transfer to a U.S. school to complete their training. To help the U.S. medical schools evaluate the transfer applicants, the Association of American Medical Colleges conducts the Medical Sciences Knowledge Profile (MSKP), a two-day examination designed to assess the knowledge of medical sciences of students seeking advanced placement. The use of test results and the criteria for advanced placement vary among medical schools. However, transfer to a U.S. school is not easy.

United States as well as international students who complete their undergraduate medical education in a foreign country must (as stated earlier) pass the FMGEMS or Parts 1 and 2 of the USMLE before entering an accredited residency program in the United States. All of these measures are designed to discourage U.S. citizens from seeking medical undergraduate education abroad, to restrict the number of alien IMGs, and to assure the quality of IMGs who train and practice in the United States.

In the current atmosphere of questioning whether the United States has too many physicians, training of IMGs is under scrutiny. Because Medicare is the primary source of funding for graduate medical education, the government has a critical stake in how many residents are trained. Throughout the 1990s, efforts were made to develop policy that would reduce the overall numbers of physicians being trained, redistribute the emphasis in training from specialization to primary care practice, and develop ways to attract physicians to underserved areas after training. Under such policy considerations, the practice of training IMGs who return to their respective countries after training is questioned. Yet, historically, IMGs have filled a very real void in hospitals and clinics that have not attracted U.S. medical graduates. As Medicare funding for residency training slots is withdrawn, hospitals may still find it desirable to maintain those slots and fill them with alternatively funded IMGs rather than give up their residency training programs. Such an approach would simply skew the ratio of IMGs to U.S. medical graduates even further. In 1997, IMGs accounted for 26 percent (6,257) of the 24,516 first-year residents. Of the 6,257 IMGs, 41 percent, or 2,565, were foreign-born, non-U.S. residents (Greene, 1999).

SUMMARY

Medical education has undergone massive changes over the years. It has evolved from apprenticeship to a highly complex system of academic, clinical, and continuing education. Many professional organizations and government bureaus have an oversight capacity over the process. Those who have the stamina to complete the rigorous training are not then left to their laurels. The oversight process continues through credentialing organizations.

The basics of medical education are also changing. Medical students must learn business skills and computer skills in addition to receiving scientific and clinical training. Many medical schools have incorporated more "caring" into their training by offering electives in "spirituality and medicine" and interpersonal relationship training to enhance the patient-physician relationship. Like all other areas of medicine, medical education will continue to experience changes in the coming years. The case study for this chapter describes one medical school's approach to medical education today.

CASE STUDY 4.1: IN THE HEALTH CARE COMMUNITY

Medical School, 1999*

The University of Tennessee College of Medicine traces its origin to 1851, as the Medical Department of the University of Nashville. It has been located in Memphis since 1911. The College of Medicine is a member of the Association of American Medical Colleges and is accredited by the Liaison Committee on Medical Education.

The UTM (University of Tennessee, Memphis) College of Medicine still follows the Flexner model of medical education (emphasizing training in the sciences), while incorporating into its model a more humanistic approach. The first two years emphasize study of the basic sciences. Clerkships in various areas of medicine are the major focus of the third and fourth years. From the very first year, student physicians participate in a "Longitudinal Community Program . . . to prepare students for their roles and relationships as physicians with individual patients, patients' families, and the local community" and to assess needs, design interventions, and evaluate the interventions. Curriculum changes target earlier contact to patient care and greater exposure to ambulatory care. Students experience integration of computers into their training both in computerized course testing and a fully computerized USMLE.

Applicants to the UTM College of Medicine submit undergraduate transcripts (a minimum 3.5 grade point average is required), MCAT scores, references, and a personal statement. Applicants also take part in a personal interview as part of the admissions process. As a state institution, the UTM College of Medicine gives priority to state residents and children of alumni. The college has increased its enrollment of minority students and holds close to national averages for the number of female students.

The goal of the UTM College of Medicine is to prepare students for the practice of medicine through accumulation of scientific knowledge and the acquisition of skills and professional attitudes and behavior (University of Tennessee, 1999a). The faculty works closely with students in classroom and clinical settings to mentor as well as train students. The option for an expanded academic program (essentially a five-year plan rather than a four-year plan) is available for students who might encounter personal or academic difficulties while in the program. Perhaps the most interesting portion of the UTM Statement of Educational Objectives is the "Attitude and Beliefs" area. An excerpt from this section (University of Tennessee, 1999b) states that

The graduate will have an appreciation for:

- The religious, spiritual, mental, emotional, and physical needs of patients and their families
- The qualities of integrity, compassion, empathy, and equanimity
- Social responsibility and recognition of medicine as a social good, as well as a commercial commodity
- The provision of health care to all patients regardless of one's prejudices or beliefs

In an era of medicine as big business, the medical school strives to ensure that students develop and maintain sensitive and effective relationships with patients.

A statewide Graduate Medical Education Program is also offered through the University of Tennessee, Memphis, College of Medicine, with twenty-five residency and twenty fellowship training programs. The training programs utilize various clinical facilities in Memphis, Chattanooga, Jackson, Knoxville, and Nashville.

*Information for this case study was obtained through a personal interview with the dean of the College of Graduate Health Sciences and from the University of Tennessee, Memphis, Web site (www.utmem.edu).

ACTIVITY-BASED LEARNING

Medical schools each have their own admissions criteria, although there are broad similarities among them. Access the Web site for the Association of American Medical Colleges (www.aamc.org) and compare various medical schools (AAMC, 1999c).

- Can you pinpoint the similarities and differences among a few medical schools you choose to review?

Now go to the Web site for the American Association of Colleges of Osteopathic Medicine (www.aacom.org). Choose the "Colleges" section with direct links to each of the osteopathic medical schools.

- Can you find similarities and differences in admissions criteria?
- What do you think might be the criteria by which potential medical students choose the schools to which they apply?

A QUESTION OF ETHICS

The high cost of a medical education, as well as the time that must be devoted to the entire training process, makes medicine as a profession available to only a select group of people.

- Does the medical education system inherently exclude certain populations, such as the poor and minorities?
- What changes could be instituted to make medicine as a profession available to a more diverse population?

It is generally believed that U.S. citizens who attend foreign medical schools do so because they cannot get accepted to U.S. medical schools.

- Should U.S. government funds be used to support the residency of a United States–born IMG?
- Should U.S. government funds be used to support the residency of foreign-born IMGs?

IMGs often fill residencies, and later practice medicine, in areas that are not attractive to U.S. medical graduates, such as poor urban areas. What should be done (if anything) to attract more U.S. medical graduates to positions in these areas if they are not filled by IMGs?

References

Accreditation Council for Graduate Medical Education. (2000) [On-line] Available: www.acgme.org (Accessed February 20, 2001).

American Association of Colleges of Osteopathic Medicine. (1998a). *Osteopathic medical education* [On-line]. Available: http://www.aacom.org (Accessed June 26, 1999).

American Association of Colleges of Osteopathic Medicine. (1998b). *Osteopathic Physicians* [On-line]. Available: http://www.aacom.org (Accessed June 26, 1999).

American Board of Medical Specialties. (1982). *Annual report and reference handbook, 1982.* Evanston, IL: Author: ABMS.

American Board of Medical Specialties. (1995). *Annual report & reference handbook.* Evanston, IL: ABMS is author and publisher.

American Medical News. (1977a, December 12).

American Medical News. (1977b, March 7).

American Medical News. (1991, April 22).

American Osteopathic Association. (1999). *Osteopathic medicine.* Available: http://www.aoa-net.org (Accessed July 2, 1999).

Association of American Medical Colleges. (1984). *Physicians for the twenty-first century.* Washington, DC: Author: AAMC.

Association of American Medical Colleges. (1999a). *COTH survey of housestaff stipends, benefits and funding* [On-line]. Available: www.aamc.org/hlthcare/coth-hss/stip00.htm (Accessed October 13, 1999).

Association of American Medical Colleges. (1999b, September 9). *Medical College Admission Test (MCAT)* [On-line]. Available: www.aamc.org/stuapps/admiss/mcat/geninfo.htm (Accessed September 25, 1999).

Association of American Medical Colleges. (1999c). *Medical schools of the U.S. and Canada* [On-line]. Available: www.aamc.org/meded/medschls/start.htm (Accessed October 2, 1999).

Bajaj, A. (1999a). How Medicare calculates GME payments (part 1). *JAMA, 281* (20), 1958.

Bajaj, A. (1999b). How Medicare calculates GME payments (part 2). *JAMA, 281* (22), 2156.

Barzansky, B., Jonas, H., & Etzel, S. (1998). Educational programs in US medical schools, 1997–1998. *JAMA, 280* (9), 803.

Barzansky, B., Jonas, H., & Etzel, S. (1999). Educational programs in US medical schools, 1998–1999. *JAMA, 282* (9), 840–846.

Beran, R., & Lawson, G. (1998). Medical student financial assistance, 1996–1997. *JAMA, 280* (9), 8019.

Burrow, J. G. (1963). *American Medical Association: Voice of American Medicine.* Baltimore: Johns Hopkins Press.

Citizens Commission on Graduate Medical Education. (1966). *The graduate education of physicians.* Chicago: American Medical Association.

Coggeshall, L. T. (1965).*Planning for Medical Progress Through Education.* Evanston, IL: Association of American Medical Colleges.

Commission on Hospital Care. (1947). *Hospital care in the United States.* New York: Commonwealth Fund.

Corner, G. W. (1965). *Two centuries of medicine: A history of the School of Medicine - University of Pennsylvania.* Philadelphia: Lippincott.

Derbyshire, R. C. (1969). *Medical licensure and discipline in the United States.* Baltimore: Johns Hopkins Press.

Ebert, R., & Ginsberg, E. (1988). The reform of medical education. *Health Affairs, 7* (2, Suppl.).

Fishbein, M. (1947). *A history of the American Medical Association, 1847–1947.* Philadelphia: Saunders.

Flexner, A. (1910). *Medical education in the United States and Canada.* New York: Carnegie Foundation for the Advancement of Teaching.

Flexner, A. (1940). *I remember.* New York: Simon & Schuster.

Greene, J. (1999, June 14). Is the U.S. training too many physicians? *American Medical News,* pp. 9–10.

Johnson, V. (1947). The Council on Medical Education and Hospitals. In M. Fishbein (Ed.), *A history of the American Medical Association, 1847–1947.* Philadelphia: Saunders.

Krakower, J., Williams, D., & Jones, R. (1999). Review of US medical school finances, 1997–1998. *JAMA, 282* (9), 847–854.

Liaison Committee on Medical Education. (1999, July 29) [On-line] Available: www.lcme.org (Accessed September 25, 1999).

Ludmerer, K. M. (1985). *Learning to heal, the development of American medical education.* New York: Basic Books.

Martin, S. (1998, July 27). New Medicare residency funding rules combat oversupply. *American Medical News,* p. 8.

Miller, R., Dunn, M., & Richter, T. (1999). Graduate medical education, 1998–1999. *JAMA, 282* (9), 855–860.

Moskowitz, D. B. (1999). *1999 health care almanac & yearbook.* New York: Faulkner & Gray.

National Resident Matching Program. (1999). *About the NRMP* [On-line]. Available: eraspo6.aamc.org/nrmp/abounrmp/indes.htm (Accessed October 13, 1999).

New York Academy of Medicine. (1988). *Clinical education and the doctor of tomorrow.* New York: Author.

Norwood, W. (1944). *Medical education in the United States before the Civil War.* Philadelphia: University of Pennsylvania Press.

Packard, F. R. (1963). *History of medicine in the United States.* New York: Hafner.

Resident Work Hours. (2001). AMA Member Communications [On-line]. Available: www.ama-assn.org/ama/pub (Accessed February 28, 2001).

Robinson, J. (1999). The new face of medical education. *JAMA, 281* (13), 1226.

Shryock, R. H. (1960). *Medicine and society in America, 1660–1860.* New York: New York University Press.

Shryock, R. H. (1966). *Medicine in America.* Baltimore: Johns Hopkins Press.

Stevens, R. (1971). *American medicine and the public interest.* New Haven, CT: Yale University Press.

Stevens, R. (1989). *In sickness and in wealth.* New York: Basic Books.

University of Tennessee. (1999a). *College of Medicine, admissions information* [On-line]. Available: www.utmem.edu/medicine/admissions.html (Accessed September 25, 1999).

University of Tennessee. (1999b). Educational objectives for the program leading to the M.D. degree. Brochure printed for the 2003 schedule of classes.

United States Medical Licensing Examination. (1999a). *USMLE eligibility requirements* [On-line]. Available: www.usmle.org/oct98.news.pencil.htm (Accessed October 15, 1999).

United States Medical Licensing Examination. (1999b). *USMLE news—CBT testing schedule* [On-line]. Available: www.usmle.org/oct98/news.pencil.htm (Accessed June 29, 1999).

Womack, N. A. (1965). The evolution of the National Board of Medical Examiners. *JAMA, 192* (June 7).

Yom, S. (1998). On the brink: The costs of medical education. *JAMA, 280* (21), 1878.

Young, J., & Coffman, J. (1998). Overview of graduate medical education: Funding streams, policy problems, and options for reform. *Western Journal of Medicine, 168*(2), 428–437.

CHAPTER

5

Professions in Health Care

Chapter Objectives

After completing this chapter, the reader should have an understanding of:

- The multiple participants in the provision of direct and indirect patient care.
- The differences in training and credentialing of health care service providers.
- The tensions that may exist among health care service providers.
- The difficulties in coordinating care among various providers, given cost and payment restrictions.

INTRODUCTION

Physicians historically gained control of health care delivery through licensing and credentialing. They had the knowledge regarding diagnosis and treatment of disease and the authority (often sole authority) to act on that knowledge. Rapid changes in the health care market (managed care, cost containment incentives, the rise in corporate medicine, the introduction of information systems technology) have drawn attention to the question of whether new forms of health care delivery reduce physician authority and raise the professional discretion of other health care providers—and whether those changes in authority are appropriate.

The dominance of physicians in health care can be explained by

- The division of labor in health care delivery that requires that all other health care professionals work under "orders" given by the physician (Friedson, 1985)
- The amount of knowledge physicians have, particularly in comparison to the patients they treat (Folland, Goodman, & Stano, 1993; Phelps, 1992; Starr, 1982)
- The capitalist economy, which promotes the freedom of practice and economic dominance of physicians (Friedson, 1985)

The free market assumes participation of consumers based on the premise of "buyer beware" while professions operate on the basis of the buyer believing in (trusting) the professional (Torres, 1991). This difference stems from the fact that professionals are deemed to have knowledge or expertise not available to the layperson. Professionals not only possess complex knowledge, but the knowledge is viewed as critical to the social welfare. Most persons would agree that physicians fit the criteria of "professional." Occupations acquire professional status over time. The state gets involved in establishing boundaries (licensing of the practitioner), which other occupations cannot cross. The profession must be in continuous movement to ensure its status in legislation as competing occupations vie for control of protected areas of performance (Torres, 1991).

Deprofessionalization occurs with the reduction in the knowledge gap between physicians and consumers that is fostered by the increase in consumer education and the computerization of knowledge (Friedson, 1985). Deprofessionalization also occurs as more and more physicians assume salaried positions in organizations and as new professions emerge with authority to treat patients independently of physicians.

Professional oversight, utilization review, and the formation of institutional review committees have become the norm in the provision of health care. The result is more formal control and supervision of individual physician practices—indirectly by corporate structures, but more directly within the profession by peers who occupy formal reviewer roles (Friedson, 1985). Current review is based on formal research and authoritative opinion of medical researchers and elite practitioners. Researchers and administrators employ a macroview of providing health care to the population, while practitioners employ a microview of the individual patient. Conflicts occur and practitioners are often limited in their freedom to choose a particular mode of care because resources are controlled by administration. Constraints on clinical judgment are generated by professional standards, and practitioners are forced to justify any moves outside those standards. Computers can add a level of control by monitoring practice habits and flagging "deviant" behavior.

Other medical specialists (nurse practitioners, physician assistants, etc.) are assuming roles previously played by physicians, thus reducing physician control and autonomy. The emergence of the health care team in patient treatment often requires deferment of judgment by the physician to a more technically skilled physiotherapist, pharmacist, or inhalation therapist (McKinlay & Stoeckle, 1988). Physicians' affiliation with medical specialty organizations has weakened the political power of the American Medical Association (AMA). The oversupply of physicians (in some areas) has added to competition and also results in a loss of power in the marketplace. Physicians have unionized in some parts of the country in order to regain some power. All of this is evidence that physicians are being divested of control in the delivery of health care services.

The questions of physician control and the limits of practice placed on other health care providers are not new. Struggles between the professions for areas of exclusive privileges are as old as the professions themselves. Legal practice parameters change as professions lobby state legislatures. Accepted standards of practice often change with reimbursement decisions made at the federal level by the Health Care Financing Administration (HCFA). While we attempt to describe the functions of various health care professionals in this chapter, we recognize that these functions are changing with time and may vary from state to state.

Countless health professionals provide direct patient care and/or work in support of those providing direct patient care. As the provision of health care changes and technology is adopted, categories of personnel also change. The health professionals discussed in this chapter do not constitute all health care professionals but are representative of the critical distinctions among health care providers.

NURSES

Nurses are "the hearts and hands of health care" (Friedman, 1991) and continue to be the largest group of health care professionals. Nursing is unique in that it encompasses the only group of health care professionals that is predominantly female. While the majority of nurses still work in hospitals, nursing practice is shifting to a focus on disease prevention and modification of lifestyles. This shift in focus results in more nurses working in community clinics, doctors' offices, long-term care facilities, schools, and patients' homes (Health Resources and Services Administration [HRSA], Division of Nursing, Bureau of Health Professions, 1999). Experienced nurses are also being recruited by insurance companies, peer review organizations, managed care organizations, and pharmaceutical companies. Some have their own independent practices. The nursing profession is undergoing change in educational and training programs and in the tasks that nurses perform.

Nursing began as a helping profession in the United States with training programs associated with general hospitals. The pattern that developed dominated the nursing field until after World War II: Nurses were trained for three years in special schools associated with hospitals. On successful completion of the course of study, the graduating student was awarded a diploma, and on passing the state licensing examination the nurse became a registered nurse (RN). Only about 24 percent of RNs in 1996 were graduates of hospital diploma schools of nursing (American Association of Colleges of Nursing, 1999). The percentage, however, is decreasing as the number of graduates from two- and four-year college programs is rising. This changing scene will be discussed after we briefly examine the various types of nursing programs.

Hospital diploma school programs typically had a large service emphasis; that is, the training was heavily weighted in favor of on-the-job training rather than academic training. From the beginning, these programs served as a form of labor exploitation because much of the students' time was spent on the wards caring for patients, and the student nurses received no compensation, save perhaps room and board. As these programs evolved, they began to adopt stronger academic components; in some states, the students took some of their courses at local colleges and universities. However, the number of diploma programs has declined significantly, from 80 percent of all programs in 1960 to only 7 percent in 1996 (Moskowitz, 1999).

During World War I, a number of university nursing programs were developed that granted a baccalaureate degree instead of a diploma. On passing the same state licensing examination taken by the diploma school graduates, the baccalaureate graduate also became an RN. Baccalaureate programs experienced a rapid rise, from 15 percent of all programs in 1960 to 35 percent in 1996 (Moskowitz, 1999). Graduates of baccalaureate programs constituted nearly 32 percent of the total registered nurse population in 1996. Enrollment in these programs, as in the other nursing degree programs, has fluctuated from 1980 through the turn of the twenty-first century as health care has gone through various streamlining efforts as a result of cost containment. Enrollment in baccalaureate programs is a mix of first-time enrollees (31 percent), those from associate degree programs (59 percent), and enrollees from diploma programs (10 percent) (HRSA, Division of Nursing, Bureau of Health Professions, 1999).

A third type of nurse training program began to develop during the 1950s in community colleges. These programs last two to two and a half years and grant an associate degree to the student. On passing the same state licensing examination taken by the diploma school and college or university graduate, the student becomes a registered nurse. Associate degree programs have also experienced a rapid rise, from only 5 percent of all programs in 1960 to 58 percent in 1996 (Moskowitz, 1999). As mentioned earlier, many of the RNs from these programs eventually go on to college or university programs to also earn a bachelor's degree. Approximately 34 percent of the total number of practicing RNs in 1996 held an associate degree as a terminal degree (HRSA, Division of Nursing, Bureau of Health Professions, 1999).

There are, as we have illustrated, three basic pathways to becoming an RN. Each has an academic component, each uses hospital facilities for clinical training, and all graduates become registered by taking a common state examination administered by the state board of nurse examiners. The diploma programs and associate degree programs are credited for providing more clinical experience than the baccalaureate programs. Some people have criticized the baccalaureate programs for not providing sufficient clinical training, leaving hospitals to augment the training by providing in-services to new employees. There are, of course, great variations among programs, with strong and weak programs in each pathway. The baccalaureate approach is distinctive in that it provides the additional educational requirements that are necessary if an RN wishes to pursue a graduate degree. Because of the debate over the comparative operational competencies of the graduates from the different types of programs, there have been attempts to categorize the programs. The data to support the various categorization attempts are far from conclusive because of the great variability among programs within each pathway and the variability of admission requirements by the programs. Nurses, whether trained at the diploma, associate degree, or baccalaureate level, have similar roles and functions in hospitals and generally receive the same salary.

Members of the nursing profession have been embroiled in a long and unproductive controversy among themselves over what is adequate educational preparation for nursing. Since 1964, the American Nurses Association (ANA) has advocated that only nurses with baccalaureate degrees be called professional nurses. However, because most nurses enter the profession with either an associate degree or a diploma, in 1985 the ANA called for the establishment of two levels of nursing practice: a level called *professional nurse* for those nurses holding a baccalaureate degree and a level called *technical nurse* for those holding an associate degree. Efforts to change state licensing laws to reflect this difference have not been successful.

There is clearly a movement on the part of nurse leaders to close the diploma schools because, they believe, nurse training should be part of an educational system and not under the control of a hospital or of any other profession. Diploma schools are closing, and although professional pressures are operative, the cause is primarily cost. The costs of diploma education can no longer be buried in general hospital costs and covered by insurance payments. Those programs that have survived are often affiliated with a college or university offering the academic courses supplementing the hospital training that results in an associate or bachelor's degree upon completion. The difference between the diploma and the other degrees is evident only in the fact that the diploma student sits for the state exam and licensing before completing the academic portion of training.

The views of nurse leaders vis-à-vis diploma education have to some extent spilled over into the classroom, and baccalaureate students frequently are persuaded to view their roles in nursing as more professional than those of diploma or associate degree students—that is, to view themselves as leaders in nursing and as people having a deeper theoretical understanding of nursing practice than the others. When baccalaureate graduates have not been able to gain perspective on this in work situations, the issue has sometimes led to conflicts with the diploma nurses, as well as with hospital administrators. An experienced diploma nurse is not likely to feel kindly toward a recent graduate from a baccalaureate program who expresses such views, nor is a hospital administrator, who is concerned more with nursing performance. On the other hand, baccalaureate graduates feel a lack of recognition for their additional training when they are treated no differently from graduates of shorter programs. This lack of consensus over issues concerning the educational preparation of nurses has caused disarray within the nursing profession.

Part of the search for professional identity has led nursing to decrease its participation in certain functions that were historically a part of nursing, such as nutrition, medical social work, medical records, and some therapies. A great deal of this change was, of course, necessary because of the growing complexity of the health field. No longer could a nurse have all the knowledge and skills necessary to cover these functional areas. Specially trained people emerged to cover these functions. But spinning off these functions to other personnel raised the question, What is nursing? Bedside nursing was historically a key nursing function; in a very real sense, it was more fundamental to nursing than all of the other functions. Now, however, a great portion of bedside nursing is being taken over by the licensed practical nurse (LPN) and nursing assistants. If bedside care and other things are given up, what is left to legitimize nursing as a profession?

This question has led nurse leaders to identify different roles. Accepting the proposition that the diploma nurse is a disappearing breed, nurse leaders have begun to see the associate degree nurse as a technical nurse capable of handling whatever functions remain for patient care in the hospital and doctor's office, and the baccalaureate nurse as the leader and teacher. The National Advisory Council on Nurse

Education and Practice (NACNEP) initiated an examination of nurse workforce issues in 1994 and describes the role of nursing in the future as follows: " to manage care along the continuum; to work as peers in interdisciplinary teams; and to integrate clinical knowledge with knowledge of community resources" (HRSA, Division of Nursing, Bureau of Health Professions, 1999, p. 1). The council identifies the baccalaureate education as providing "the critical thinking and problem solving skills; sound foundation in a broad range of basic sciences; knowledge of behavioral, social and management sciences; and the ability to communicate and analyze data" (p. 1)—skills most appropriate for nursing's future.

Nurse leaders are even beginning to recognize the professional nurse as being one who earns a master's degree (9 percent of the 1996 nursing workforce) as a specialist in a clinical area of nursing (e.g., pediatrics, public health, medical-surgical nursing, intensive care) or in a health services management area; or as one who holds a doctorate (about 1 percent of the 1996 nursing workforce), not in sociology or higher education but in one of the developing doctoral programs in nursing, health administration, or health services research. Just as in other areas of health care delivery, professional nursing is no longer concerned only with "sick care" but also with "wellness." Others argue that there is a unique role for nursing that relates to helping people cope with conditions that medicine is unable to cure or help: the growing area of chronic care.

Changes in health care require health professionals to function in teams, and physicians and nurses are now working in a more collaborative, rather than adversary, environment. Change is very prominent in the large teaching hospitals, where nurses today are doing things that neither they nor physicians ever thought would be nursing functions. Nurses are performing tasks that are new, as well as some functions that were once done by physicians. Though the *theory* of nursing may not have taken such events fully into account, nursing is being *operationally* redefined. There is, of course, no ironclad definition of what a nurse or a physician is. The terms and the things they describe are human devices applied to a world that is forever changing.

A significant attempt to address nursing issues was the formation of the National Commission on Nursing in 1980. This was an independent commission composed of leaders in the fields of nursing, hospital administration, medicine, government, academia, business, and hospital trustees. The commission concluded that nurses should be given more responsibility for patient care and be involved along with physicians in decisions affecting patient care. The commission recommended that nurses be included in policy making in hospitals and be responsible for resources to ensure high-quality care (National Commission on Nursing, 1983). Nurses have continued to struggle to expand their role in the changing, more technological atmosphere of health care. They have taken advanced training either to specialize in a certain clinical area (ICU, NICU, psychiatry, operating room, etc.) or to provide more independent care (nurse practitioners, nurse-midwives, etc.).

Strains between physicians and nurses continue to exist as the nursing role expands and the relationship with physicians becomes more of a collaborative partnership, with nurses being a part of the clinical decision-making process. Designed to ease some of the friction, in 1983 the AMA House of Delegates adopted a statement that nurses should not be expected to blindly follow all medical orders and that a nurse may take action contrary to standing orders to protect a patient in an emergency if a physician is not available. The resolution was sending a message to physicians that the nurse has a responsibility to use judgment too.

Factors Affecting the Supply of Nurses

Throughout the 1980s and 1990s, there has been conflicting information about a national nursing shortage. The severity of the shortage depends upon the geographic location and type of nurses needed. Although the national shortage was much discussed in the 1980s, changes in hospital reimbursements resulted in many hospitals releasing nurses in an attempt to downsize and reduce costs. The downsizing resulted in the use of other personnel, such as nursing assistants, to pick up some of what had traditionally been nursing's responsibility. But hospitals also found themselves working with patients who were older and more critically ill as many of the less acute cases were handled on an outpatient basis. The current nursing shortage is mainly in large urban hospitals providing high-tech care to sicker patients—a shortage of highly skilled nurses.

Wages and working conditions contribute to the shortage. The wages of hospital nurses compare poorly to the wages of female professional and technical workers in other fields. Although the starting salaries of nurses are now comparable to those of other college graduates, the maximum average salary is much lower. Women who plan to work a number of years do not find the pay raises and career ladders in nursing that exist in many other professions women now enter. In other words, women today have many more career options in which the economic rewards are greater, their contributions are better recognized, and the hours are more regular. In addition to the low pay and difficult hours for nurses, there are other dissatisfactions: short staffing, which prevents nurses from giving optimal care; superiors (especially physicians) who do not listen to or respect nurses' professional abilities; and a lack of authority to make decisions they feel qualified to make. Those who remain in nursing have more options to work in other clinical sites, such as medical practices, HMOs, ambulatory surgical centers, home care, and so on. (American Association of Colleges of Nursing, 1999).

Clinical Specialists in Nursing

Just as we see with physician education and practice, coping with new knowledge has forced specialization in nursing. A nurse with a baccalaureate degree may undertake graduate study toward a master's degree and/or a doctorate in a variety of clinical areas to develop the needed special competence for teaching, for supervision, and for advanced practice. In addition to training in such clinical specialties as pediatrics, obstetrics, medical-surgical services, and psychiatry, a number of specialized programs have been developed, such as those for the nurse practitioner and nurse-midwife, that train nurses to work on their own in private practice or as equals on a health care team. Some of these programs are described in more detail later in this chapter.

Licensed Practical Nurses

Licensed practical nurses (LPNs) provide nursing care to patients under the direction of a physician, dentist, podiatrist, optometrist, or registered nurse. Their responsibilities are similar, to but more limited than, those of a registered nurse. Most LPNs can administer medications, take vital signs, treat bedsores, prepare and give injections, insert catheters, and the like. Their responsibilities differ by state regulations. Some states, such as Ohio, certify LPNs to administer intravenous therapy after specific additional training (Central School of Practical Nursing, 1998).

The LPN developed from the nursing shortage that followed World War II; hospitals began to hire LPNs in place of more expensive RNs whenever possible. However, this trend subsided as technological procedures increased and patients who were admitted to hospitals were sicker. LPN training takes twelve months on average to complete and is usually part of public vocational school programs, although some LPN programs are run by hospitals, community colleges, or community agencies. In 1995, the most recent year with available data, there were over 1,200 schools offering LPN programs and over 44,000 graduates of such programs (Moskowitz, 1999). Often there is no carryover credit for LPNs. If they wish to go on to other nursing programs, they must start from the beginning with no transfer credits.

Nursing Education Approval and Accreditation, and the National League for Nursing

Nursing programs—LPN, diploma, associate degree, and baccalaureate degree—must be approved by an agency of state government if graduates are to be permitted to take the licensing examination. The *state board of nurse examiners* is typically the name of the state agency that handles this. The National League for Nursing (NLN) provides a mechanism for academic accreditation over and above the state approval process. The NLN focuses principally on educational nursing programs—from LPN, diploma, and associate degree programs to baccalaureate and advanced degrees. Some disagreement exists with the ANA about accreditation of continuing education programs. RNs who are graduates from NLN-accredited programs normally can have their licenses endorsed by other states (reciprocity).

Graduate programs in nursing can be professionally accredited by the NLN. Approval of graduate programs is usually beyond the scope of state government authority. Specialty subcomponents of a master's program are sometimes accredited by a nurse specialty body, in addition to being accredited by the NLN.

The American Nurses Association

The ANA is a professional association for RNs that establishes and implements nursing political and legislative programs, promotes a professional and equitable work environment for nurses, and develops standards that ensure high-quality patient care. It also approves organizations for providing continuing nursing education. The ANA works to increase nurses' pay and improve their conditions of employment. It actively lobbies lawmakers and regulators whose decisions have an impact on nursing concerns. Its current focus is on improving working conditions for nurses, particularly the stress nurses encounter under staff shortages and mandatory overtime. With the focus on cost containment, the professional organization is concerned with the quality of care rendered to patients in this nurse shortage environment.

The American Nurses Credentialing Center has provided certification programs for the ANA since 1973. The certification programs are similar to those in other areas of medical care, administering exams and requiring documentation regarding formal and continuing education for each level of certification. The newly reorganized and implemented certification process offers two certifications: (1) "RN,C" (RN, certified) for the RN who has received a diploma or an associate degree and passes the certification exam and (2) "RN,BC" (RN, board certified) for the RN who has received a bachelor's degree and passes the appropriate exam. Among the goals of the credentialing program is the desire to educate the public regarding the value of professional nursing and credentialing. Certification is voluntary at this time and has no connection to state licensure (American Nurses Association, 2000).

Public Health and Community Nursing

Public health nursing, with its focus on preventing disease and promoting health in the community, offers an alternative to hospital care of the sick. It also provides nurses with an opportunity to work more independently than in the hospital. For the most part, public health training is generalized to enable a single well-trained nurse working in the community to recognize and cope with multiple problems that may arise in a family. Generalized training is based on the premise that people and families, rather than diseases or physical situations, should be served. There is some specialized training in such areas as industrial or full-time clinical nursing.

Most state health departments have separate bureaus or divisions of public health nursing, in which public health nurses are employed as advisers to local health departments, boards of education, voluntary health agencies, and other state agencies. They also may conduct in-service training and promote services that are available through the local public health nursing programs.

At the local level, public health nurses are employed by local health departments, where their primary tasks relate to disease prevention and health promotion; and by agencies such as visiting nursing associations, which are concerned primarily with rendering home nursing care to the sick. When employed outside of a public health department, the public health nurse is frequently called a community nurse. The nomenclature, however, is not precise. Some public health departments also call their public health nurses community nurses.

As the health care system becomes increasingly complex, with a proliferation of public, private, and proprietary health service agencies that target specific population groups, there is some concern that the health of the entire community is not being addressed. Health departments and others, for example, are often affected by reimbursement mechanisms and the growth of federal- and state-mandated categorical programs that promote a narrow focus of services. The fact that many nurses without public health preparation work in community settings has resulted in some confusion about what public health nursing is. The Public Health Nursing Section of the American

Public Health Association defines the purpose of public health nursing as improving the health of the entire community (American Public Health Association, Public Health Nursing Section, 1981). To accomplish this goal, public health nurses work with groups, families, and individuals, as well as in multidisciplinary teams and programs, identifying subgroups within the population who are at high risk of illness, disability, or premature death, and directing resources toward these groups.

NURSE PRACTITIONERS

An expanded role for nurses is that of the nurse practitioner, who is trained to serve as the regular health care provider for children and adults during health and illness. The nurse practitioner obtains medical histories, performs physical examinations, diagnoses illness and disease, orders laboratory tests, prescribes medications (in collaboration with physicians in some states and independently in others), provides education and counseling, and assumes responsibility for medical management of cases with emphasis on primary care. Typically, nurse practitioners graduate from a two-year master's program in one of many specialty areas. They are employed in both urban and rural areas in settings such as community-based clinics, physicians' offices, home health agencies, nursing homes and hospices, hospitals, and independent nurse practitioner offices. The most important reasons nurses give for becoming nurse practitioners are the chance to have a greater influence on patient care and the opportunity for additional learning.

Many nurse practitioners choose settings where populations are underserved for health care services. Statistics indicate that a large number of nurse practitioners are in rural states, and the majority practice in clinics providing direct primary care. They practice independently and have a collaborative arrangement with a physician, who cooperates in the management of patients' health care problems when necessary. It is assumed that a nurse practitioner functioning "interdependently" has a physician available for ready consultation and can refer patients easily.

The role of the nurse practitioner has been well accepted by the community, but less so by physicians and other health providers. Nurse practitioners have an expanded role in health care, with greater independence than nurses have, including third-party reimbursement. Since January 1998, Medicare has reimbursed nurse practitioners directly for independent patient care. Some states have extended prescription-writing privileges to nurse practitioners (American Academy of Nurse Practitioners, 1999). Some physicians, in the current climate of physician oversupply and increased physician competition, view these developments as intrusions on their turf and oppose extended independent privileges to nurse practitioners, while other physicians welcome the opportunity to work alongside them.

NURSE-MIDWIVES

The number of nurse-midwives is increasing in the United States, totaling about 6,700 in 1999. Approximately 5,700 of them are in clinical practice. The number of deliveries by nurse-midwives has also increased every year since 1975. Certified nurse-midwives delivered over 258,000 babies in 1997—8.47 percent of all vaginal births that year (American College of Nurse-Midwives, 1999).

Midwives delivered most newborn Americans until World War I, when medical advances and the acceptance of hospital deliveries resulted in a dramatic decline in the practice of midwifery. Early midwives were not professionally trained or licensed, but apprenticed with other practicing midwives. However, that has changed, and currently there are forty-seven accredited nurse-midwifery education programs in the United States, most offering a master's degree. About 4 percent of midwives have a doctoral degree. The American College of Nurse-Midwives (ACNM) accredits the education programs. According to the ACNM:

- Nurse-midwifery practice is legal in all fifty states and the District of Columbia.
- Thirty-one states mandate private insurance payment for services, and Medicaid reimbursement is mandatory in all states.
- Most certified nurse-midwife–attended births occur in hospitals; only 2 percent occur in freestanding birthing centers and 1 percent in the home.

- The primary workplace of most nurse-midwives is an office or clinic environment.
- Nurse-midwives have prescription-writing privileges in all fifty states.
- Visits to the nurse-midwife include annual exams, reproductive health visits, and visits outside the maternity cycle.

Nurse-midwives tend to offer personalized, family-centered, low-intervention maternity care. They have low cesarean section rates and low infant mortality rates—both an indication of quality care and a result of the fact that nurse-midwives refer high-risk cases to physician specialists.

Even though nurse-midwives have physician backup, there is considerable opposition from physicians to nurse-midwives opening their own practices. In many instances they and their collaborative physicians have been refused hospital privileges, the authority to admit and care for private patients. However, a midwife-attended birth costs about 50 percent less than a physician-attended birth. This difference in cost has led managed care organizations and clinics in underserved areas to embrace the concept of midwife deliveries. Specialists with busy obstetric practices have also recognized the value of midwife deliveries in low-risk pregnancies. Collaboration is now more common, although some stress remains over the scope of midwife practices in more competitive environments.

CERTIFIED REGISTERED NURSE ANESTHETISTS

Certified registered nurse anesthetists (CRNAs) became the first clinical nursing specialists in the late 1800s, as a response to the growing need surgeons had for anesthetists. Today, there are more than 27,000 CRNAs providing 65 percent of the 26 million anesthetics given to patients in the United States each year (American Association of Nurse Anesthetists, 2000).

CRNA training requires a registered nurse to attend an accredited nurse anesthesia education program to receive an extensive education in anesthesia. Entry into the program requires a bachelor's degree in nursing or another appropriate baccalaureate degree from an approved nursing program, a license as a registered nurse, and a minimum of one year of acute care nursing experience. CRNA programs range from twenty-four to thirty-six months of graduate course work, including both classroom and clinical experience. All nurse anesthesia education programs now offer a master's degree in nursing, allied health, or biological and clinical sciences. Upon graduation, the nurse must pass a national certification exam to become a CRNA and pass a recertification program every two years thereafter (American Association of Nurse Anesthetists, 2000).

All states permit CRNAs to practice. Although CRNAs can be found in various practice settings (hospitals, freestanding surgical centers, etc.) and in various geographic areas, they are the sole anesthesia providers in more than 70 percent of rural hospitals in the United States.

There is much debate about the propriety of allowing CRNAs to practice independently of physician supervision. The Health Care Financing Administration (HCFA) eliminated Medicare requirements that CRNAs be supervised, saying there were no studies indicating negative patient outcome when CRNAs were unsupervised. The American Society of Anesthesiologists and the AMA argue that there is potential increased risk to patients. The HCFA has left it to the states to determine whether CRNAs should have physician supervision (American Medical News, 2000).

PHYSICIAN ASSISTANTS

Physician assistants (PAs) are licensed to practice medicine with supervision by physicians. As members of the health care team, PAs "conduct medical exams, diagnose and treat illness, order and interpret tests, counsel on preventive health care, assist in surgery, and in most states can write prescriptions" (American Academy of Physician Assistants, 1999; p. 1).

Statistics gathered by the American Academy of Physician Assistants for 1999 indicate that there are more than 40,000 PAs, practicing in at least sixty specialty fields. More than half report that their primary specialty is one of the primary care fields: family/general practice medicine (38 percent), general internal medicine (9 percent), general pediatrics

(3 percent), and obstetrics/gynecology (2 percent). Other prevalent areas of practice for PAs include general surgery/surgical subspecialties (20 percent), emergency medicine (10 percent), and the subspecialties of internal medicine (7 percent). More than one-third (38 percent) of all respondents work in a hospital, another third (35 percent) work in solo or group practice offices, about 12 percent work in some type of federally qualified health center or community health facility, and about 13 percent work for a government agency.

The PA profession was started in the mid-1960s in response to a perceived doctor shortage in order to increase access to medical care and reduce the cost of the services. Dr. Eugene Stead started the first PA training program at Duke University, forming a first class in 1965. Originally, most PA programs were designed to attract hospital corpsmen or medics who were leaving the armed forces. Because many of these people had some formal training and usually a considerable amount of experience, it was felt that their talents could be effectively employed in civilian health care. Within ten years, fewer than half of PAs had a military background, and today the vast majority are men and women with no military experience.

Physician assistants are educated in intensive medical programs accredited by the Commission on Accreditation of Allied Health Education Programs. There are currently 120 accredited programs, but a growing interest in the profession has resulted in many new programs being formed. All must become accredited. Education consists of classroom and laboratory instruction in the basic medical and behavioral sciences, followed by clinical rotations in internal medicine, family medicine, surgery, pediatrics, obstetrics and gynecology, emergency medicine, and geriatric medicine. State licensure requires graduation from an accredited physician assistant program and passage of the national certifying exam, developed by the National Commission on Certification of Physician Assistants in conjunction with the National Board of Medical Examiners (American Academy of Physician Assistants, 1999).

To remain certified, PAs must take 100 hours of continuing medical education every two years and pass a recertification exam every six years. Certified PAs carry the title "PA-C." PAs are licensed to practice in all fifty states and have prescribing authority in forty-six states. Physicians have had mixed responses to the growth in the numbers of PAs in practice, depending largely on the degree of competition in their health care environment. Many patients view their PA as their primary care provider and have a continuing relationship with the PA for their care. PAs are not simply seen as an occasional fill-in for the doctor. PAs refer patients to a physician and/or closely consult with a physician in complicated cases; otherwise the physician acts only in a supervisory role.

PHARMACISTS

Pharmacy is an ancient profession. Certainly it was prominent in seventeenth-century England; the practitioners were apothecaries who ran shops and compounded various drugs and medications. The pharmacist today, however, is rarely called on to compound a drug or medication, which now comes packaged from the manufacturer. Pharmacists have become part of the health care delivery team, with an emphasis on more direct patient care, particularly in counseling patients about medication use, possible adverse affects, and other medication-related concerns.

There are approximately 201,700 pharmacists in the United States with the numbers increasing by about 2,200 annually (National Association of Boards of Pharmacy, 2000). Pharmacists are the third largest group of health care professionals, exceeded only by physicians and nurses. Most pharmacists entering the workforce today choose to practice in community pharmacies, and a substantial number take positions within the pharmaceutical industry. This trend has left a shortage of pharmacists available to work in the hospital setting. Community pharmacists make higher salaries than hospital pharmacists and spend more time on patient care functions.

Hospital pharmacy is an expanding area. Pharmacists and hospitals are responsible for systems of total control of drug distribution, designed to ensure that each patient receives the appropriate medication in the correct form and dosage at the correct time. They are also an authoritative source of drug information for physicians, nurses, and patients. There are a number of specialized areas within hospital pharmacy, such as nuclear pharmacy, drug and poison information, and intravenous therapy. Hospital pharmacists are seeking to change the pharmacy from a *supply* department, which is a product-oriented technical function, to a patient-oriented clinical service in which the pharmacy would be a department of drug experts who would be more involved in monitoring and counseling on matters relating to drugs.

There are eighty-one schools of pharmacy in the United States accredited by the American Council on Pharmaceutical Education. In 1998 over 33,000 students were enrolled in first-degree pharmacy programs. Among them, 12.3 percent were minority students and 64.4 percent were women. An additional 4,245 students already holding a Bachelor of Science (BS) degree in pharmacy were enrolled in Doctor of Pharmacy (PharmD) programs (American Association of Colleges of Pharmacy, 1999).

Students are accepted in pharmacy schools after graduation from high school. There are two first professional degree programs that usually qualify graduates for the licensure examination. Thirteen accredited programs offer a baccalaureate degree program, which is customarily a five-year program that awards the BS in pharmacy. The PharmD program is offered as the first professional degree (usually a six-year program) at eighty colleges/schools of pharmacy. Sixty-one programs offer the PharmD as a post-BS degree (American Association of Colleges of Pharmacy, 1999).

Pharmacy graduates must pass the North American Pharmacist Licensure Examination (NAPLEX), developed by the National Association of Boards of Pharmacy, before practicing pharmacy in all states. Each state also requires applicants to take a special examination on the legal aspects of pharmacy practice in that state (Multistate Pharmacy Jurisprudence Examination), and some also require the disease state management examinations. License transfer between states is possible for pharmacists under a uniform licensure agreement recognized by all states (National Association of Boards of Pharmacy, 2000).

Some professional organizations in pharmacy have urged that training be extended to a one-year residency after graduation. The additional experience would better prepare new pharmacists to function as true members of the health care team. There is no clear consensus on the residency issue and therefore no current requirement for credentialing or licensing (American Society of Health System Pharmacists, 2000). A six-year program (two years of liberal arts, three years of pharmacology, and one year of medical school) plus a one-year clinical residency has become the norm in most pharmacy schools that offer the PharmD.

DENTISTS

There are about 162,000 practicing dentists in the United States (1996 figure) who diagnose and treat diseases, injuries, and malformations of teeth, gums, and related oral structures (America's Career InfoNet, 2000). Most of the nation's dentists (approximately 92 percent) are in private practice, and about 79 percent are general practitioners. Of the more than 31,000 dental specialists, most are practicing orthodontics or oral surgery. Approximately 67 percent of private practitioners work in solo practice, while 21 percent work with one other dentist and 12 percent with two or more dentists (American Dental Association, 1999a). The average net income for all dentists was about $123,000 in 1997 (America's Career InfoNet, 2000).

Much like medical school, the first two years of dental school training are focused mainly on academic study, with the last two years devoted to clinical experience. Graduates from dental schools are awarded either a DDS (Doctor of Dental Surgery) or a DMD (Doctor of Dental Medicine), depending on the school. There are fifty-five U.S. dental schools, for which the American Dental Association is the accrediting agency. In addition, there are a number of postgraduate opportunities in dentistry. Some consist of residencies to qualify for credentialing as a specialist; others consist of advanced study for a combined master's degree or doctorate. The first-year class entering dental school in 1996–97 was about 38 percent female and about 35 percent minority students. The numbers of women and minority practicing dentists are growing (American Dental Association, 1999a).

To be licensed, candidates must pass a national written examination *and* a clinical examination conducted by licensed dentists from the individual states or from a regional grouping of states. Specific requirements may differ among the states. Thirty-four states have reciprocal agreements, or licensing by credentials. Credentialing in a specialty requires examination by a chosen specialty board, much like medical board certification (American Dental Association, 2000b).

The American Dental Association (ADA) was founded in August 1859, at Niagara Falls, New York, by 26 dentists representing various dental societies in the United States. Today it has more than 141,000 members, 54 constituent (state-territorial) and 529 component (local) dental societies, and it is the largest and oldest national dental association in the world. The ADA's Commission on Dental Accreditation is the accrediting agency for dental educational and dental auxiliary educational programs in the United States. Its accrediting authority is granted by the U.S. Department of Education. The ADA formally recognizes eight specialty areas of dental practice: dental public health, endodontics, oral and maxillofacial pathology, oral and maxillofacial surgery, orthodontics and dentofacial orthopedics, pediatric dentistry, periodontics, and prosthodontics.

The widespread use of fluorides has dramatically reduced the incidence of tooth decay in children and has changed the nature of dental practice. Since the 1970s, tooth decay in American children has declined, and more time and effort are now spent on other dental problems, such as the management of periodontal (gum) disease and cosmetic dental procedures. Because of the success of preventive dentistry, growing older populations will retain their teeth longer and require regular dental care, contributing to a growing need for dental services. However, the number of graduating dentists is declining. Shortages exist in some rural areas and in some dense urban areas, while an oversupply exists in some of the major suburban areas—much like the distribution of physicians.

Dental Hygienists

Each state has its own specific regulations regarding the responsibilities and regulation of dental hygienists' services. In general, however, dental hygienists do general patient screening procedures, take dental x-rays, remove dental plaque calculus from the surfaces of the teeth, provide oral hygiene education, and provide support services to the dentist as necessary. Dental hygienists are licensed by the state. Licensure requires graduation from an accredited institution and passing scores on the National Board Dental Hygiene Examination and a state or regional exam (American Dental Association, 2000a).

Dental hygiene education involves a minimum of a two-year college education. The majority of community college–based programs award an associate degree. University-based dental hygiene programs offer baccalaureate degrees along with the dental hygiene training. There are approximately 250 dental hygiene education programs in the United States accredited by the American Dental Association. Approximately 95 percent of the students enrolled in dental hygiene programs are women, with minority students representing approximately 12 percent of the total enrollment. There are approximately 100,000 practicing dental hygienists in the United States, most employed in general dentist practices (American Dental Association, 2000a).

Dental Assistants

The responsibilities of the dental assistant vary according to the setting in which she or he works. Primarily the dental assistant works with the dentist in providing dental treatment, acting as an integral member of the team. In addition, the dental assistant may take and develop x-rays; take the patient's medical history, blood pressure, and pulse; provide patient education; and participate in office management tasks. Most dental assistants receive their training in community colleges or technical institutes in programs that take nine to eleven months.

Dental assistant programs receive credentialing through the Commission on Dental Accreditation of the ADA (approximately 245 programs are currently credentialed in the United States). Individual dental assistants might choose to become nationally certified by taking the Dental Assisting National Board examination. State regulations vary, and some states offer licensure and accreditation; other states do not require licensing for dental assistants (American Dental Association, 1999b).

OPTOMETRISTS

An optometrist is a Doctor of Optometry (OD—not to be confused with the DO, the degree conferred to a Doctor of Osteopathy). The optometrist's training is quite different from the training of the ophthalmologist, who is a medical doctor (MD) with a specialty in medical and surgical treatment of eye diseases.

The optometrist is trained and licensed by the state to examine the external and internal structure of the eyes; diagnose eye diseases and vision conditions; prescribe eyeglasses, contact lenses, and low-vision aids; and provide vision therapy services. Optometrists serve as a major point of entry into the vision care system and may refer patients to ophthalmologists or other physicians for treatment of ocular and systemic diseases. Optometry differs from ophthalmology in that optometrists provide the vast majority of primary care services for eye care but are limited in the amount of treatment they may provide. The nature of these limitations sometimes causes tension between the ophthalmology and optometry professions. In some states, optometrists are licensed to prescribe medications and perform laser therapies for certain eye diseases. In other states, optometrists are limited to diagnosis of disease for referral to ophthalmologists. The differences across states are often the results of the lobbying strengths of the professional organizations.

Historically, most optometrists were self-employed, mostly in solo practice. However, optometrists today work in private practices, multidisciplinary medical practices, hospitals, teaching institutions, research positions, community health centers, and the ophthalmic industry. There were about 41,000 active optometrists in the United States in 1996. The number of practicing optometrists is expected to grow in the early years of the new millennium, as indicated by a growing enrollment in schools of optometry. The percentage of women in schools of optometry has increased from 47 percent in 1990 to 53 percent in 1995 (America's Career InfoNet, 2000; Moskowitz, 1999).

Today optometrists are trained at seventeen schools of optometry, which are accredited by the Council on Optometric Education. The four-year postgraduate degree consists of classroom and clinical training, including training in the basic sciences. Unique to the education of optometrists is the advanced study of optics (the science of light and vision) and extensive training in lens design construction, application, and fitting (American Optometric Association, 1997). The curriculum emphasizes a comprehensive, holistic approach to patient care. Most state licensing boards now accept for licensure the results of a national board examination and also require continuing education as a condition for license renewal, but there is increasing concern in optometry, as in other professions, that participation in continuing education courses is no guarantee of competency in practice and of incorporating the latest developments into daily practice. One way an optometrist demonstrates clinical proficiency is by becoming a Fellow of the American Academy of Optometry, which requires careful examination of clinical skills. Fellows of the academy can be awarded *diplomate* status in specialty areas (e.g., contact lenses, binocular vision, and perception) following further tests.

PODIATRISTS

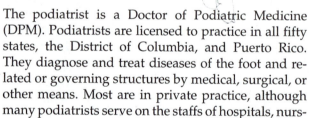

The podiatrist is a Doctor of Podiatric Medicine (DPM). Podiatrists are licensed to practice in all fifty states, the District of Columbia, and Puerto Rico. They diagnose and treat diseases of the foot and related or governing structures by medical, surgical, or other means. Most are in private practice, although many podiatrists serve on the staffs of hospitals, nursing homes, medical schools, armed forces, and health departments (American Podiatric Medical Association, 2000).

Candidates for admission to colleges of podiatry are expected to complete a baccalaureate degree. About 95 percent of all first-year entering students have a bachelor's degree (students with exceptional promise and a minimum of ninety college credit hours are sometimes admitted without the degree); about 10 percent have a master's degree. Training in one of the nation's seven colleges of podiatry accredited by the Council on Podiatric Medical Education is four years in length. The first two years are devoted to the basic medical sciences, the third and fourth years to clinical experience. Upon graduation, the candidate qualifies to take a state board examination and obtain a license to practice in about one-third of the states; two-thirds require an additional year of postdoctoral work before licensure. There are over 11,000 active podiatrists in the United States and three specialty areas of podiatry: podiatric orthopedics, podiatric surgery, and primary podiatric medicine. Certification requires a written and oral examination and demonstrated experience in the specialty (American Podiatric Medical Association, 2000).

CHIROPRACTORS

The word *chiropractic* is derived from Greek words that mean "done by hand." The profession of chiropractic evolved in the United States in the late 1800s and focuses on the treatment of illnesses by manipulation (particularly of the spinal column), physiotherapy, and dietary counseling and *without* the use of drugs or surgical intervention. Chiropractors use standard procedures and tests to diagnose conditions, and they rely heavily on x-ray of the skeletal system as a diagnostic tool.

Chiropractic education consists of four years of study at a chiropractic college after completion of a bachelor's degree. The first two years of chiropractic education emphasize the biological sciences and clinical disciplines. The last two years emphasize practical studies, with about half of the time being spent in college clinics. Upon graduation a Doctor of Chiropractic (DC) degree is awarded, but in order to practice, graduates must obtain a license by passing an examination given by state chiropractic boards. The Council on Chiropractic Education accredits fifteen chiropractic colleges in the United States and has joint accreditation agreements with colleges in Canada and other international locations (American Chiropractic Association, 1999). There were about 43,500 chiropractors in the United States in 1996, and the numbers are projected to grow through the year 2006 (America's Career InfoNet, 2000).

The AMA and AHA previously opposed insurance coverage, hospital-admitting privileges, and physician referrals to chiropractors, maintaining that

there was no scientific evidence of chiropractic's curative powers. Policies have changed, and some physicians do refer patients to chiropractors if they are unable to successfully treat certain back problems. Medicare, Medicaid, state workers' compensation programs, and most private health and accident policies authorize reimbursement for chiropractic services. Some managed care organizations have also approved chiropractors as the primary care gatekeepers for patients who choose that option. Reimbursement policies and competition for patients continue to feed the tension between chiropractic and medical doctors.

ORIENTAL MEDICINE PRACTITIONERS

Oriental medicine includes a variety of therapies; however, acupuncture is probably the most widely known. Acupuncture originated in China more than 2,500 years ago, but its entry into U.S. medicine is more recent. Thirty-eight states and the District of Columbia license, certify, or register acupuncturists, twenty-two of them to practice independently.

Currently there are more than fifty schools of acupuncture in the United States, and several medical schools include acupuncture training in their curriculum. Accreditation of programs is administered by the American College of Acupuncture & Oriental Medicine (ACAOM), and the National Certification Commission for Acupuncture and Oriental Medicine (NCCOAM) administers certification of the acupuncturist. There are currently over 10,000 licensed acupuncturists working in the United States (American Association of Oriental Medicine, 2000).

According to the American Association of Oriental Medicine (2000), this is how acupuncture works:

> Science has determined that human beings are complex bioelectric systems . . . energy circulates throughout the body along well-defined pathways. Points on the skin along these pathways are energetically connected to specific organs, body structures, and systems. If this energy circulation is disrupted, optimum function is affected and this results in pain or illness. Acupuncture points are stimulated to balance the circulation of energy, which influence the health of the entire being.

While acupuncture has long been categorized as "alternative medicine," it is making its way into mainstream medicine. The World Health Organization of the United Nations has issued a provisional list of forty-one diseases amenable to acupuncture treatment. The American Osteopathic Association, the American Chiropractic Association, the American Veterinary Medical Association, former Surgeon General C. Everett Koop, and the National Institutes of Health have in various ways recognized the promise of acupuncture treatment. In April 1996 the Food and Drug Administration reclassified acupuncture needles from experimental status to a Class II medical device (American Association of Oriental Medicine, 2000).

THERAPISTS

Therapy is most often linked with rehabilitation or development of skills lost through injury or illness. Many services today are designated as therapies, and it is impossible to include them all in this discussion. However, the two most widely known—physical and occupational therapy—are described here.

Physical Therapists

Physical therapists work mainly with strengthening of the joints and muscles. Treatment performed includes therapeutic exercise, cardiovascular endurance training, therapeutic pain relief, and training in activities of daily living. Physical therapists are trained to evaluate the patient for treatment needs, and thus they work as part of the health care team for developing a case management approach.

There were approximately 114,000 physical therapists employed in the United States in 1996 (America's Career InfoNet, 2000). They work in hospitals, private physical therapy offices, sports facilities, nursing homes, home health agencies and a variety of other settings. Although historically there has been a shortage of physical therapists, a new interest in physical therapy as a career in the 1990s has increased the number of physical therapists in practice (American Physical Therapy Association, 1999). At the same time, new regulations from the Health Care Financing Administration have restricted payment for physical

therapy services through the Medicare program and, in effect, decreased the employment options and salary ranges for many physical therapists.

Some 173 colleges and universities offer professional education in physical therapy. The minimum requirement is a four-year bachelor's degree program; after the year 2002, however, a master's degree will be required. After graduation, candidates must pass a state-administered national exam to be licensed to practice (American Physical Therapy Association, 1999).

The physical therapy assistant (PTA) is trained to work under the supervision of a licensed physical therapist to provide direct patient care, transport patients, and prepare and maintain physical therapy equipment. There are over 250 educational programs, most often in community colleges or junior colleges offering an associate degree, graduating 5,000 PTAs annually. Over half of the states require licensing, registration, or certification of PTAs. The major difference in training of PTAs from that of the physical therapist is the physical therapist's ability to work independently in providing therapy and in the training to evaluate the patient and provide a treatment plan (American Physical Therapy Association, 2000).

Occupational Therapists

The occupational therapist works to help people regain and build skills lost to illness or injury, or to develop skills blocked by developmental or psychological impairment. The primary objective is to develop skills that help people live independent, productive, and satisfying lives and avoid institutionalization or long-term care.

There were more than 57,000 occupational therapists in the United States in 1996 (America's Career InfoNet, 2000) providing independent hands-on care to patients. Occupational therapists are trained in a four-year baccalaureate program, complete a supervised fieldwork program, and pass a national certification exam. All fifty states regulate the practice of occupational therapy. A related profession, the occupational therapy assistant, completes a two-year associate degree program and works under the direction of the occupational therapist.

Candidates for occupational therapy vary greatly: The needs may stem from such impairments as arthritis or other chronic illnesses, head or spinal cord injuries, burns, head trauma, stroke, and developmental disabilities (American Occupational Therapy Association, 2000).

ALLIED HEALTH PERSONNEL

The term *allied health* includes a large number of health-related areas of work that assist, facilitate, and complement the work of physicians and other health professionals. The AMA's Committee on Allied Health Education and Accreditation (CAHEA) had worked collaboratively with various specialty societies, allied health organizations and societies, and educational associations to accredit allied health programs, but this responsibility was turned over to an independent, nonprofit agency, the Commission on Accreditation of Allied Health Education Programs (CAAHEP) in 1995. CAAHEP accredits 18 allied health professions in more than 100 institutions, including universities and colleges, academic health centers, junior and community colleges, hospitals, and others (CAAHEP, 2000). Among the more familiar allied health professions accredited by CAAHEP are athletic trainer, emergency medical technician-paramedic, medical assistant, ophthalmic medical technologist/technician, physician assistant, respiratory therapist, and surgical technician.

There are many other allied health programs accredited by bodies other than CAAHEP, such as programs in physiotherapy, occupational therapy, health education, medical dietetics, dental hygiene, and graduate programs in health administration. In addition, a large number of other allied health occupations have no formal program accrediting process at this time, except that some of them are parts of regionally accredited academic institutions. There is a shortage of many allied health personnel, especially in rural geographic areas and inner-city urban hospitals. Although many new graduates choose the hospital as their first place of employment, many later go into outpatient or other nonhospital settings where the pay is better and the work conditions more appealing.

HEALTH ADMINISTRATORS AND HEALTH PLANNERS

The health sector is large and complex. It is labor intensive—a heavy user of people—and requires a large amount of money to fuel its operations. Skilled health administrators are much in demand to run the hospitals, nursing homes, primary care centers, managed care organizations, health departments, mental health centers and hospitals, home care agencies, and other health care facilities. "To run" means to plan the services and their provision, to assemble or secure the resources, and to manage the use of those resources so that the purposes of the organization are fulfilled. Planning is, of course, an essential part of every administrative job, but in large organizations the planning function is frequently delegated to someone whose planning skills are well developed, to allow that person to focus on planning only, and to advise the administrator of what he or she should adopt as the planned course of action for the organization. In recent years, because of the complex interrelationships and dependencies between health agencies and government, the competitive nature of health care delivery, and the increased awareness of health care consumers, planning has become known as strategic planning and often includes a strong consideration of marketing.

Historically, the top administrator in most large health institutions was a physician or a nurse. Few were trained for their administrative roles. Even today, one finds health administrators and health planners who grew or fell into their jobs, whose academic preparation was not geared to either of these roles. In recent years, however, health care organizations have turned increasingly to people who have academic training in health administration or health planning. The necessity for specially trained health-oriented people, and not just any business administration or planning program graduate, stems from the complex nature of the health sector and the historical context within which the organizations and health professions operate. People are needed who understand not only planning and administration, but also the special aspects that apply to the health field—the constraints under which health professionals operate and the culture of health care professionals.

The time-honored doctrine of the doctor-patient relationship is increasingly experiencing interference from many arenas. The good health administrator must know how to orchestrate that intercession without altering the confidentiality of the doctor-patient relationship and without affecting the ability of the physician to render the best care for the patient. Well-trained health administrators and health planners are sensitive to these special circumstances and are able to apply their administrative or planning skills in that context so that the aims of the organization are achieved in terms of seeing that the highest-quality service is delivered.

The academic training of health administrators and health planners traditionally took place in a number of settings. Some were trained and awarded a master's degree by schools of public health, which were geared initially to the training of a variety of public health workers, of which public health administrators were only one type. Some were trained in schools of health administration, which were geared primarily to the training of hospital administrators. In fact, until about 1970, most of these schools were known as schools of *hospital* administration. The name change was designed to reflect the recognition by the schools that they were training not only hospital administrators, but also administrators for other kinds of health services organizations. Today, health administration programs are associated with a variety of organizational units of colleges and universities, including schools of public health, business administration, and health and human services, among others.

Baccalaureate programs in health administration are accredited through the Association of University Programs in Health Administration (AUPHA), on the basis of self-study and peer review. As of November 1998, twenty-two undergraduate programs in health administration were certified by AUPHA (1999). The Accrediting Commission on Education for Health Services Administration (ACEHSA) was organized in 1968 to replace the program conducted by AUPHA for accrediting master's programs. As of November 1998, there were sixty-seven accredited graduate programs in health administration in the United States and Canada. Accreditation is a rigorous process of self-study documentation, site visits and reporting by a peer panel, and review by the commission of the program's mission, curriculum, and faculty (AUPHA, 1999).

Doctorate programs in health administration and/or health planning do not currently have accrediting programs from AUPHA or ACEHSA, but fall under accreditation processes for the specific colleges or divisions of the universities granting the degrees.

The field of higher education is experiencing a great deal of change that is affecting the training of health administrators (as well as other health care professionals). Particularly at the master's level, new programs are becoming available in growing numbers through distance learning, condensed executive programs, Web-based programs, and combined degree programs. Some are accredited and some are not. It is the responsibility of the prospective student to determine the quality of such programs by inquiring about accreditation status.

SUMMARY

The definition of a "profession" is somewhat debatable, and the description of the various health-care personnel provided here is certainly not all-inclusive. Some may even debate the appropriateness of inclusion of some personnel. The goal, however, is not to place the label of *professional* on some personnel and withhold it from others. The goal is to make the reader aware of the various persons involved in patient care—directly or indirectly—and to provide a background for understanding the complexity of health care delivery. Conflicts exist at various levels—government, institutions, and individuals—over what professional might deliver certain levels of care. In a competitive and cost-conscious environment, alternative delivery processes are attractive, yet quality must be the overriding consideration.

ACTIVITY-BASED LEARNING

Many different professions are described in this chapter. Most professionals receive credentialing or simply affiliate, through membership, with a national professional organization. General information about education and licensing is available on Web sites for these organizations, but often individual state regulations guide the professionals more specifically.

- Interview a health care professional (other than a physician) to hear the story of the individual's education, licensing, credentialing, and so on, in order to learn about the differences or challenges that the professional faced in practicing in your local area.

A QUESTION OF ETHICS

- Is it the government's role, through licensing and regulation, to ensure the competency of health care professionals? Can licensing and regulation be an indicator of quality, or is it simply a process to protect the domain of certain health care providers?
- What is the individual's responsibility when choosing a health care provider, and what information regarding the provider should be made available to the individual consumer to help determine the provider's competency?
- Is health insurance reimbursement for "alternative medicine" increasing consumer choice or simply a matter of providing less expensive health care treatment?

References

American Academy of Nurse Practitioners. (1999). Public Relations Information: *What is a nurse practitioner?* [On-line]. Available: www.aanp.org (Accessed Feb. 27, 2001).

American Academy of Physician Assistants. (1999). *AAPA general information* [On-line]. Available: www.aapa.org (Accessed April 3, 2000).

American Association of Colleges of Nursing. (1999). *Nursing school enrollments lag behind rising demand for RNs, AACN survey shows* [On-line]. Available: www.aacn.nche.edu/media/news release (Accessed March 21, 2000).

American Association of Colleges of Pharmacy. (1999, August). *Academic pharmacy's vital statistics* [On-line]. Available: www.aacp.org (Accessed April 3, 2000).

American Association of Nurse Anesthetists. (2000). *AANA information.* [On-line]. Available: www.aana.com (Accessed April 3, 2000).

American Association of Oriental Medicine. (2000). *Historical view and purpose of AAOM* [On-line]. Available: www.aaom.org/aboutaaom.html (Accessed March 24, 2000).

American Chiropractic Association. (1999). *About chiropractic* [On-line]. Available: www.amerchiro.org/about_chiro (Accessed March 24, 2000).

American College of Nurse-Midwives. (1999). *Basic facts about certified nurse-midwives* [On-line]. Available: www.midwife.org/press/basicfac.htm (Accessed April 2, 2000).

American Dental Association. (1999a, August 31). *ADA fact sheets, dentistry* [On-line]. Available: www.ada.org/prac/careers/fs-dent.html (Accessed April 4, 2000).

American Dental Association. (1999b, August 31). *Dental assisting* [On-line]. Available: www.ada.org/prac/careers/br-dass.html (Accessed April 14, 2000).

American Dental Association. (2000a, January 11). *Dental hygiene* [On-line]. Available: www.ada.org/prac/careers/fbr-dhyg.html (Accessed April 14, 2000).

American Dental Association. (2000b, February 21). *Licensure by credentials, reciprocity, endorsement or criteria* [On-line]. Available: www.ada.org/prac/careers/fs-dent.htm (Accessed April 4, 2000).

American Nurses Association. (2000). *About the American Nurses Credentialing Center* [On-line]. Available: www.nursingworld.org/ancc/anccinfo.htm (Accessed September 29, 2000).

American Occupational Therapy Association. (2000). *About us* [On-line]. Available: www.aota.org/about.asp (Accessed March 24, 2000).

American Optometric Association. (1997). *So you want to be an optometrist* [On-line]. Available: www.aoanet.org/career-guidance.html (Accessed April 14, 2000).

American Physical Therapy Association. (1999). *The physical therapist: A professional profile* [On-line]. Available: www.apta.org/about (Accessed March 24, 2000).

American Physical Therapy Association. (2000). *The physical therapist assistant: A profile* [On-line]. Available: www.apta.org/about (Accessed April 21, 2000).

American Podiatric Medical Association. (2000). *Podiatric medicine: The physician, the profession, and the practice* [On-line]. Available:

www.apma.org/careers.html (Accessed February 27, 2001).

American Public Health Association, Public Health Nursing Section. (1981). *The definition and role of public health nursing in the delivery of health care.* Washington, DC: Author.

American Society of Health System Pharmacists. (2000). *Council on Educational Affairs* [On-line]. Available: www.ashp.org/public/hq/policy/ (Accessed March 24, 2000).

America's Career InfoNet. (2000). *Occupation report* [On-line]. Available: www.acinet.org/acinet/oc (Accessed April 4, 2000).

Association of University Programs in Health Administration. (1999). *Health services administration education: Directory of programs 1999–2001.* Washington, DC: Author.

Central School of Practical Nursing. (1998). *What is an LPN?* [On-line]. Available: www.cspnohio.org (Accessed April 2, 2000).

Commission on Accreditation of Allied Health Education Programs. (2000, April 7). *About CAAHEP* [On-line]. Available: www.caahep.org (Accessed April 14, 2000).

Folland, S., Goodman, A., & Stano, M. (1993). *The economics of health and health care.* New York: Macmillan.

Friedman, E. (1991). Nursing: Breaking the bonds? *JAMA, 264*(24), 3117–20; 3122.

Friedson, E. (1985). The reorganization of the medical profession. *Medical Care Review, 42*(1), 11–35.

HCFA drops supervision requirement from CRNAs. (March 27, 2000). *News at Deadline,* American Medical News, p. 4.

Health Resources and Services Administration, Division of Nursing, Bureau of Health Professions. (1999, September 16). *Basic workforce report executive summary* [On-line]. Available: www.hrsa.dhhs.gov/bhpr (Accessed March 21, 2000).

McKinlay, J., & Stoeckle, J. (1988). Corporatization and the social transformation of doctoring. *International Journal of Health Services, 18*(2), 191–205.

Moskowitz, D. (1999). *The 1999 health care almanac & yearbook.* New York: Faulkner & Gray.

National Association of Boards of Pharmacy. (2000). *Competency assessment* [On-line]. Available: www.nabp.org/competency (Accessed April 3, 2000).

National Commission on Nursing. (1983). *Summary report and recommendations.* Chicago: Hospital Research and Educational Trust.

Phelps, C. (1992). *Health economics.* New York: HarperCollins.

Starr, P. (1982). *The social transformation of American medicine.* New York: Basic Books.

Torres, D. (1991). What, if anything, is professionalism?: Institutions and the problem of change. *Research in the Sociology of Organizations, 8,* 42–68.

CHAPTER

6

Ambulatory Care

Chapter Objectives

After completing this chapter, the reader should have an understanding of:

- The definition of ambulatory care.
- The variety of settings for the delivery of ambulatory care.
- The importance of ambulatory care services as a part of the U.S. health care system.

INTRODUCTION

Ambulatory care covers a wide range of services for the noninstitutionalized patient and in its most basic description is simply care that does not require an overnight stay by the patient. Office-based physicians provide the majority of ambulatory care. An estimated 787.4 million visits were made to doctors' offices in 1997, or about 3.0 visits per person (Woodwell, 1999). More than 50 percent of those visits were made to primary care specialists (family practice, pediatrics, and internal medicine). However, there are a number of other ways ambulatory care is delivered, and they are described in this chapter.

In recent years the number and type of ambulatory or outpatient facilities have increased to allow more patients to receive treatment outside of the more costly acute care hospitals. Because of advances in technology and technique, many of the procedures formerly done in hospitals can now be performed on an outpatient basis. More familiar ambulatory care facilities, such as hospital outpatient departments and community health centers, have expanded to include surgery centers, diagnostic imaging centers, cardiac catheterization laboratories, and other freestanding facilities. Some facilities are for-profit and are operated by chains, either independently owned or affiliated with a hospital. In other cases, nonprofit health care systems with hospitals have expanded their ambulatory facilities as part of an integrated, cost-efficient way to provide care. When we address health care comprehensively, it is also important to recognize pharmacies, dental care, and "alternative" care such as chiropractic as fitting into what we categorize as ambulatory care. We look now at just a few of the major types of ambulatory care.

MEDICAL PRACTICE

Extraordinary changes are taking place in the practice of medicine in the United States. The sheer number of physicians has more than doubled since 1970. Women, who made up only 9.7 percent of the physician population in 1970, now account for 22 percent of all physicians. A larger percentage of female (47.4 percent) than male physicians (31 percent) are in primary care specialties (American Medical Association, 1999).

After decades of "business as usual," physicians are now faced with a decline of professional autonomy, increased competition among themselves, and changes in the methods of payment for their services. Although much of this change can be attributed to cost containment efforts that seek to provide more efficient, effective medical care, and to the alternative delivery systems that have developed, the growing supply of physicians is also a major factor.

There were 756,710 physicians in the United States in 1997, or 282 physicians for every 100,000 people— more physicians than ever before (American Medical Association, 1999). While the focus in the 1960s was concern over a shortage of physicians, current discussions focus on whether there is an oversupply of physicians (see Table 6–1). The majority of physicians are in office-based patient care (60.6 percent in 1997). Not everyone agrees that we have an oversupply, but there is general agreement that there is an imbalance in primary care versus specialty care physicians, and a shortage of physicians practicing in certain geo-graphic areas. Although the sheer numbers of physicians in primary care specialties increased in the 1990s, the overall percentage of physicians in primary care dropped from 36.5 percent in 1980 to 34.6 percent in 1997 (American Medical Association, 1999).

The increase in the U.S. physician-population ratio intensifies competition and is one reason why physicians join large group practices or accept salaried positions with hospitals and managed care organizations (Table 6–2). An adequate supply of physicians fosters easy access to care. The level of our knowledge and technology affects the number of physicians needed. New knowledge and new technology permit physicians to do what was previously not possible, and they increase the need for more physicians.

Table 6–2 Practice Type for Physicians (Nonfederal), 1997

Employment Status	Percent
Self-employed, solo	25.9
Self-employed, group	30.7
Employee	
HMO	2.7
Group practice	11.1
Private hospital	7.3
Medical school, academic center	7.0
State and local government	9.6
Unknown	1.1
Independent contractor	4.7

Source: Data from the American Medical Association Center for Health Policy Research (Moran, 1998).

Table 6–1 Physician Supply for Selected Years, 1960–1997

Year	Total No. of Physicians	Physicians/100,000 People	Total Population/Physician
1960	260,484	142	703
1970	334,028	161	623
1980	467,679	202	494
1985	552,716	228	440
1990	615,421	244	404
1995	736,279	280	359
1997	756,710	282	363

Source: American Medical Association, 1996, 1999.

Determination of need is complex and, one might say, elusive. Need is affected by the age characteristics of the population (the elderly having greater needs), by the existing health problems that are recognized by the population as problems, by public decisions about which health services should be covered by insurance or government programs, and by the level of investment that should be made in research and facilities. The need for physicians is also affected by the extent to which physicians are willing to use other health workers, by the population's willingness to accept other practitioners, and by the expectations of the population regarding health care services delivery. Thus, there is no more consensus on the correct number of physicians than there is consensus on the amount of money to spend on health care.

About 40 percent of physicians in 1996 were in the primary care areas of internal medicine (18.9 percent), family and general practice (12.3 percent), and pediatrics (8.5 percent). The majority of U.S. physicians are under forty-five years old. More than 20 percent of practicing physicians are women, about 23 percent of physicians are international (foreign) medical graduates, and 62 percent of all physicians are board certified in their specialty. The average annual income for physicians in 1996, after expenses and before taxes, was $199,000. While over 60 percent of all physicians provide office-based patient care, an increasing number of physicians are hospital based or engaged in other professional activities, such as research, teaching, and administration (American Medical Association, 1998).

The Development of Medical Practice

The practice of medicine brought neither financial wealth nor social prestige in early America. Medicine was practiced by a wide array of individuals, from those who had studied medicine in Europe to persons with little or no medical training. Most families cared for themselves. Many medical practitioners found it difficult to support themselves solely from medical practice and were forced to resort to a second occupation. Most patients who were treated by physicians remained at home, and their physicians spent many hours traveling to visit them with a horse and buggy

for transportation. The hours spent traveling severely limited the number of patients a physician could attend. As transportation and roads improved, physicians were able to travel between patients more quickly; patients were also more able to visit the doctors' offices.

Most physicians essentially practiced alone and had little need for hospitals. Medical societies were few and tended to draw only the most elite members of the profession—that is, the ones who had more formal training and who were seeking to upgrade the educational process and the overall quality of medical practice.

The practice of medicine began to change significantly as hospital use increased. In the late nineteenth century and early 1900s, the number of hospitals grew rapidly as hospital sanitation improved, hospital infections decreased, and antiseptic surgery was introduced. Urban life that accompanied industrialization (working away from home and having smaller living accommodations) also contributed to the increased use of hospitals, although well-to-do families still preferred treatment in their homes. Around this time and as a result of these developments, "hospitals moved from the periphery to the center of medical practice as well as medical education" (Starr, 1982).

As hospitals became a necessary part of medical practice, medical practitioners increasingly sought access to them, to admit their patients and to continue treatment. Physicians did not become employees of the hospitals, but rather used the hospitals as one of the tools necessary for patient care. Sometimes they established their own hospitals, particularly when they encountered resistance to joining the staffs of existing institutions, which were frequently dominated by the professional elite. Hospitals had no control over the patient's treatment. This was solely the responsibility of the individual physician.

Solo Practice

Historically, most physicians were in the *solo practice of medicine*; that is, they practiced alone. Now however, more than half of all physicians work in group practices, and an increasing number of physicians choose direct employment arrangements (American Medical Association, 1998). The advantages of solo practice, however, are hard to dispute from an individual standpoint. They include:

- Greater autonomy for the physician.
- A more personal patient-physician relationship.
- Little bureaucracy for both the patient and the physician.

Risks, however, are great for the solo practitioner. Among them are:

- Financial risks.
  - Investing in facilities and equipment.
  - Attracting a sufficient patient base.
- Administrative responsibilities (hiring staff, contracting insurance, etc.).
- Long hours.
  - Providing scheduled care convenient to patients, usually including evening and weekend hours.
  - Covering for emergency care.
- Limited access to capital .
- Difficulty in contracting in a market-driven environment.

Group Practice

A rapidly growing number of physicians are in group practice—either in a group made up of physicians of the same specialty or in a multispecialty group. Group practice is normally defined as consisting of three or more physicians (two physicians are usually referred to as a partnership) who have organized to practice together, typically sharing offices, personnel, equipment, and other expenses. Groups can, however, be much larger, even numbering in the hundreds (see Table 6–3). How they are paid varies from fee for service, to salary, to share of the group's income. The income of group practice physicians tends to be a little higher than that of solo practitioners because of economies achieved by the group from the sharing of support personnel and other resources. Financial risk is also shared, such as the raising of capital and investment in facilities and equipment. The appeal of group practice also comes from other than economic advantages, including:

- More peer interaction (ease of consultation and intellectual stimulation).

Table 6–3 The Largest Medical Group Practices (in Terms of Number of Physicians) in the United States in 1998

Group	Location	No. of Physicians
Mayo Clinic	Rochester, MN	1,147
Henry Ford Medical Group	Troy, MI	1,100
Emory Medical Care Foundation	Atlanta, GA	1,020
University of Iowa College of Medicine	Iowa City, IA	990
Cleveland Clinic Foundation	Cleveland, OH	990
University of Wisconsin Medical Foundation, Inc.	Madison, WI	886
Group Health Co-Op of Puget Sound	Seattle, WA	800
Emory Clinic	Atlanta, GA	795
Medical College of Wisconsin Physicians & Clinics	Milwaukee, WI	750
UT-MED	Galveston, TX	650
University of Miami Medical Group	Miami, FL	576
Baylor College of Medicine	Houston, TX	570

Source: Moskowitz, 1999. © Faulkner & Gray, Inc., reprinted with permission.

- More-flexible time (shared emergency coverage, vacation coverage, administrative responsibilities)
- Availability of a professional manager (appropriate staffing allowing physicians to relinquish direct concern for the financial aspects of patient care)

Group practice, however, is not without its disadvantages. In making the decision to share risks, costs, and administrative responsibilities, the physician also loses some individual autonomy. Group decisions are made regarding office hours, office locations, staffing, and capital investments. Although there are advantages to sharing financial risk, group practice places an additional risk on physicians—legal and ethical risk. The peer group is expected to be aware of each physician's medical practice habits and decision-making capabilities, and act as a standard-bearer for each member of the practice. If a member of the group is sued for malpractice, other members of the group may be held liable if there is any indication that the group was aware of the shortcomings of the sued physician.

Another difficulty often shared in group practice situations results from the financial structure of the organization. Particularly in multispecialty practices, it is often difficult to formulate an income distribution policy that satisfies all parties. Fee structures, capitation rates, and operational expenses vary greatly with the specialty of the physician. Some specialties require a high use of technology and years of intensive training. Other specialties rely more on cognitive skills, greater time spent with the patient, and less use of technology. Various models have been developed to address income disbursement.

Historically, group practices consisted of independent physician-owners (often called "partners") sharing office space and personnel, but each tracking their own income and expenses. This model was somewhat easy to follow in the atmosphere of fee-for-service medicine. As groups became larger, some practices went to a combination of physician-owners and employed physicians. Physician-owners act as the board of directors and hire additional physicians as the need arises. Hired physicians may be offered a share in ownership after an initial period of employment or may stay on as employees indefinitely. As managed care and capitated payment structures have become more prominent, so too has the employed-physician model.

Why would a physician choose to be an employee of a practice rather than a partner or owner? The advantages are many. Employed physicians need not invest in the organization, and thus they carry limited financial risk. They have more defined working hours, few if any administrative responsibilities, and little legal risk for actions of other physicians, yet they have access to greater resources of equipment, facilities, and peer interaction. The disadvantages, however, include limited income potential, an atmosphere of greater regulation and review, and limited input into management decisions. The security of an employed position often outweighs the limitations for many new physicians entering practice in today's uncertain health care environment.

Some larger group practices follow scheduling patterns that make it difficult for the physician to build a continuing relationship with his or her patients. However, most group practices do try to have each patient followed by a specific physician, particularly in primary care specialties. So, while there is some risk of loss of the physician-patient relationship, often a group practice setting provides many advantages to the patient. The patient can get a wider range of care—a type of one-stop shopping—from one medical practice. The medical record is available to all of the patient's physicians without duplication of the information. The patient benefits from improved emergency coverage and, often, a better-informed staff to aid the patient in understanding his or her diagnosis and treatment, as well as the costs, insurance benefits, and financial responsibilities surrounding his or her care.

The Controversy over Contract Practices

Although contract (employed) and group practices are commonplace today, are growing, and are accepted by organized medicine as appropriate and ethical ways to deliver medical care, many individual practitioners initially resisted what they perceived to be an unwise trend. These trends are represented today by salaried group practices and health maintenance organizations (HMOs). When they first appeared, they were seen as a threat to other practitioners. The cry of unethical practice was heard, and the organizations that represented the aggrieved physicians—the state and local medical societies and the AMA—went to battle. The controversies seem at first to be economic—that is, a threat to the incomes of the protesting physicians—but some very real issues lie behind the protests. To understand the resistance to salaried physician groups, it is important to define contract practice and group practice, and then look at the storms that surrounded their development.

Certain industries (e.g., railroads, mining, lumbering, steel) traditionally employed company doctors to do preemployment health examinations, to treat occupational injuries, and in some instances to develop employee medical programs. These physicians were mostly salaried—that is, under contract. Medical societies opposed this type of practice (except when physicians were under contract to serve the military), which they regarded as exploitation because doctors bid against each other for the contracts, thus reducing the price of their services. The opposition of the medical profession over time discouraged employers from expanding medical services, except in remote areas where physicians were generally unavailable.

Another type of contract practice emerged when mutual benefit societies, employee associations, unions, and fraternal orders flourished among immigrants in the early 1900s. These were often social organizations, and sometimes they made life insurance policies available to members. Some also contracted with physicians to provide medical care for their members (and sometimes the members' dependents) for a fixed yearly fee per member—thus, a capitation method of payment. These "benefit societies" thrived in the industrial areas of several states despite the opposition of most physicians. Although many of these contract physicians felt they were not paid enough for their services, some needed this type of contract, especially if they were younger and trying to establish their practices. Many local medical societies complained about poor-quality care by these contract practitioners, and there may have been some validity to their complaints.

The medical societies were also concerned about contract doctors undercutting them economically, doing work for less than they would normally charge on a fee-for-service basis. The AMA, which was as interested in upgrading the medical profession and preserving the independence of doctors as it was in improving medical education, also objected to contract practice. As Starr (1982) notes, the AMA in 1907 could see "no economic excuse or justification" for this type of practice, and it objected "to the unlimited service for limited pay and the 'ruinous competition' it 'invariably' introduced" (p. 208). This type of contract practice declined over time as the supply of physicians decreased and there were enough patients for a physician to earn a living without resorting to contracting. However, it began to rise again with the development of HMOs posing a threat to the traditional form of fee-for-service solo practice, which many physicians still feel serves the best interests of the patient and the physician.

Group practice has been a part of the American scene for a long time. The founding of the Mayo Clinic in Rochester, Minnesota, at the end of the nineteenth century is generally cited as the beginning of organized group practice as we know it today, although there were some antecedents. Mayo was followed by other groups, among them the famous Ross-Loos Clinic in Los Angeles, which served the city water department employees and others under contract. Some group practices operated on a loose fee-for-service basis as in solo practice, but as the groups became organized, many paid their member physicians a salary, sometimes also a percentage of the net business income or a bonus. MacColl (1966) notes that the quality of care in many of the early groups "was reasonably good, but there were others which did not reflect much credit on either the organizers or the physicians involved" (p. 12).

During the early period of group practice development, the AMA was somewhat ambivalent about it. Where groups existed, physicians outside the groups often expressed concern about the quality of care the groups provided, as well as concern about the competition from lower fees the groups sometimes charged. Then, in 1932 the Committee on the Costs of

Medical Care, a national committee, issued a report titled *Medical Care for the American People.*

The committee was a prestigious group, chaired by a former AMA president, Dr. Ray Lyman Wilbur, who was at the time in President Hoover's cabinet as Secretary of the Interior. The committee recommended, albeit with some medical and dental member dissent, that medical care should be provided by organized group practices and that "the costs of medical care [should] be placed on a group payment basis, through the use of insurance, through the use of taxation, or through the use of both these methods. This is not meant to preclude the continuation of medical services provided on an individual fee basis for those who prefer the present method" (U.S. Department of Health, Education, and Welfare, 1970, p. 120). As noted, the report was published in 1932, and it galvanized the opposition of the AMA to both group and salaried practice.

In 1933 the AMA declared that groups of physicians in salaried practice were considered unethical (U.S. Department of Health, Education, and Welfare, 1970)

> when there is solicitation of patients either directly or indirectly . . . when there is competition and underbidding to secure the contract . . . when compensation is inadequate to secure good medical practice . . . , when there is interference with reasonable competition in a community . . . when free choice of physicians is prevented.

This change on the part of the AMA reflected widespread concern within the profession. The concern was professional as well as economic, although critics all too frequently focus on the economic component, ignoring the professional objections.

The AMA's involvement in state and local disputes generally stemmed from questions and issues raised by state and local medical societies. Typically, the latter had a problem for which they needed advice, and they turned to the AMA. The AMA's Judicial Council got involved whenever an aggrieved physician appealed an adverse decision rendered by the state medical society. A focal point has been the AMA's *Principles of Medical Ethics,* which serves as a guide to state and local medical societies. This document was developed by physicians from the states and adopted by local state society representatives in the AMA House of Delegates.

The AMA became directly involved in a local issue in the late 1930s and was found guilty of restraint of trade in 1941. The case involved the AMA and the Medical Society of District Columbia (MSDC) in their actions relating to the Group Health Association (GHA) of Washington. Opposition to the GHA by the DC Medical Society arose almost immediately after the GHA was organized in 1937. The society notified "all the physicians in the area that the plan was unethical. The GHA's salaried physicians were expelled from the Society, and a list of 'reputable physicians' was circulated to all the hospitals for their guidance" (MacColl, 1966, p. 140). The MSDC and the AMA were subsequently indicted, found guilty, and fined for having conspired to monopolize medical practice. The GHA physicians were later admitted to the society and had no subsequent difficulty over hospital privileges. In other parts of the country, specifically Seattle and San Diego, the local medical societies and not the AMA were the defendants in similar cases, and in each case the medical societies lost in their efforts to block development of group health plans. After the AMA fine in the GHA case, the AMA disengaged from "further legal entanglement." Local societies were left to interpret or misinterpret the code of ethics (MacColl, 1966).

The objections to group practice at times took on rather nasty characteristics. In metropolitan New York, for example, the Health Insurance Plan (HIP) was established in the mid-1940s as a demonstration project for national health insurance. HIP, the fiscal agent, contracted with medical groups, paying each group so much for each person on its list. How the group divided the money was up to the group. In return for the capitation payment, the group was responsible for providing comprehensive physician services, prevention, and treatment. For hospital care, most HIP subscribers were at that time covered by Blue Cross. Though the local medical societies might not have been able to keep HIP physicians from joining, they could ostracize them socially. As late as the 1960s, HIP physicians were denied hospital privileges.

The intensity of local medical feeling did not need AMA fuel. HIP, at its inception, had proclaimed itself a demonstration project for a national system, and there were many physicians in New York who were accustomed to government systems before coming to the United States. In addition, the economic pressures on physicians in New York City were considerable because many believed in the 1950s that New York City had an oversupply of medical practitioners. At every turn, non-HIP physicians challenged HIP physicians. Blue Shield, which was sponsored by the medical profession, used paid salesmen and advertising, but when HIP did this, "the charge of unethical conduct was raised. Ben E. Landis, one of the HIP physicians, took the matter to the Judicial Council of the AMA, which ruled in his favor, finding that HIP was a legally organized plan and had as much right to advertise as did Blue Shield so long as the personal qualifications of the physicians were not promoted" (MacColl, 1966, p. 139). By the late 1970s in New York, all wounds were healed, and HIP physicians were fully accepted by medical societies and hospitals. The AMA's Judicial Council, in addition to the Landis case, also reversed, on appeal, the earlier expulsion from the Los Angeles County Medical Society of the developers of the Ross-Loos Medical Group.

Opposition to contract practice, group practice, and salaried practice has all but disappeared. Organized medicine no longer opposes them, and each of these forms of practice is growing. The change came about partly as a result of effective legal challenges against organized medicine, but perhaps more importantly as a direct result of a recognized physician shortage in the 1950s that would ensure fee-for-service, solo practice physicians an ample number of patients to maintain a good income, regardless of the presence of contract and group practice. By this time, group practice had also evolved and now was seen by its advocates as a way to regularize their hours, get easy consultation, and afford ownership of expensive technology that they could not justify, economically, by themselves but could justify on a shared basis. All forms of medical practice could thus live together in harmony.

Group practices are expanding in size, and increasingly they compete for patients with one an-other, with solo practitioners, and with hospital-based physicians. Many groups now contract with managed care plans. Even though they compete with hospital ambulatory clinics, these groups can have considerable influence on hospitals because they control the admission of a significant number of patients to a particular hospital. The 1990s saw groups affiliating with hospitals to form integrated systems of care in order to survive in a much more competitive environment. The balance of influence is much harder to identify in a dynamic health care system, which has seen hospitals, physicians, and insurance plans all operating under the same umbrella organizations.

Medical Practice Costs and Financing

The costs to maintain a medical practice, which in many ways must function as any other business or organization, are considerable. As in most service organizations, the greatest expenses are wages and benefits, including those of physicians, clinical personnel, and office personnel. Additional expenses are incurred for facilities (rent, lease, or real estate), office and medical supplies, medical equipment, liability insurance, and other expenses. Depending on the specialty of the medical practice, malpractice insurance can be one of the largest expenses incurred. Increasingly, physicians' offices are investing in computer systems, not only for the business function of the practice, but to maintain clinical records.

At one time, medicine was the highest-paid profession in the United States. Given the state of the health care environment and the growth in computerization, telecommunications, and Internet industries, medicine may no longer be as attractive a career as it once was. The average physician's net income (after expenses, before taxes) reached $199,000 in 1996. Specialists with the highest average earnings were surgeons, radiologists, and obstetrician-gynecologists. Lowest average earnings were found among psychiatrists, general/family practitioners, and pediatricians (American Medical Association, 1998).

In a fee-for-service atmosphere, concern over increased health care costs centered on the possibility of overservice. A number of U.S. and Canadian economists advance what is called the target income hypothesis. This hypothesis contends that physicians set their sights on a given income level, and that they adjust their fees to reach it. When the demand for services is down and threatens attainment of the desired income, physicians raise fees. When fees are decreased (as in the cost containment environment), physicians provide more services, which could be for the purpose of augmenting income rather than for more comprehensive and appropriate medical care. Supporters of this hypothesis point to the rise in physician incomes despite increased competition for patients and reduced third-party payments per patient encounter. Surgery is often cited in this regard, particularly accusations of unnecessary surgery being performed simply to compensate for decreased fees per procedure.

Others argue that the more critical factors in rising physician incomes may be increased demand and productivity resulting from the provision of additional, appropriate diagnostic and therapeutic services as a result of new knowledge and new technology; fear of possible malpractice suits (the practice of defensive medicine); a more educated population seeking medical care with higher expectations for improved outcomes; and a rapidly aging population with correspondingly increased morbidity. Managed care has tried to curb overservice through capitated payment mechanisms; however, charges have been made of an overcorrection and fears that some patients might actually be underserved because of the costs involved in providing needed services. (See more on the costs and financing of health care in Chapters 2 and 3.)

Malpractice and Professional Liability

Medical professional liability (medical malpractice liability) continues to be an important issue. Questions arise regarding whether physicians have overused tests as a defense against possible malpractice charges and whether patients have used charges of malpractice to demand perfection rather than prevent negligence and/or incompetence. Malpractice insurance is a significant expense to medical practitioners. Premium rates are highest for obstetrician-gynecologists and surgeons, which is a direct reflection of claims filed.

As a defense to malpractice claims, physicians have become more careful. They are keeping better records so that they can defend themselves in court. They are improving their communication skills to enhance the physician-patient relationship and to help patients to understand better the risks involved in procedures because there are fewer lawsuits when the physician-patient relationship is good. Physicians may try to reduce the risk of lawsuits by practicing "defensive medicine," ordering more diagnostic tests than may be necessary to confirm a patient's diagnosis but also adding to the rising costs of medical care.

The adoption of standards of care by some specialty groups and medical societies may reduce the number of malpractice actions. For example, the American Society of Anesthesiologists adopted a standard in 1990 that requires its members to use certain devices to measure the level of oxygen in the blood, which it estimates could have prevented serious injury or death in almost one-third of the cases in which anesthesiologists have been accused of malpractice. In Maryland, as another example, obstetrician-gynecologists' premiums were reduced about 35 percent when they agreed to follow certain standards of care, such as specific procedures for handling breech deliveries and hypertension during pregnancy. In addition, some states have passed laws to penalize patients who make frivolous claims.

Both hospitals and the government are increasing efforts to identify doctors with a history of malpractice. In 1990 the federal government established a National Practitioner Data Bank to keep track of doctors who have been successfully sued for malpractice, who have been disciplined for incompetence, and/or who have had hospital privileges revoked. Hospitals are required to access the data bank prior to granting hospital privileges to physicians. Unfortunately, this information is not available to patients when they are choosing a doctor.

About half of the states limit the amount or type of damages that can be recovered in malpractice suits. Still, the average annual malpractice premium for physicians in 1996 was $14,000. Premiums for specialties such as obstetrics and gynecology (average $35,200) and surgery ($21,700), are much higher

(American Medical Association, 1998). Since 1990, premiums have been somewhat consistent and in some states have dropped. More than half of all doctors in private practice are insured by physician-owned companies, usually state medical societies, which try to keep premiums at a minimum.

Primary Care Physicians

A primary care physician was defined in 1975 by the Coordinating Council on Medical Education (CCME) as one who provides an individual or family with continuing health surveillance, along with the needed acute and chronic care he or she is qualified to provide and referral service to specialists as appropriate. General practitioners and family practitioners fall within this category, as do pediatricians, internists, and obstetrician-gynecologists, although not everyone would agree about these last three.

The pediatrician typically limits his or her clientele to children and adolescents; the internist typically does not handle some things that a family practitioner might handle, such as obstetrics and pediatric problems. Obstetrics and gynecology has more recently evolved as a primary care specialty for categorical care for obstetric and/or gynecological problems, with female patients going directly to OB-GYN practitioners without referral.

The definition of primary care specialties developed by the CCME leaves much to be desired. Other specialties handle a considerable amount of routine primary care that in other settings might be handled by a family practitioner or other health professionals. Prior to the growth of managed care and the gatekeeper concept, many people had the tendency to self-diagnose and self-refer to a specialist—psychiatrist, surgeon, dermatologist, orthopedist—when, in fact, the family physician or other primary care practitioner might well handle many of the problems. For example, some patients frequently used ophthalmologists and orthopedic surgeons when optometrists and podiatrists might well have sufficed.

Part of the recent emphasis on primary care physicians is economic. The rising costs of health care make the principal payers want a mechanism to control costs. They believe that one way to control costs is to decrease the use of specialists by encouraging primary care physicians to treat mild illnesses rather than refer patients to expensive specialists. When specialists and primary care physicians treat patients with comparable illnesses, specialists hospitalize patients more often, write more prescriptions, and order more diagnostic tests (Greenfield et al., 1992). Of course, when an illness is complicated or severe, treatment by specialists is appropriate. Primary care medicine provides the majority of preventive services, such as counseling about healthy lifestyle changes, immunizations, and regularly screening for detection of illnesses before they become serious, all of which are becoming more important in maintaining good health.

Managed care organizations use primary care physicians as "gatekeepers" to prevent the unnecessary use of specialists. Medical students are being encouraged to enter primary care fields by the increased payment for their services by Medicare and some insurance companies using the Resource Based Relative Value Scale (see Chapter 3 for more details).

Before the American College of Surgeons (ACS) was established, and for many years after, the general practitioner did everything, including general surgery. In some communities in the United States, particularly in the more remote areas, family practitioners still provide a wide range of services because of the limited availability of specialists.

The American Academy of General Practice, the predecessor of the American Academy of Family Physicians (AAFP), found in a 1969 survey that 39 percent of its members performed major surgery. Estimates in 1973 were that the percentage was down to 20 to 25 percent (*Medical World News*, 1973). Though physicians in general or family practice may be doing less major surgery overall, 88 percent of them were reported in 1982 to be performing some ambulatory surgery, which generally consists of the less complicated surgical procedures (American Medical Association, 1982). With managed care organizations placing emphasis on ambulatory care, and particularly on care delivered by the primary care physician, the percentage of surgical procedures, particularly minor surgery, performed by practitioners other than surgeons is difficult to determine. The American College of Surgeons has long sought to curb surgery by those not specializing in surgery. However, the content of family practice residencies requires some training in a variety of other specialty areas, including surgery. *General practice* is now an antiquated term that referred to the practice of medicine after one year of internship and no participation in a specialty residency. Today, the Accreditation Council for Graduate Medical Education (ACGME) states that the transitional year (first year of general residency replacing the internship) is *not* meant to be a complete graduate medical education program for the practice of medicine (ACGME, 1999).

The controversy can be seen as a professional debate stressing the importance of strict qualifications for those engaged in surgery or as an attempt on the part of specialists to protect their domain both economically and professionally.

The Appeal of Specialization

Physicians specialize for many reasons. People in general have always held specialists in high regard—as physicians who could do things that general physicians could not do and whose special skills warranted a higher fee. Often, the medical school faculty physicians were considered the best of these specialists. There has always been a certain aura that surrounded the physician—a mystique that was even more pronounced for the specialist, who had knowledge and skills that saved lives, eased pain, and improved functioning.

The medical student must choose the area of medicine she or he will practice. Many factors may enter this decision process, but because most members of the faculty are specialists, the pressure to respond to one of those specialty role models is ever present. Specialization has a certain intellectual appeal, which enables the curious to know more and more about the problems that afflict the human being. Because the problems are complex, the curious specialize in order to understand them.

Other factors may enter. A person's own medical history or that of the family frequently channels a physician's interest. For some specialties, very high incomes are ensured; for others, more orderly personal lives are possible because of fewer emergencies and more regular hours.

Most of the factors that affect the location of the primary care physician also influence the specialist's choice of practice location. Hospital access, however, may be even more critical for the specialist, in terms of the supportive services that may be necessary for the effective practice of her or his specialty. Studies have also shown that specialists tend to locate in areas close to the place where they did their residency because the new specialist is familiar with the clinicians in the area and tends to know and be comfortable with other specialists for referrals. At the same time, because the new specialist is known by many of the local physicians, the new specialist can anticipate some helpful referrals. Notwithstanding the pull to practice in urban settings, during the past decade the overall increase in the supply of specialists, the spread of technology, and the disadvantages of urban life have influenced the movement of new specialists to outlying areas.

Medical Society Memberships

Most physicians find it valuable to belong to the county or city medical society in the area in which they practice and to their state medical society. Not all physicians elect to join the AMA, for a variety of reasons. Many disagree with the AMA's policies (although the association probably truly represents the views of its members), others are more interested in their specialty society, and still others are concerned about the rising costs of membership, particularly in view of the many other memberships a physician feels he or she must maintain.

Membership in the local and state societies is more vital for the practicing physician. These organizations enable the physician to meet his or her colleagues, to learn about the skills and abilities of other physicians for the purpose of referring patients to him or her, and to facilitate an intellectual interchange among physicians, which has always been a key element in the continued learning process. Medical societies provide an organizational focus for representation of medical viewpoints about matters affecting the health of the population and about other matters of interest or concern to them. In addition, if any government, industry, or other body wishes to communicate something to the medical community, the medical society is perhaps the most effective vehicle. Finally, membership often enables the physician to receive such financial benefits as group life, health, and malpractice insurance.

Physicians often belong to other medical societies, depending on their interests and specialties. Among the many other societies is the National Medical Association (NMA), an association representing the special interests of African-American physicians (see www.nmanet.org).

Rural and Inner-City Medical Practice

However one chooses to define primary care physicians, rural areas and inner cities have had considerable difficulty in recruiting and retaining them. The lack of appeal of rural practice stems from fear of professional isolation: lack of professional interactions, inaccessibility of hospitals, absence of consultation and continuing medical education opportunities, lack of career opportunities for spouse, and cultural deprivation (no theater, no concerts, no lectures, limited adult education activities, etc.). The physician today and his or her spouse are urbanites by virtue of their long periods of education and training in urban professional settings, and the adjustment to rural living, though sometimes inviting in moments of idyllic dreaming, has not been successful in most cases. There seems to be greater chance of retention if the physician is originally from a rural area, but no one yet has devised a generally valid formula for the successful establishment of rural practices. Professional as well as personal isolation are factors that are very real. Government-sponsored health plans have adjusted payments to rural physicians and facilities to increase the attractiveness of rural practices. Medical schools and residency programs have established training centers in rural outreach clinics, and student loan programs have offered loan reductions for services to rural areas. Still, rural areas struggle to maintain health services to what is often a deprived socioeconomic population.

There is some ambiguity in the word *rural.* One federal agency set the definition at a population of 35,000 or 50,000. Other agencies have used other, usually lower, figures. For those rural regions of 35,000 to 50,000 that have recruited physicians, the reasons for their successes are several: There are more physicians available, and the supply/demand factor operates to secure a more even distribution; the large urban settings are congested and are plagued by high costs and high crime rates; the assets of urban life are not as remote as our road networks improve; the small communities have sought to make their areas attractive to primary care and other physicians by developing for their communities the best hospital facilities their communities can support, and sometimes more than they can support. These small communities, however, do not face the levels of sparse population scattered across a large geographic area that are problematic in a truly rural area.

Inner-city problems are somewhat different. In large cities, the poor have not always used private doctors. Hospital outpatient departments and emergency rooms have served as the primary source of care. As people moved to the suburbs, the physicians went where their paying patients were. The outmigration of physicians and lack of interest from new physicians are a result of the high cost of office and parking spaces, transportation hassles, and crime. In addition, the cities are far more litigiously inclined, and malpractice insurance rates are generally higher. The movement of physicians out of the cities has become a matter of concern because the poor under Medicaid are entitled to private physician care, but the availability of private physicians is limited. Managed care programs for Medicaid recipients are attempting to provide more comprehensive and continuous care to underserved populations, but the insufficient number of physicians practicing in areas where the Medicaid population resides continues to be a problem.

HOSPITAL OUTPATIENT DEPARTMENTS

Hospitals offer ambulatory care services in clinics where people with nonurgent medical problems can receive treatment. Clinics are separate from emergency department services, but the emergency department often handles nonurgent patients during hours when the clinics are not open. Clinics may be general or specialized (e.g., in diabetes, oncology, women's health). Historically, only hospitals with teaching programs or those in areas (usually urban) where patients *could not* or would not go to doctors' offices had clinics, and they served mostly those with low incomes. The situation has changed since competition among hospitals has increased and inpatient reimbursement has decreased. Hospitals are establishing and expanding clinics, some of them in the community away from the hospital (freestanding). These clinics also attempt to attract middle-income persons to provide the hospital with additional income and to "feed" patients to their hospitals for admission.

COMMUNITY HEALTH CENTERS

Community neighborhood health centers began to develop in the late 1960s, with funding initially from the Office of Economic Opportunity and later from the U.S. Department of Health, Education, and Welfare (HEW). These centers provided primarily comprehensive ambulatory services for a defined population of poor people. The poor had always received large amounts of care from health departments and in hospitals. The larger hospitals, and particularly medical school hospitals, had long histories of care of the poor on both an inpatient and an outpatient basis. But the outpatient care was often demeaning: There were impersonal, crowded surroundings, and long waits on hard benches. The neighborhood health center was designed to overcome these demeaning features by providing a broad range of primary and secondary ambulatory care services by salaried physicians and other health professionals, by emphasizing prevention, having available a wide range of supporting nonmedical services, and providing these services in the neighborhoods in which the people lived. Important, too, was the concept that the people who were served, the consumers, should be involved in the control of their centers.

When possible, the centers were financed on a fee-for-service basis by Medicare and Medicaid and other

vendor payments and by government grants. As with so many other government programs, priorities shifted and funding tapered off. In addition to decreased funding, community health centers faced other problems. The demand for services far exceeded their availability because these centers were the only source of medical care for the poor in many rural areas and in many inner-city neighborhoods. Many of these centers provide prenatal and obstetric care for low-income women who are considered high risk and who might otherwise not have access to care.

Much of the focus of community health centers has turned to primary health care. The centers provide a more limited range of services and refer patients to clinics and hospital centers for more specialized care. Many of these centers have developed with support from one of several federal programs: the National Health Service Corps, the Rural Health Initiative, Health Underserved Rural Areas program, and the Appalachian Regional Commission. Such support augmented local organizational efforts and local building of the facilities. While the original concept of the typical federally supported center often had two family practitioners and one dentist, many centers are now staffed by nurse practitioners and physician assistants who provide primary care.

The supporting services vary from center to center. Some, in very remote areas, have implemented telemedicine to link primary care providers with specialists who are able to "examine" the patient and provide consultation without physically being in the remote site. Telemedicine is a fairly new concept made possible by advances in technology. Health care providers in remote areas who use telemedicine are equipped with monitors that make it possible to transmit medical information to a "home base" (emergency room, hospital specialty department, etc.) where consulting physicians receive vital diagnostic information regarding the patient. In some cases the consultant is able to see the patient on a TV monitor. The consultant is therefore able to assist in or direct the patient's care. Studies are under way to determine the effectiveness of possible applications of telemedicine in a variety of settings.

The long-term survival of community health centers depends on attaining financial resources from grants and cooperative ventures with larger medical centers, and on finding ways to attract and retain quality professional personnel and implement new technologies within limited funding opportunities.

AMBULATORY SURGERY CENTERS

Technology and reimbursement patterns have increased the amount of surgery performed on an ambulatory basis. Hospitals all over the country are experiencing a rise in the number of surgical patients who come into the hospital and go home on the same day, cases that previously required at least an overnight stay in the hospital, if not a two- or three-day stay. In many cases, ambulatory surgery is not optional; third-party payers require that many procedures be done on an outpatient basis. The move to outpatient treatment can significantly affect a hospital's use of beds and its overall organization.

Many surgeons, however, have been accustomed to performing a limited amount of ambulatory surgery in their offices, depending on their facilities, support services, and self-imposed limits. One of the major limits was anesthesia. The surgeon typically provided only surgery requiring a local anesthetic, not a general anesthetic, because board-certified anesthesiologists should administer general anesthesia. Advances in technology make it possible to perform an increasing number of surgical procedures on an outpatient basis and with general anesthesia. During the 1970s, a number of freestanding—that is, not hospital-based—surgical centers began to develop in several parts of the country.

After the American College of Surgeons began to approve freestanding surgical centers in 1981, the number of facilities increased rapidly throughout the country. In 1999 there were over 2,700 freestanding outpatient surgery centers, up from 2,400 in 1996. Some 5.7 million surgical procedures were performed at such centers, up from 4.3 million in 1996 (Ferreter, 2000). The most common procedures performed at these ambulatory surgical centers are in ophthalmology, gynecology, otolaryngology, orthopedics, and plastic surgery. The rapid growth of ambulatory surgery has been due to a demand by insurance companies and government to provide surgery at lower costs. Surgery centers are able to function at lower costs because they incur lower overhead costs than hospitals. Even with the growth of freestanding centers, however, hospitals perform some 84 percent of all outpatient surgery and freestanding surgical centers perform only about 16 percent (Hall & Lawrence, 1998).

Freestanding surgery centers are able to compete effectively with hospitals because Medicare now covers many procedures on an outpatient basis only. Surgery centers also affiliate with HMOs and preferred provider organizations (PPOs), thereby competing with hospitals for a certain flow of patients. Hospitals have responded to the growth of ambulatory surgery centers by establishing their own freestanding centers, by affiliating or going into partnership with some of the freestanding centers, and by aggressively marketing and expanding their own hospital-based outpatient surgical services.

Freestanding surgical centers may be independently owned, some by surgeons who are competing with the very hospitals in which they perform their more complicated surgical procedures. Some independently owned facilities are small, single-specialty centers with fewer physicians than those owned by hospitals and corporate chains. The development of ambulatory surgical centers in an area depends on such factors as state regulations, certificate-of-need requirements, competition, and reimbursement policies (Henderson, 1992).

EMERGENCY CARE

When considering emergency treatment, most people still think of the hospital emergency room. However, changes have taken place even in this area of health care delivery on the basis of costs, competition, and quality of care. Many communities have tried to provide care to the uninsured in more suitable settings, recognizing that emergency rooms are overburdened with treatment requests that could better be served in a primary care setting. Managed care companies try to address this issue by requiring that the primary care provider (gatekeeper) be the initial contact even in emergent cases, mandating that primary care physicians provide twenty-four–hour contact options for their patients. The emergency care described in the sections that follow is just a sampling of the care that is available, and it may vary greatly in local communities.

Hospital Emergency Departments

The emergency room (ER) or emergency department (ED) is still the most familiar setting for emergency care and is the most appropriate for most acute and all life-threatening medical situations. The hospital ER has at its disposal all of the resources of equipment and specialty care provided by the hospital. It also has the referral mechanisms in place for care not available in-house. Although each hospital may have its own method for staffing the ER, most hospitals today either directly employ physicians trained and certified in emergency medicine (a new and growing specialty area of medicine) or contract with emergency medical groups for continuous coverage. In very specialized areas of care, area physicians may be on call to provide care rather than such care being available in-house.

Although most hospitals do have emergency rooms or emergency departments, there is no general mandate to have an ER. However, if a hospital does have an emergency department, it must treat all patients who present for care, regardless of ability to pay. The mandate to treat is defined as a requirement to stabilize the patient. A 1986 federal "antidumping law" states that hospitals cannot inquire about patients' insurance status before providing emergency care ("Patient Dumping," 1999). The statute often places ERs in a difficult situation because many managed care organizations refuse to pay for emergency care without prior authorization. An ER also places stress on the hospital's financial status because most acute trauma cases are very expensive to treat and many patients requiring such treatment are uninsured or underinsured and unable to pay for this very expensive care. ERs also face financial stress in that they are often used as a primary source of care by patients who have no regular source of care because they have no, or very inadequate, insurance.

The emergency room is considered an outpatient service of the hospital. Patients most often are provided care and return home on the same day. Those requiring additional care are either admitted to an inpatient service of the facility or referred to another appropriate facility.

Freestanding Emergency Centers

Freestanding emergency centers (urgi-care centers) provide episodic emergency care twenty-four hours a day for non-life-threatening problems. It is estimated that there are over 5,000 such centers in the nation. They provide primary care on a "walk-in" or appointment basis, as well as more acute care. Sometimes they are storefront operations located in large shopping malls, but more often they are fully equipped clinics that provide a wide range of care for non-life-threatening situations. Like the ambulatory surgical centers, they provide the opportunity for physicians and for-profit organizations to compete with hospitals and office-based physicians for patients. They provide a treatment option to the use of hospital emergency departments and other practitioners whose location or appointment systems are inconvenient for patients. Unlike medical clinics provided by hospital outreach programs, urgi-care centers are often a cash-and-carry operation, requiring payment at the time of service (cash, check, or credit card) and not billing insurances. Patients are given proper documentation to submit to any insurance plans they may have for reimbursement after payment is made to the center.

Ambulance Services

Ambulance services are provided by a variety of agencies. Depending on the community, services may be provided by police and fire departments, hospitals, volunteer groups, and private ambulance companies. Considerable effort has been made in recent years to train ambulance crews in dealing with the kinds of emergencies they are likely to encounter and in connecting ambulance services via sophisticated communications equipment to emergency facilities to provide care swiftly to the patient at the point of contact. Many communities have paramedic teams and emergency medical technicians (EMTs) as part of their ambulance services who are able, in communication with the hospital emergency room staff, to provide treatment prior to the patient's arrival in the emergency room.

On the other hand, ambulance services can also provide routine transport for patients being transferred from the hospital to more appropriate sites of care, such as a rehabilitation center, nursing home, or home care. Transport can also be arranged for a bed-bound patient from home to physician visits or other ambulatory care. Costs and reimbursement policies for ambulance services vary by insurance company and reason for transport and can be a financial burden to patients required to pay out of pocket. Some community ambulance companies provide free services to individuals who become annual "members" of the ambulance service by making an annual contribution to the ambulance corps.

FAMILY PLANNING CENTERS

Family planning centers were first established in 1970 when Congress passed Title X of the Public Health Service Act, which provided federal funding for establishing family planning services on the local level. Depending on the state and geographic area, local health departments, hospital agencies, or voluntary agencies established the centers, which typically provided gynecological examinations, breast or cervical cancer screening, contraceptive information and supplies, and other services related to reproductive health care. Many centers have expanded their services to include genetic screening; routine child health screening; and sexually transmitted disease diagnosis, treatment, and follow-up. During the early 1980s, federal funding became less available as the Reagan administration cut back on many health and social services, so funding now comes from a combination of federal and state funds, private donations, fund-raising, and sliding-scale client fees.

CLINICAL LABORATORIES

Physicians may require a variety of laboratory analyses to facilitate diagnosis and treatmentof their patients. Some physicians do their own tests or have their own technicians to carry out whatever tests are desired. However, some tests are very complicated and require rather costly equipment. For these tests, as well as some of the simpler tests, the physician may have an arrangement with the nearby hospital or may use a freestanding clinical laboratory run by a pathologist or by a registered medical technologist. Sometimes the physician sends the patient to the lab; sometimes the physician sends the specimen to the lab. In rural settings, doctors may have to mail the specimen to a lab, or the lab may arrange for periodic pickup of specimens.

Although there is state licensing of clinical laboratories and federal monitoring of those labs that work across state lines, there has been concern over the years about the quality of laboratory analyses. Periodically, studies are completed that call into question the accuracy of clinical lab results. This is, of course, a serious matter because a physician treats a patient on the basis of lab reports.

The Clinical Laboratory Improvement Amendments of 1988 (CLIA '88)—changes to the Clinical Laboratory Improvement Act of 1967—brought much-needed regulation to laboratories to ensure the quality of test results. CLIA '88 brought standards to freestanding and office-based laboratories similar to those imposed on hospitals and reference laboratories by CLIA '67. Laboratories must be registered, must be open to periodic inspection, must perform proficiency testing, and must follow staffing guidelines in order to be paid by government programs for their services. These requirements have helped to improve the quality of laboratory findings, which ultimately lead to higher-quality treatment planning. Although not foolproof, CLIA '88 is a move in the right direction (Health Care Financing Administration, 1998).

VOLUNTARY HEALTH AGENCIES

Many national health agencies operate state, and sometimes local, chapters. These agencies are typically oriented toward special disease and are financed largely by charitable contributions. Some of the more prominent agencies include the American Heart Association, American Cancer Society, the Arthritis Foundation, American Diabetes Association, and Mental Health Association. Some of these agencies provide direct service (e.g., diagnostic services, clinical consultation), some support research, some help finance needed services, and most conduct some health education activities to educate the population about the health problem of their concern.

SUMMARY

The move from inpatient to outpatient care has become more predominant since changes in reimbursement in the Medicare system in the early to mid-1980s. However, it is important to note that several types of care have always been found in outpatient settings. Key among those services are physician services, but

dentistry, pharmacy, and visiting-nurse services have also historically been ambulatory services.

As new technology develops, we will continue to see new forms of care in all settings. Although hospitals have been the focal point of health care delivery in the past and continue to consume the largest portion of health care expenditures, the hospital is no longer synonymous with the *health care system*. The *system* is more diverse and more complex than ever before and, at least for the near future, continues to change in its functions, size, and scope of services. To highlight the changes taking place in ambulatory care, this chapter's case study tells the story of one medical practice.

CASE STUDY 6.1: IN THE HEALTH CARE COMMUNITY

Lehigh Valley Eye Center*

Lehigh Valley Eye Center, like many medical practices today, grew through the addition of physicians, integration of services, and merger of independent practices. Perhaps the best way to trace the history is to begin with one of its divisions: Lehigh Valley Ophthalmic Associates (LVOA).

In 1978, after medical school in Philadelphia and residency training in New Jersey and Philadelphia, Dr. Thomas Burkholder established a solo practice in ophthalmology in his hometown of Allentown, Pennsylvania. His patient base and referrals from area optometrists grew, and in 1985 the solo practice became a group with the addition of Dr. Mark Staffaroni. Both of these general ophthalmologists cared for a large number of patients for a wide range of medical and surgical eye care but recognized that some of their patients needed specialized care, particularly for advanced glaucoma and diseases of the retina. Most such patients were referred to Wills Eye Hospital in Philadelphia, over sixty miles away. A needs assessment conducted in the late 1980s resulted in a decision to expand the practice to include

both a retina subspecialist (the position currently held by Dr. Alan Listhaus) and glaucoma subspecialists (the position currently held by Dr. Howard Kushnick). Shortly afterward, a pediatric ophthalmologist (Dr. Mark Trachtman) also joined the group.

By 1992, with a complement of five physicians, LVOA employed some twenty-five staff members equally divided between front-office personnel and clinical staff. In 1989 the offices moved to a 7,000-square-foot state-of-the-art office in a building housing an ambulatory surgery center, where most of the ophthalmic surgery was performed. Physicians also held privileges to practice at three local hospitals. Income to the practice was based on fee-for-service contracts with many different insurance plans, including some managed care plans. Within the next two to three years, an optometrist was hired, as well as a physician specializing in ocuplastics (the position currently held by Dr. Frank Baloh). Although expansion of the group provided almost full-service ophthalmic care, the physicians felt there was a gap in comprehensive care because they had no cornea specialist.

(continues)

---

*Information for this case was obtained through personal interviews with the administrator and physicians of Lehigh Valley Eye Care and from organization documents.

(continued)

Fairgrounds Eye Associates, a two-physician practice in the same building as LVOA, consisted of a general ophthalmologist and a cornea specialist. The practice had its own manager, front-office staff, and clinical support staff, totaling approximately eight employees. Payers and hospital affiliations were similar to those of LVOA.

The two groups explored common needs and joined under the umbrella corporation of Lehigh Valley Eye Care in 1995. Although the groups identified common needs and a common mission, the merger was not easy. Each practice had its own management, employees, computer systems, retirement plan, and so on. Consolidation meant major compromises, elimination of some procedures and policies and adoption of others, job redesign for most employees, and even elimination of some positions. The reengineering process is continuous.

The umbrella corporation is Lehigh Valley Eye Care. Six physicians (previously owners of the individual practices) make up its board of directors. The board makes strategic management decisions for the overall business. Under its direction are the two ophthalmology practices and a retail optical division, which is about to open its second location. The physicians answer to the board. A practice manager is responsible for coordination between the divisions and operations of the two practices. A manager experienced in the retail optical business coordinates the activities of the optical division (see Figure 6–1).

Billing for all divisions is centralized, as are the computer systems. The pension plan, benefits package, policies, and procedures are merged. Medical records, appointment schedules, and phone systems remain separate and are areas for possible additional consolidation. The total number of staff members has grown accordingly. Four people staff the billing office. Staff members are trained to cover across locations, but clinical and front-office personnel do not cross areas of expertise.

Although growth has been apparent over the years for this medical practice, the challenges are

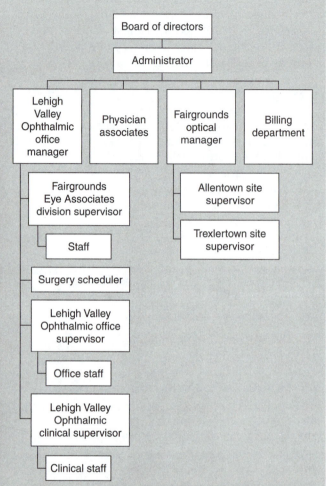

Figure 6–1 Lehigh Valley Eye Center Organizational Chart

not as obvious. Managed care has had a significant impact, forcing a difficult balance between costs and quality. The incentive to become a full-service practice was spawned by a desire to provide care that patients might otherwise have to access by long trips to Philadelphia. However, providing full-service care requires additional capital for physical space, equipment, and staffing. Although payment still tends to be fee for service for specialty physicians, those fees

(continues)

(continued)

are drastically discounted by managed care contracting. The billing department estimates that some 65 percent of the revenue is currently derived from managed care contracts, including some Medicare managed care contracts.

The geographic area is highly competitive in terms of insurance plans offered. Medical practices must manage a wide range of billing functions in order to service all of their patients. It is also a highly competitive health care arena, causing a shortage in the pool of qualified allied health and support staff.

Lehigh Valley Eye Care poses a significant presence in the Lehigh Valley area, but it differs significantly from either of its original components. While the practice has been able to survive and grow in a highly competitive environment, each of the component practices has lost some of its "personality" and unique patient relationships. And the challenges are not yet over. The Lehigh Valley area remains a center of change as the community itself grows and experiences changes in hospital systems and other integrated forms of care.

ACTIVITY-BASED LEARNING

- Identify a group medical practice in or near your community and determine its characteristics: number of physicians, single or multispecialty practice, and history of its development and growth. Does the story sound similar to the one presented in this chapter's case study of the Lehigh Valley Eye Center? In what ways is it similar and/or different?

- Identify an ambulatory surgery center in your community and determine its ownership and/or affiliation. Research the following: the year it first opened, procedures most commonly performed, number of operating rooms, and number of physicians performing procedures in the facility.

A QUESTION OF ETHICS

- It has been said that an increased number of physicians is related to an increase in the utilization of health care services—a concept known as *physician-induced demand*. Is the utilization of health care, in your opinion, related to greater access to care for those who previously could not get care, or do physicians provide unnecessary care in order to maintain their income in a competitive environment?

- The move from inpatient to outpatient care is driven by cost containment, as well as by new technologies. Are there risks to care provided in the ambulatory setting?

- Many freestanding ambulatory care facilities came into being as an opportunity to capture payments diverted from inpatient services. Does the ownership structure or profit motive of an ambulatory care facility have any bearing on the quality of its services?

References

Accreditation Council for Graduate Medical Education (June, 1999). *Program requirements for the transitional year* [On-line]. Available www.acgme.org/req (Accessed February 28, 2001).

American Medical Association. (1982). *SMS report, Socioeconomic Monitoring System.* Chicago: AMA.

American Medical Association. (1996). *Nonfederal physicians in the United States and possessions by selected characteristics* [On-line]. Available: www.ama-assn.org/physdata (Accessed February 17, 2000).

American Medical Association. (1998). *Socioeconomic characteristics of medical practice 1997/1998.* Chicago: Author.

American Medical Association. (1999). *Physician characteristics and distribution, 1999.* Chicago: Author.

Ferreter, M. (2000). Taking their cut. *Modern Physician*, 4(1), 40.

Greenfield, S., Nelson, E., Zubkoff, M., Manning, W., Rogers, W., Kravitz, R., Keller, A., Tarlov, A., & Ware, J. (1992, March 25). Variations in resource utilization among medical specialties and systems of care. *JAMA, 269*(12), 1624–1630.

Hall, M., & Lawrence, L. (1998). *Advance data: Ambulatory surgery in the United States, 1996* (Vital and Health Statistics, Vol. 300). Hyattsville, Maryland: National Center for Health Statistics.

Health Care Financing Administration. (1998, July 23). *CLIA: General program description* [On-line]. Available: www.hcfa.gov/medicaid/clia/progdesc.htm (Accessed April 24, 2000).

Henderson, J. (1992, May 18). Surgicenters cut further into market. *Modern Healthcare*, pp. 108–110.

MacColl, W. A. (1966). *Group practice and prepayment of medical care.* Washington, DC: Public Affairs Press.

Medical World News. (1973, September 21).

Moran, M. (1998, March 9). More physicians are employees. *American Medical News*, pp. 7–8.

Moskowitz, D. (1999). *1999 health care almanac & yearbook.* New York: Faulkner & Gray.

Patient dumping: Hospitals caught between feds, HMOs. (1999, February 19) *American Health Line.*

Starr, P. (1982). *The social transformation of American medicine.* New York: Basic Books.

U.S. Department of Health, Education, and Welfare. (1970). *Medical care for the American people: Final report of the Committee on the Costs of Medical Care.* Chicago: University of Chicago Press.

Woodwell, D. (1999). *National ambulatory medical care survey: 1997 summary.* Hyattsville, MD: National Center for Health Statistics.

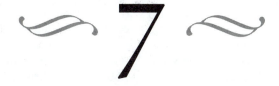

CHAPTER
7

Hospitals

Chapter Objectives

After completing this chapter, the reader should have an understanding of:

- The historical development of hospitals.
- Characteristics and functions of hospitals.
- Developments in the health care environment that have imposed changes on hospital functions.
- The response of hospitals to environmental changes.
- Competitive and regulatory influences on hospitals.

INTRODUCTION

Although, in their very early history, hospitals were considered a place to die, advances in medical knowledge transformed hospitals into the centers for medical care and cure. The hospital became the focus of medicine for acute patient care and the center for medical education. Physicians provided the bulk of their services in hospitals, laboratories were located in hospitals, nurses were employed by hospitals, and research was conducted in hospitals. Since the hospital was the focus of care, it naturally follows that hospitals have also experienced the greatest amount of

change over the last two decades. Technology, developments in drug therapy, cost containment efforts focusing on efficiency and efficacy, and a competitive environment have all changed the structure and function of hospitals as we see them today. The history and transition of hospitals are the focus of this chapter.

HISTORY OF HOSPITALS

Religions and wars had a great deal of influence on the development of hospitals, particularly because the earliest conception of a hospital was as a facility for care of the poor and infirm. One of the earliest hospitals in what was to become the continental United States was established in 1658 in New Amsterdam, now New York City. It consisted of several houses and accepted soldiers and slaves; civilians were not accepted until 1791. The first hospitals in the continental United States that were built specifically to care for the sick in the general population were voluntary hospitals. They were based on the British voluntary hospitals that flourished in the provincial centers outside of London in the eighteenth century. They differed from the earlier royal hospitals in Britain in that they were maintained by voluntary contributions, and the consulting physicians served without pay; the royal hospitals were maintained by both municipal governments and voluntary contributions, and their physicians were salaried.

The initiative in founding voluntary hospitals came largely from laypeople and depended on gifts and subscriptions from donors who, for religious or humanitarian reasons, felt some responsibility for those less fortunate. The wealthy and social elite governed the hospitals. The success of these hospitals depended on the willingness of the wealthy to help the poor because poor sick people were virtually all of the hospital's patients. It was still preferable to endure illnesses at home, if possible, and the wealthy were better able to do this. Britain's first voluntary hospital was established in 1720; numerous reports of success of this and similar hospitals made their way to the United States and influenced the development and administration of U.S. hospitals.

The Pennsylvania Hospital, in Philadelphia, was the first permanent hospital for civilians in the continental United States and was a voluntary hospital. During the nineteenth century the United States experienced dramatic growth in territory, population, and industry. New York became the largest and most influential city. Municipal and state hospitals were becoming permanent, and the role of hospital leadership passed from Pennsylvania Hospital to hospitals in New York and Boston.

Because Boston was an important seaport, confronted with many sick and injured seamen with no homes or families to care for them, the city opened the Boston Marine Hospital in 1804 to accommodate about thirty patients. This hospital was possible because Congress, in 1778, enacted a law requiring that 20 cents a month be withheld from the wages of each seaman on U.S. ships to support seamen's hospitals in seaports. This was the first compulsory health insurance law in the U.S. In addition, Boston, like many other U.S. cities, had an almshouse that functioned mainly to give food and shelter to the poor but that also provided a few beds for the poor who were sick. In addition to the lack of facilities for the sick poor, there was a lack of training opportunities for physicians in New England. In a period when medicine was beginning to make relatively significant advances, hospitals were important centers for the dissemination of new knowledge. It was there that a variety of cases with similar clinical symptoms could be studied. Hospital experience was becoming indispensable for the training of new physicians, but few of them could afford to study in Philadelphia or London and Paris.

These facts were very much on the minds of a number of the distinguished Bostonians who met in 1810 to consider the establishment of a general hospital for the sick poor, needy pregnant women, and the insane. People who could afford it still preferred to be cared for at home. Supporters of the hospital petitioned the General Court (the Massachusetts legislature) for a hospital charter. The problems of the poor and insane were described, but the concluding paragraphs emphasized the need for medical students in New England to have hospital training. They cited the advantages that physicians from Philadelphia or New York had because hospital training was available to them.

The hospital was incorporated as the Massachusetts General Hospital in 1811. This voluntary hospital was a corporation composed of contributors with twelve trustees, four of whom were to be appointed by a board composed of the governor, lieutenant governor, president of the senate, speaker of the house, and the chaplains of both houses. Thus, the state had a share of control from the beginning. The legislation also granted, as an endowment, the Province House (an unproductive estate that was initially considered and then rejected as a possible temporary hospital), on the condition that the corporation raise an additional $100,000 in private subscriptions—the concept of matching funds for the establishment of a hospital. The legal owner of the hospital was the corporation, which met once a year, but the trustees managed the institution. Government regulation or interference was not a problem because the trustees were all Federalists with many friends at the state capitol.

The hospital design included kitchens, laundry, a small sickroom for dying patients, morgue, storerooms, large wards to care for the sick, smaller rooms, water closets (lavatories), and accommodations for nurses and doctors. The water closets made the Massachusetts General Hospital the first U.S. hospital to have interior plumbing. The hospital, noted for its imposing structure and utility of interior design, was completed and ready for patients in 1821. At this time the structure of the American hospitals was superior to that of their European counterparts, mainly because American architects were able to design new buildings rather than remodel old ones.

Finances were a major problem for the Massachusetts General Hospital. The operating expenses exceeded the income from endowments; thus, although only half of the hospital beds were occupied, many deserving persons were turned away because of a lack of operating funds. In 1825 the Boston trustees proposed a successful method of increasing operating funds called the free bed subscription. People who contributed $100 would support one patient in the hospital free of expense during the following year. People and organizations responded well to the idea, and the drive for free bed subscriptions became an annual event. Because of these subscriptions, the hospital was able to give free care to about 40 percent of its patients, which was comparable to the percentage of free beds at the Pennsylvania Hospital during the same period.

An important source of money for the hospital during the early 1800s was the Massachusetts Hospital Life Insurance Company, which, by an 1824 agreement, gave the hospital one-third of all its profits over 6 percent and frequently lent money to the hospital. In addition, as the reputation of the hospital increased, many citizens remembered it generously in their wills.

The hospital's board of trustees met monthly to deal with matters that ranged from ratifying the decisions of the superintendent concerning wages for attendants, building repairs, and purchase of supplies to selecting personnel and investing the corporation's capital. The admission policy of the hospital followed the precedent set by the Pennsylvania and New York hospitals in forbidding the admission of incurable patients. The reasoning was that the institution was intended to cure disease; if incurable patients were admitted or kept in free beds, there would

soon be no room for treating and curing diseases. Therefore, those people with chronic or incurable diseases, except mental disorders, could not be admitted as free patients. If patients were classified as incurable after a reasonable period of time, they were discharged, to the almshouse if they had nowhere else to go. In case of accidents, patients were admitted immediately.

The visiting committee, one of the subcommittees of the board, inspected the hospital routinely and had the power to adjust rates and extend free care. The demand for free beds was so great that the trustees limited the free patient's hospital stay to four weeks unless the attending physician or assistant authorized additional time. In certain instances, the visiting committee reduced or eliminated patient charges. Sometimes they canceled small debts of poor patients and even occasionally paid their fares home. On the other hand, the committee, after consulting with the physician or surgeon, sometimes ordered incurable patients to be taken to the almshouse.

One very persuasive reason for establishing a hospital was to provide care for the mentally ill. The care of the insane had been studied in Pennsylvania and New York. In contrast to the Pennsylvania Hospital, the Massachusetts General Hospital housed its insane patients in a separate building from the beginning. One of the first activities of the board was to purchase an estate overlooking the Charles River, which was designated for the insane and named the McLean Asylum. The patients came from towns and villages throughout New England. The asylum was under the direction of the hospital trustees, but the financial accounting was separate. By this time bleeding and purging were no longer used in the treatment of the insane, and there was an emphasis on keeping the patient usefully occupied in a strict routine. The asylum had both a resident and an attending physician.

The Massachusetts General Hospital, like the Pennsylvania and New York hospitals, was a teaching hospital. It provided practical clinical instruction for the students of the Harvard Medical School. Lecturers in surgery and medicine at the medical school were supplemented with classes at the hospital. In time, the hospital also became the leading New England center for medical research, largely because it had an adequate number of patients to study.

Hospitals moved westward with the population. They appeared along the Mississippi River as navigation increased. In New Orleans, St. John's Hospital (later known as Charity Hospital) was founded in 1736 from an endowment left by a French sailor. It began serving about 24 people, but today Charity Hospital has 3,500 beds. The increased navigation along the Ohio River prompted the township trustees of Cincinnati to rent a house to care for the sick and indigent. In 1821 the Ohio legislature established a hospital to provide facilities for the sick poor, boatmen, and the insane, and to train medical students. At first the hospital was also used as an orphanage and almshouse. Later, the orphans, insane, and paupers were transferred, and the hospital today is known as the Cincinnati General Hospital.

The first hospital west of the Mississippi River was established because of the efforts of the Catholic bishop of St. Louis. John Mullanphy, an Irish-American trader and merchant in St. Louis, gave some land and had a three-room log cabin built on it. Four Sisters of Charity journeyed from Emmitsburg, Maryland, to St. Louis to run the hospital. The sisters used one corner of the kitchen for sleeping; the other two rooms were used for patients. The hospital opened on November 28, 1828, and the cabin was used for four years. By 1832, John Mullanphy and other citizens had provided a two-story brick building, which later became the City Hospital of St. Louis. In 1845, St. Louis built a new hospital that became the official City Hospital, and the old St. Louis Hospital operated by the Sisters of Charity was renamed the Mullanphy Hospital.

In May 1856, when the City Hospital was destroyed by fire, the patients were transferred to the Mullanphy Hospital. During the Civil War the Mullanphy Hospital took in the sick and wounded. The need for a larger hospital had been apparent for some time, and by 1874 the Daughters of Charity of St. Vincent de Paul (formerly the Sisters of Charity) took possession of a new and larger building, financed in part by the sale of the property given to the Sisters of Charity by John Mullanphy.

Mullanphy Hospital was the first private institution in the West to establish a regular nursing school, and the first hospital in the United States to establish a maternity hospital and foundling asylum. Mullanphy Hospital was also a teaching hospital for the Washington University Medical School. After a tornado virtually destroyed the hospital in 1927, a larger institution was built at a new site and was named De Paul Hospital to honor St. Vincent de Paul, who was instrumental in establishing the Daughters of Charity of St. Vincent de Paul.

The design and management of hospitals was largely influenced by Florence Nightingale, although she is more widely known for her reforms in the nursing profession. In the 1850s the relationship between filth and disease was recognized, and sanitary measures for preventing disease were accepted. At that time the prevalent theory of disease was that a vaporous emanation from humans could "enter into the putrefactive condition," causing disease. The germ theory of disease was yet to come.

In Nightingale's design, the dangerous emanations were quickly and continually removed by proper ventilation. The dominating theme of the Nightingale ward was pure air. To deprive the sick of pure air "is nothing but manslaughter under the garb of benevolence," according to her. Her ideal ward, described in *Notes on Hospitals,* was oblong with windows on each side extending from two feet from the floor to one foot from the ceiling. Windows should make up one-third of wall space, and there should be one window for every two beds. The wards should be 111 to 128 feet long, 30 feet wide, and 16 to 17 feet high. These dimensions were all calculated to provide the optimal flow of air. There should be thirty to thirty-two patients in the ward, each bed with 8 by 12 feet of "territory to itself." The water closets, lavatory, and baths, independently ventilated, should be located at the far end of the ward. The head nurse's room should be at the entrance to the ward with a window onto the ward so that she could see all of the patients. Behind the nurse's room Nightingale called for a room for cleaning and storing dishes, washing vegetables, and the like. Fireplaces in the center of the ward would serve for both heating and further ventilation. Each ward should open onto a long corridor. Wards designed on these principles were used in the United States and Britain.

Scientific Advances Influencing Hospital Care

Advances in science and medicine during the mid-nineteenth century revolutionized medicine and had a great impact on hospitals. Hospitals became important centers for disseminating new knowledge and places where all classes of society could benefit from treatment.

Surgery was radically changed with improved ways to deaden pain during operations. Until the mid-1800s, operations were limited mainly to amputating, repairing wounds, setting fractures, reducing dislocations, suturing muscles and tendons, and removing kidney stones and some tumors. Pain was somewhat lessened by the administration of large doses of brandy, wine, opium, henbane (a plant extract resembling belladonna), by constricting of the limb above the portion to be amputated, and by hypnotism. Morphine was not introduced into general practice until 1844. In 1846, ether was first used for an operation at the Massachusetts General Hospital. From that date forward, operations could be performed on the inner cavities of the body without pain, but most patients died nonetheless from subsequent infection.

In 1865 an English surgeon, Joseph Lister, dramatically reduced surgical infections by using carbolic acid sprays during surgery. Lister postulated that microorganisms in the air caused infection. Later he realized that the organisms were also present on hands and instruments and insisted on the use of antiseptics on hands, instruments, and dressings. His introduction of antiseptic procedures was based on the work of the French chemist Louis Pasteur, who, in opposing the theory of spontaneous generation, showed that organisms found in putrefying materials originated from the organisms found in the air. The introduction of antiseptics so revolutionized surgery that the history of surgery can be divided into two periods: pre-Listerian and post-Listerian.

Before Lister, Oliver Wendell Holmes, a physician at Harvard, observed that puerperal (childbed) fever was a contagious disease that was transmitted by the unclean hands and clothing of doctors and midwives (from other women having the disease or from patients with infections) to women undergoing childbirth. During the same period, Ignaz Semmelweis, a Hungarian doctor, also concluded that unclean hands and clothing, as well as unsanitary hospital conditions, transmitted childbed fever, which killed 12 mothers out of every 100 in the Vienna General Hospital where he worked. By introducing antiseptic methods, Semmelweis was able to reduce the maternal mortality resulting from childbed fever to only 1 to 2 percent. He was ridiculed for his work, however, and it was not until Lister's work that Holmes and Semmelweis received professional recognition for their work.

The work of Semmelweis, Lister, and Holmes provided some evidence that microorganisms cause human diseases, but it was Robert Koch, a German physician, who firmly established the germ theory of disease, in 1876. Since the sixteenth century it had been thought that something could be transmitted from a sick person to a well person that caused the well person to become sick. After microorganisms were discovered, it was generally believed that they caused disease, but there was no proof. Koch studied anthrax, a disease of cattle that occasionally occurs in humans. He established that anthrax bacteria were always present in the blood of animals with the disease, and that if blood from an infected animal were injected into a well animal, the well animal would develop anthrax. Koch also grew the bacteria in nutrients outside the animal's body and found that, when those cultured bacteria were injected into a well animal, that animal also developed anthrax. On the basis of this and other experiments, Koch proved that specific bacteria produce specific diseases.

Using Koch's methods, investigators isolated and identified bacteria that caused a wide variety of contagious diseases. Once the causative agents were identified, cures were possible either by immunization with killed bacteria or blood serum from recovered animals, or by other methods.

Koch used the microscope to identify disease-causing bacteria, and Rudolph Virchow used it to study diseased body tissue. In 1893 the first real hospital laboratory was set up in Paris, and laboratories soon became an integral part of every hospital. In the first part of the nineteenth century, other instruments, such as the stethoscope, clinical thermometer, and sphygmomanometer, were introduced to aid in the diagnosis and treatment of disease. Toward the end of the century, Wilhelm Roentgen's discovery of the x-ray had an important impact on medical care.

The Johns Hopkins Hospital

The Johns Hopkins Hospital in Baltimore became world renowned because it incorporated many of the advances in hospital design and function, medical education, and medical care. In 1867 a Baltimore businessman, Johns Hopkins, endowed the city with $7 million to be divided equally for the funding of a university and a hospital. The university and the hospital were to form two separate corporations with separate boards of trustees, but there was some liaison between the two because several men sat on both boards. Johns Hopkins purchased the thirteen-acre site for the hospital and pledged $100,000 a year toward construction costs while he lived. He died within a year, but the income from the $2 million that he also willed the hospital amounted to approximately $120,000 a year. The construction was to be financed only from the income; after the hospital was completed, the income was to be used for maintenance.

This was to be no ordinary hospital. Hopkins stipulated that the hospital's staff should be surgeons and physicians of the highest character and greatest skill and that the facility should be used as a teaching hospital for the university's medical school and should provide care to the indigent sick of the city and state free of charge without regard to sex, age, or color. There should be space for a limited number of paying patients, and the income from their care should be applied to the care of the poor. Although the administration of the hospital was to be nonsectarian, a religious spirit should be apparent. In addition, a training school for female nurses should be established. The hospital trustees interpreted Hopkins's mandates as meaning they should build the best hospital in the world.

After much study of the best design, along with consideration of what was known at the time about the spread of disease, the building began in 1877 with construction of the administration building and the two paying-patient wards. It continued for twelve years because only the income from the endowment could be used. Each time the income was exhausted, construction ceased until enough income was accumulated to begin again. Finally, in 1885 the hospital was opened for patients.

An important function of the hospital was its integration with the medical school's curriculum. The clinical methods established at the hospital enhanced research and promoted improved teaching of future physicians. The nurse training school introduced a two-year course of systematized instruction at the hospital rather than the usual practice of placing nursing students with private families during the second year. A very generous endowment, international consultation, early recruitment of leading clinicians, and careful planning resulted in a hospital with a worldwide reputation for excellence to which others would look for many decades for the latest and best in medical care and training.

Increased knowledge, new technology, and societal pressures caused hospitals to modify and develop as the decades advanced. Hospitals changed in many ways. For example, when the principles of the germ theory of disease were understood and aseptic techniques were practiced, and as a result hospital infections began to decrease, the type of patient changed. It became advantageous for sick people, regardless of their financial status, to be treated in hospitals. The number of separate paying-patient wards and expensive private rooms increased, and this change in turn altered the way in which hospitals were financed. In addition, as the number of paying patients increased, there was an increasing patient demand for privacy, which led to the replacement of the large paying-patient wards with semiprivate rooms accommodating two to four patients. This development forced changes in the nursing supervision of patients and also increased construction and operating costs. Infection control also affected hospital planning. No longer was it necessary to have separate buildings or separate floors for certain conditions. With the introduction of iron and steel for construction, along with the development of elevators, hospitals could be built with multiple stories and occupy less ground space, a most fortunate development as city populations grew and land prices rose.

Changes in the U.S. hospital have been dramatic. "Nevertheless, the modern hospital's basic shape had been established by 1920. It had become central to medical education and was well integrated into the career patterns of regular physicians; in urban areas it had already replaced the family as the site for treating serious illness and managing death. Perhaps most important, it had already been clothed with a legitimizing aura of science and almost boundless social expectation" (Rosenberg, 1987).

Hospitals are still evolving in response to technological developments, societal needs, pressures from special interest groups, and a competitive environment.

MODERN HOSPITALS

The environment in which hospitals function is changing dramatically, forcing them to make significant changes in how they are organized and how they operate. Following World War II, the federal government encouraged the construction, expansion, and renovation of hospitals by providing grants under the Hill-Burton Act (Hospital Survey and Construction Act of 1946). The legislation provided federal aid to states under the Public Health Service Act for surveying hospitals, planning construction, and authorizing grants for the construction. Grants were designed under a formula taking into account greater need for hospitals in the poorest states. Those who received grants were required to provide matching funds, and the institution, once in operation, was required to provide a specified amount of care to those who could not pay. The results were impressive: New hospitals were built, and existing institutions were expanded and upgraded. However, the "planning" portion of the legislation fell short, and some areas of the country remained without hospital care while other areas became "overbedded" ("Hospital's Expenses for Providing Care," 1996; Stevens, 1989).

Simultaneously, the rapid growth of health insurance, followed by the introduction of Medicare and Medicaid, increased the demand for health care (Custer and Musacchio, 1986). Government also facilitated growth by allowing nonprofit hospitals to issue tax-exempt bonds for construction and acquisition of capital-intensive new technologies. These developments were in large measure dictated by the development of antibiotics and other new drugs, new anesthetics, new instrumentation, and new knowledge

that permitted physicians to treat what was previously untreatable, as well as to treat other patients more effectively.

By the late 1960s and early 1970s, concern began to mount over the rapidly rising cost of health care. Many states passed certificate of need (CON) legislation to prohibit the construction or expansion of hospitals unless they could prove that more beds were needed. As health care costs continued their dramatic climb, government and others encouraged shorter hospital stays and more outpatient services. Corporations, seeking to contain costs incurred by their employees, began to require second opinions about the necessity for surgery before the surgery would be covered by insurance, and they modified their health insurance policies by requiring higher copayments and deductibles. They began to review the length of and necessity for inpatient hospital stays, and they encouraged their employees to join cost-effective health maintenance organizations (HMOs) and other alternative delivery systems. A number of state governments started to control the rates charged by hospitals. Then, in 1983 the federal government tried to slow the cost spiral by implementing prospective payment to hospitals for Medicare patients. These patients accounted for about 40 percent of hospital revenues.

As government and businesses moved to control health costs, hospitals were transformed from expanding institutions with little regard for costs (because they were largely reimbursed for them) into institutions with a declining number of patients, in an environment that had become very competitive and in which the payers were questioning the efficiency and quality of their services.

To understand this shift in emphasis, one first needs to understand the basic structure of the hospital field as it developed in the second half of the twentieth century, which will be the focus of the remainder of this chapter.

HOSPITAL CHARACTERISTICS

The community hospital is the hospital with which we are most familiar. The community hospital is defined as nonfederal, short-term (average length of stay less than thirty days), general and specialty care provider whose facilities and services are available to the public (Healthcare InfoSource, 1998a). It provides a variety of diagnostic and therapeutic services for both medical and surgical cases. Excluded from the definition of community hospital are "hospital units in institutions such as prison and college infirmaries, facilities for the mentally retarded, and alcoholism and chemical dependency hospitals" (National Center for Health Statistics, 1999, p. 277–280). At its most advanced development, the community hospital handles almost every kind of case; it is truly a *general* hospital. But there are, and always have been, compromises of this ideal. In the early part of the twentieth century, it was easier for a hospital to approach the ideal because the limits of our knowledge and technology did not suggest or permit the sophisticated differentiation that we now find.

Mental health patients and tuberculosis patients were separated, and if one goes back far enough, one finds other contagious diseases isolated in special hospitals. In some communities, obstetric and gynecological cases were reserved for special women's hospitals; eye, ear, nose, and throat (EENT) cases went to EENT hospitals; and there were hospitals for children with special services for severe cardiac and orthopedic problems. Many of these private hospitals later evolved into larger for-profit or nonprofit community hospitals.

Today the differentiation from, and compromises on, the ideal model of a general hospital are dictated largely by technology and cost. Some medical care requires highly trained clinicians whose skills cannot be maintained unless those clinicians are employed in a large hospital with a high volume of cases. Open-heart surgery is one example. A cardiac surgeon cannot maintain his or her skill working solely in a rural twenty-five–bed general hospital. Cost is another issue, and a related one, for highly specialized services typically require extensive support from other hospital services. An open-heart surgery team requires, among other things, skilled technicians, diagnostic imaging, and sophisticated laboratory support. None of these could be justified clinically or economically in a small general hospital. Thus, general hospitals today are almost always compromises on the ideal, with the smaller hospitals tending to compromise more than the larger ones.

Differentiation in hospital services and structures is even more difficult to describe since the 1980s. Competition and restructuring has led to unprecedented partnering among hospitals, so much so that it is difficult to describe the "average" hospital or even to categorize hospitals. We therefore simply present some of the characteristics of hospitals today.

Hospital Ownership

Hospital ownership can be described in broad terms as falling into three major categories: nonprofit, for-profit, or government. These broad categories today may be somewhat less definitive when we consider integrated systems with umbrella for-profit organizations owning hospitals that are nonprofit. Whatever the ownership configuration, understanding the major categories is still a worthwhile endeavor.

In 1997 there were 5,057 community hospitals (down from 5,134 in 1996 and continuing a downward trend since 1980). Of those, 3,000 were nonprofit, 797 were for-profit, and 1,260 were government hospitals. The downward trend in the number of hospitals is largest in the number of government hospitals, with slower decreases in the number of nonprofits and a somewhat consistent number of for-profits (National Center for Health Statistics, 1999).

Nonprofit Hospitals

Nonprofit (voluntary) does not mean that the hospital cannot make a profit; rather it means that there are restrictions on what can be done with the profit. Profits must be turned back into the hospital's operation rather than distributed to shareholders. The nonprofit hospital does not have shareholders; rather it has a board of trustees who serve on a voluntary basis, receiving no pay, to guide and govern the hospital. The nonprofit organization is exempt from paying taxes, but it must follow certain criteria to qualify and remain nonprofit. Tax-exempt status must be granted on each of the government levels separately. The federal statutes (501[C][3]) require that the hospital serve those unable to pay for services and be nonrestrictive toward physicians; that is, the facility cannot limit participation to a particular group of physicians to the exclusion of other qualified physicians. The nonprofit hospital's earnings also cannot be used for the benefit of any individual. Earnings must be turned back to the hospital's operations or used for the benefit of the community. State requirements are similar to federal requirements, but each state may have specific definitions of *charitable* or of the use of revenues. Local tax-exempt status usually means property tax exemptions, and qualifications again may differ from locality to locality. All levels of tax exemption, however, do require some level of charity care or community service on the part of the hospital.

The reliance on community business, industrial, and professional leaders to serve on hospital boards has long-standing historical roots. These people were the very ones who could provide leadership in raising funds to support the hospital, and in a great many cases they underwrote hospital deficits with personal checks. Though the latter practice has declined sharply, community leaders still tend to dominate hospital boards because of their ability to exercise influence on behalf of the hospital, because of the valued entrepreneurial skills that they apply to hospital work without cost to the hospital, and because of their positions, in which they can readily allocate some of their working time to hospital activities.

Church-affiliated hospitals are often the most readily recognized nonprofit hospitals. They are different only in that they are owned, or heavily influenced by, the churches or church groups that sponsor them. A large number of Protestant denominations and Catholic orders and dioceses own and operate hospitals. Their roles in this field have deep historical roots. Though rooted in a religious denomination, none is discriminatory in terms of access to care (save the limitation dictated by whether or not one's physician has admitting privileges), although a church hospital may be sensitive to the special spiritual or dietary needs of the denomination that sponsors it. It might be noted, with regard to Jewish-sponsored hospitals, that the sponsorship is not by the synagogue or other official body, but by the Jewish community.

Churches are tending to lessen the extent of their control on their hospitals. This trend is reflected in the makeup of their boards, on which nonchurch members serve and fewer church officials and ministers serve. This may be a reflection of the increased secularization in U.S. society, as well as recognition of the need for many other talents for the successful direction of a hospital. On the other hand, it may also be a necessity, given the decreased numbers of persons joining religious orders and able to carry out the work of the orders directly.

For-Profit Hospitals

Unlike the nonprofit hospital, the for-profit hospital does operate with the goal of making a profit to distribute to its shareholders. The shareholders elect a board of directors to govern the hospital. Board members may or may not be compensated for their services. Responsibilities are somewhat the same as those of the nonprofit's board of trustees. For-profit organizations do not qualify for tax exemption, although they may provide some charity care. Because of the responsibility to shareholders/owners and the burden of paying taxes, for-profit organizations often operate more efficiently, with an eye to cost effectiveness. For this reason, for-profit health care organizations are often criticized for paying more attention to the bottom line than to quality of care. Competitive pressures and reduced reimbursement rates, however, have made both for-profit and nonprofit hospitals more aware of the bottom line. Studies bring mixed results as to the quality of care provided by each. Accreditation, outcomes research, and a more watchful consumer eye make it difficult for any hospital to remain in operation if not providing quality care.

Among the investor-owned hospitals, the corporately owned hospital is perhaps the most visible and controversial. A number of corporations have developed that build, own, and/or operate general and specialty hospitals all over the United States. Most of the firms are small, but some are quite large. Columbia/HCA, for example, which is based in Nashville, Tennessee, owns 320 hospitals in the United States. Quorum Health Group owns 22 hospitals and has 237 hospitals under contract management. HealthSouth, a network of rehabilitation hospitals, owns 73 facilities, and Tenet Healthcare Corporation owns 129 hospitals (Health InfoSource, 1998a). Most of the investor-owned hospitals are members of the American Hospital Association (AHA) and are accredited by the Joint Commission on Accreditation of Healthcare

Organizations (JCAHO). Some are community general hospitals; some are specialized institutions—psychiatric, drug dependency, rehabilitation, and so on. The controversy, again, is focused on the emphasis on profits versus the emphasis on quality health care delivery.

Hospital Boards

In recent years court decisions and federal regulations caused hospital boards of trustees to become more active in their oversight role. Both for-profit and nonprofit boards are responsible for:

- Establishing the hospital's mission and vision
- Hiring, and evaluating the performance of, the hospital administrator (often called the chief executive officer, or CEO)
- Appointing physicians to the medical staff
- Ensuring the quality of care delivered
- Approving long-range plans and budgets
- Monitoring performance against plans and budgets

Where for-profit and nonprofit boards differ is in their ability to sell assets or discontinue operation of the hospital. Boards of for-profit hospitals may sell assets or discontinue the operation of the business and disperse the proceeds to owners. Boards of nonprofit hospitals must follow specific regulations regarding selling or transferring of assets. Any proceeds from a sale must go into a nonprofit foundation and continue to be used for charitable purposes or community needs (Griffith, 1999).

Government Hospitals

The *federal government* owns and operates general hospitals for clientele for whom it is responsible. Specifically, the federal government, through the Department of Defense, has 27 army, 19 navy, and 44 air force hospitals. Though some of these hospitals specialize, most are general hospitals. The Veterans Administration (VA) also has 144 hospitals throughout the country, to care for veterans with service-connected disabilities, as well as non-service-connected disabilities when the veteran cannot afford private

care. Some of its hospitals are psychiatric, but most are general, with strong rehabilitation medicine services. The Indian Health Service in the U.S. Public Health Service has 51 hospitals located on various Native American reservations. General hospital services are also provided by the U.S. Department of Justice for inmates of federal prisons (Health Info-Source, 1998a).

County and city hospitals exist in many parts of the country. In large urban areas, these tend to be safety net hospitals (serving the poor and uninsured), although since the advent of Medicare and Medicaid and the growth of private health insurance, these hospitals now also serve private patients. The governance of these hospitals by local government varies from the highly political to the highly professional, depending on the style or pattern of political practice in that area. In larger cities, these are frequently teaching hospitals and also hospitals with strong medical school ties. Some famous hospitals are in this group, including Bellevue Hospital Center (811 beds) in New York, Cook County Hospital (591 beds) in Chicago, and Los Angeles County & University of Southern California Medical Center (1328 beds) in Los Angeles, (American Hospital Directory, 2000).

State governments and, in some instances, local governments have been primarily responsible for establishing facilities for the care of the mentally ill. See Chapter 9 for more information on mental health and the providers of mental health services.

Hospital Size and Services

Hospitals may be large or small, teaching or non-teaching. The size of the hospital, typically indicated by the number of beds, depends on the size of the population served, the range of services provided, and whether it is used as a referral hospital. A small community may be able to justify only a small general hospital, just large enough to support the general run of cases. Smaller communities must also limit the range of services provided because the volume of patients may be so small in a specialized area of medicine that not enough patients would use the service to justify the expense of developing and maintaining it. Similarly, in such cases there would not be enough cases to enable the specialist to maintain his or her skills. In these instances, the patient would be referred to another facility that has been able to put together and maintain that service. Generally speaking, however, the larger the community served, the larger the hospital, in terms of number of beds, range of specialists, and range of supporting equipment and services.

A community hospital may also be a *teaching hospital.* Teaching hospitals are hospitals that have an approved residency program. The presence of nursing or other health professional programs in a hospital does not define it as a teaching hospital. On the other hand, a teaching hospital need not be a university hospital, but merely affiliated with a medical school accredited for medical education. Historically, most teaching hospitals were either public general hospitals for the poor or other types of general hospitals with a large number of indigent patients. These indigent patients were the ones on whom the medical students, interns, and residents learned. The patients, in a sense, paid for their care by allowing their bodies to be used for medical training purposes. The poor frequently resented this form of payment, and they often looked upon the hospital as the place where "they" experimented on patients. It was, in part, this perception by the poor that contributed to the development of Medicaid, under which all people are entitled to private care. But by that time (1966), teaching-hospital practice had changed, and all patients, paying as well as indigent, were teaching patients. Teaching hospitals became known for their advanced technology and expert practitioners and, as a result, became the centers of choice for many patients.

Hospitals can also be described as *allopathic* or *osteopathic* institutions. Although the allopathic (MD)-oriented institutions predominate in this country, the same types of hospital standards apply also to the hospitals that were established to serve osteopaths (DOs). The separation has historical roots that go back to the time when neither would relate to the other school of medicine. But times have changed, and now osteopaths serve on the staffs of allopathic institutions and MDs serve on the staffs of osteopathic hospitals. In some communities, these institutions have merged.

Children's hospitals are community hospitals dealing specifically with chronic, congenital, and/or acute childhood diseases. Whether needed surgical care is performed in these hospitals or in other institutions varies. Advances in technology and scientific medicine generally dictate a close affiliation with other hospitals in order to benefit from the latest instrumentation and the now essential supporting specialties and services.

Maternity hospitals, women's hospitals, EENT hospitals, and other specialty hospitals still retain a significant presence in health care delivery. Cancer treatment hospitals are perhaps the newest specialty hospitals on the rise.

The definitions that apply to the various hospitals are not rigid. As noted at the outset, all hospitals are in a sense compromises on the concept of the total hospital. Hospitals in each category differ from each other not only in scope of services, but also in patient mix. Whereas a specialty hospital may exist in one community, the same kind of hospital in another community may be part of a broader-based institution. Specialized hospitals sometimes developed because of the presence of a benefactor, or because a physician had a unique therapeutic approach best handled in a specialty setting. What is clear, however, is that rising costs, coupled with new technology and the interdependency of the various specialties, are dictating affiliations and mergers. Completely freestanding institutions, including the very small community general hospitals, are a dying breed.

Multihospital Systems

The future of many hospitals (especially small, rural hospitals) may well depend in large part on the concept of *regionalization,* whereby small hospitals affiliate with larger, more urban hospitals. Under regionalization, each level of hospital (the small rural hospital, the moderate-sized hospital, and the large regional referral center) provides only those services that it is able to provide efficiently and effectively. Thus, the small rural hospital provides basic general care; the moderate-sized hospital, more specialized care and equipment; and the regional hospital, the most sophisticated and expensive special types of care. Patients have access to a full range of services and are admitted or transferred to the appropriate level of hospital according to their medical needs. With this type of arrangement, hospitals avoid duplicate expensive services, obtain consultation assistance from medical personnel in larger hospitals, and have the advantages of sharing certain support services, such as human resources departments and purchasing departments. The affiliations range from an informal regional working agreement to a merger of institutions into multihospital or multi-institutional systems with a single, coordinated management structure. Many European countries have regionalized their hospital systems to provide hospital services more efficiently. The occasional hesitancy of small institutions in this country to enter into the more formal regional agreements stems from a long-standing desire for local control, coupled with a fear that the arrangements will serve the financial and occupancy rate needs of the higher-level institution at the expense of the smaller institution.

Advances in telemedicine make it possible for small rural institutions to bring needed expertise to the patient's bedside without bringing costly services into the institution. Regional affiliations make telemedicine and technology diffusion possible and plausible.

Regionalization is not the only motivation for hospital affiliations. Competition and the pressures of managed care are contributing to the affiliation frenzy. Nationwide, the numbers of multihospital systems are changing rapidly, with disassociations occurring almost as rapidly as new affiliations. One needs only to go to nationally recognized newspapers (*The New York Times, The Wall Street Journal, The Washington Post*, etc.) to read about changes in affiliation that occur on an almost daily basis. The cost effectiveness of such ventures is unknown. Promises of consolidation of services fall into low levels of priority when local needs and cultures are taken into account. The entire process is still in a high degree of uncertainty and chaos.

Hospital Statistics

The most reliable source for data about hospitals is the American Hospital Association (AHA). Each year the AHA conducts a survey of "all hospitals—registered and nonregistered, in the U.S. and its associated areas . . . with an average response rate of 89.9%" (Healthcare InfoSource, 1998b, p. 1). Not all registered hospitals are accredited by JCAHO, nor are they required to be members of the AHA. In lieu of accreditation, hospitals do have to be licensed and meet a specific list of criteria published by the AHA, such as maintaining at least six inpatient beds, an organized medical staff, continuous nursing services, a pharmacy service supervised by a registered pharmacist, a governing authority and chief executive, up-to-date and complete medical records on each patient, and so on. (Healthcare InfoSource, 1998a).

The AHA's publication *Hospital Statistics* provides useful current and trend data on hospital utilization, personnel, and finances. The *AHA Guide to the Health Care Field* provides information on individual hospitals, networks, and systems; and lists of organizations, agencies, and providers.

Other useful reports are issued periodically by the National Center for Health Statistics (NCHS) of the Centers for Disease Control and Prevention (CDC), and by the Health Care Financing Administration (HCFA). These reports and publications relate not only to hospitals but also to other components of the health field.

Hospital Organization and Administration

The governing board of a hospital not only establishes policies for the institution but also hires the administrator. The word *administrator* is used in a generic sense. Some hospitals designate the top administrative person as *president, chief executive officer (CEO)*, or *executive director*. The training and experience of the administrator may vary greatly by size and location of the hospital. Today many hospital administrators have a master's degree in health administration (MHA) or business administration (MBA). Some administrators have PhDs, while others are MDs or DOs. Whatever the formal education structure, the administrator must also possess a wide range of experience in the health care field.

The administrator is responsible for carrying out the strategic plan developed by the board and carries on the day-to-day operation of the facility. It is important for the administrator to align him- or herself with qualified personnel in finance, human resources management, and other management skills while having the ability to work with the medical staff and other clinical managers. Griffith (1999) categorizes the responsibilities of the administrator into four functional areas: to *lead, support, represent, and organize.* As such, the administrator is responsible not only for the internal functioning of the organization, but for its role, image, and responsibility in and to the community.

The organizational functioning of a hospital is not as clear-cut as it is in business and industry. The lines of authority are not precise (see Figure 7–1). Organizational lines of authority are even more difficult to define in multi-hospital systems (see Figure 7–2). The board appoints the administrator. The board also appoints the medical staff. Membership on the medical staff allows physicians to admit patients and continue to treat them and call in specialists as needed. Though the medical staff is technically accountable to the board, it has a daily functional relationship with the administrator. Nursing service is administratively accountable to the administrator but professionally accountable to the medical staff. Other personnel, such as pharmacists, lab and x-ray technicians, and dietitians, are also administratively accountable to the administrator but professionally accountable to the medical staff.

The hospital is really the physician's workshop, although some argue that it is also the center for meeting all community health needs. However, only the physician can admit a patient (except in a few circumscribed areas in which admitting and treatment privileges are held by other health professionals), and all others must act on the physician's orders. But the physician typically does not hire or fire unless, as a member of the medical staff, the physician is an employee of the hospital. Even then the physician's authority is circumscribed by a certain administrative accountability to the administrator.

Physicians are the driving force in hospitals. They ask that certain procedures be done for the patient and that certain supplies or equipment be purchased. It is up to the administrator and the nurses and others working with the administrator to cooperate to the greatest extent possible with the physicians. Since the 1980s, with additional cost containment imperatives

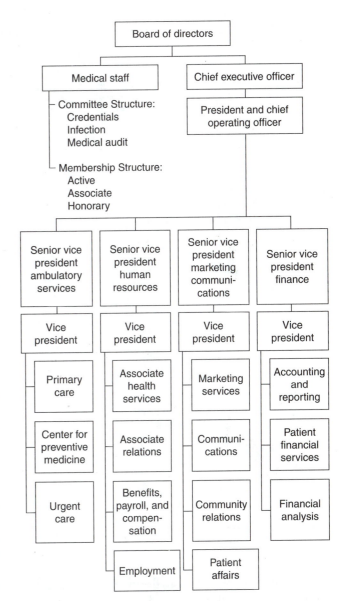

Figure 7–1 Hospital Organizational Chart

in place, third-party payers and the utilization review process have added difficulty to the hospital personnel decision-making equation. As one might guess, conflicts occur: Personality clashes, misunderstandings, and insufficient funds create problems. The various parties try to resolve differences, figure out ways to get the needed funds, and reach agreement

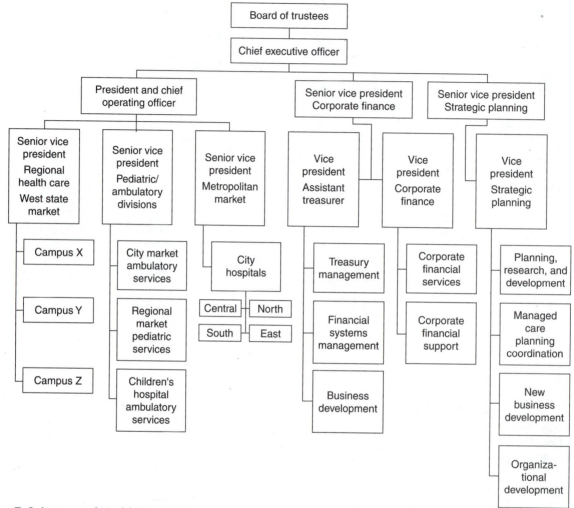

Figure 7–2 Integrated Health Care Delivery System

on outstanding issues. When the medical staff and administrator cannot resolve differences, the board must enter to decide.

Most hospitals minimize tensions between hospital governing boards and the medical staff by having a physician representing the medical staff as a member of the board. Hospitals depend on physicians to refer patients to them and fill their hospital beds. An individual physician may have admitting privileges at several hospitals. The physician and patient choose the hospital to which the patient will be admitted.

Administrators try to make their hospital the most attractive to the doctor by making the physician's dealings with the hospital convenient and pleasant. Attempting to meet this objective sometimes means obtaining equipment the physicians want or prefer. At times physicians and hospitals compete with each other as both develop and expand outpatient services, such as freestanding ambulatory and diagnostic centers, to improve their financial status.

Hospitals are changing their organizational structure to a corporate model and calling themselves *medical centers* to create fiscal flexibility at a time when greater constraints are placed upon hospitals by government programs. The corporate model permits a hospital to set up profit-making operations, such as a medical office building or a freestanding clinic, with the profits kept completely separate from hospital operations and thus not taken into account by government, insurance companies, and business coalitions as they identify hospital costs in determining how much the hospital should be paid for care. The for-profit operations, in other words, cannot be counted as an offset against losses in hospital operations, such as in care of the poor who have no insurance or Medicaid protection. The profits are then free for use as the overall governing body sees fit. Corporate restructuring is a rapidly developing phenomenon, although Congress has considered legislation to curtail such profit-making activities by nonprofit organizations, with much opposition from the AHA. To date, such mixed corporate structuring continues to operate.

Despite the varieties and complexities of hospital organization, the board delegates to the medical staff retain certain professional responsibilities. These responsibilities are typically described by the medical staff bylaws, which the board approves. More importantly, however, the smooth functioning of the hospital can be attributed to improved quality of administration, which came with the introduction of sound management practices and appropriately trained administrators.

Medical Staff Privileges

The board also grants admitting and practice privileges to physicians and others, usually on recommendation of the medical staff. Physicians apply to a hospital for staff privileges.[1] If the hospital is a closed–group practice hospital, then the only way to become part of the hospital staff is to be accepted by the medical group. Hospital bylaws define how a

physician may secure admitting privileges. Typically, in community general hospitals the physician who seeks privileges makes application to the board. The board typically seeks the advice of its credentialing committee (which includes members of the medical staff), which judges the applicant's qualifications and character and makes a recommendation. The decision about appointment to the medical staff is based on a variety of factors, including current state licensure, board certification status, medical school education, residency training, written recommendations, malpractice insurance coverage and history, and the type of privileges sought.

The Health Care Quality Improvement Act of 1986 mandated that hospitals query the National Practitioner Data Bank for information on each new appointment to the medical staff and once every two years for existing medical staff. The data bank legislation requires malpractice insurers to report "all medical malpractice payments they make on behalf of physicians and dentists." It also requires hospitals, state licensure boards, professional societies, and other health care organizations to report adverse actions they take against physicians. The purpose of the data bank is to provide protection to the public from incompetent physicians (Yessian & Greenleaf, 1997). Prior to the establishment of a national system, physicians who had lost their licenses could simply move to another state and establish a practice without their previous history becoming known to the community.

The larger and more complex the hospital is, the more precisely defined the admitting privileges are. In some remote rural hospitals, a family practitioner may be doing general medical care, reading electrocardiograms, handling obstetrics, and performing a variety of surgical procedures. The same physician in a large urban teaching hospital might be restricted to carefully circumscribed family practice privileges.

Staff privileges fall into several categories. The *active medical staff* consists of those physicians accorded

---

[1] Hospital privileges may be dictated by state law, other government regulations, or local custom. Although dentists, podiatrists, chiropractors, midwives, and others may have staff privileges in some hospitals, physicians are those most generally recognized as professionals on the medical staff. References are made to physicians' privileges for the sake of simplicity.

all rights, privileges, and responsibilities. They provide most of the care, offer leadership in various committees, and may hold a variety of medical staff offices. *Associate medical staff* members are the more junior physicians, or those who wish to become active staff when vacancies occur. They may have limited access to beds for their patients. *Courtesy medical staff* is the category for those physicians who seek the privilege of admitting only occasional patients and who do not wish to become part of the active staff, either because the bulk of their admissions are to other hospitals or because they do not have practices that necessitate frequent admission of patients. The *consulting medical staff* consists of those who serve primarily as specialty consultants to members of the active staff. In some types of cases, for example, the law, or hospital or medical staff bylaws, may require the attending physician to secure consultation, and this staff is available in the event an appropriate consultant is not on the active or associate staff.

The bylaws, rules and regulations, and offices of the medical staff organization vary from hospital to hospital. Typically, however, a *chief of staff* or *medical director* is elected by the medical staff for a fixed term and represents the staff's interests to the board and to the hospital administration. This physician is usually elected by the medical staff for a fixed term and represents the staff's interests to the board and to the hospital administration. This is the formal line for communication, particularly on major issues, but hospitals also have a wide informal mechanism that functions as the rule. Whether the physician is an employee of the hospital varies within organizations. Full-time salaried physicians, other than radiologists, pathologists, anesthesiologists, and emergency department physicians, are usually found in the larger teaching hospitals. When a hospital has divided its staff into clinical departments or services, there is typically a chief of service for each clinical area, and each chief of service reports to the chief of staff.

Clinical and Supporting Departments

The clinical organization of the general hospital varies depending on its size, the pattern of patient mix among the various specialties, and the extent of specialization of the medical staff. Except in very small hospitals, obstetrics tends to be segregated in a separate wing or on a separate floor of the hospital, along with the newborn nursery. This is done to minimize the risk of infection to the newborn and mother, and in more recent times, unfortunately, these units have become locked units to prevent abduction of newborns. Pediatric cases also tend to be segregated. The assignment of other patients to clinical services or departments varies considerably. If there is any departmental breakdown in the smaller hospitals, it tends to be into medicine and surgery, with patient assignment as appropriate.

As specialization increases in a hospital and the volume of patients increases within each specialty, there is a tendency for departments to be established with beds assigned to that specialty. When the volume of patients is sufficient to justify it, the specialty beds may be located in a separate wing or on a separate floor. The establishment of specialty services with assigned beds permits a more effective and efficient concentration of support services peculiar to that specialty (equipment, specially trained nurses, and other personnel) and contributes to the development of the specialty and its scientific work. Assignment of beds to a given specialty has clinical advantages; however, it decreases institutional flexibility in terms of bed use.

In the general hospital, the *emergency department* (sometimes called *emergency room*) and the *outpatient* or *ambulatory services* department have increased importance. Their functions and importance are described in more detail in Chapter 6.

Some of the larger teaching hospitals have departments of *family medicine*. These departments serve as family physician to a community or to an enrolled group, and they ensure admission to that hospital when necessary. The department of family medicine also serves as a training area for future primary care physicians.

Supporting the patient care services are three medically supervised departments: *anesthesiology, radiology,* and *pathology*. In smaller hospitals, the services are staffed by part-time specialists; in larger hospitals, however, the specialists work full-time. They may be paid by salary or fee for service, or the services may be contracted out to independent group practices. Both radiology and pathology are rapidly expanding departments, owing to rapidly developing technology. Anesthesiology services are often staffed by one anesthesiologist supervising a larger number of nurse anesthetists.

All hospitals have a number of other support services. Whether or not they have departmental status depends on the size of the institution and the rationale of those responsible for establishing the organizational arrangements. Some of these services are nursing, pharmacy, health information management (medical records), and dietary. Larger hospitals also have such services as inhalation therapy, physical therapy, occupational therapy, and medical social work.

Increasingly, hospitals are seeking new ways to cope with rising costs. *Shared services*—services shared with other hospitals—such as laundry, purchasing, and computer services, are methods of cost control. Whether a hospital participates in a given shared service or purchases the service from an outside firm depends on whether the hospital's needs can be adequately met and whether it is economically advantageous. Some hospitals find it advantageous to contract to outside firms for services such as food, security, and housekeeping, and even for nurses and other personnel.

Hospital Licensure and Accreditation

Hospitals are licensed to operate by state governments. Each state has its own requirements, but all states' requirements are similar. Originally, the various states focused their attention for licensure on hospital physical plants—for example, fire safety, heating, space allocations, and sanitation. Now, however, states have moved beyond this and are beginning to pay more attention to professional standards, often by defaulting to Joint Commission accreditation (see the next section) as a criterion for licensure.

We noted in Chapter 4 that the American College of Surgeons (ACS) suppressed its 1919 hospital inspection report because the conditions it found were so poor. The ACS and the American Medical Association (AMA), however, have worked consistently for reform of hospitals. Though they were concerned, as

were the states, with physical plants, these professional bodies were also concerned with matters relating to quality of care. Their efforts at reform culminated in 1952 with the initiation of a hospital accreditation program by the Joint Commission on Accreditation of Hospitals (JCAH).

Joint Commission on Accreditation of Healthcare Organizations

The history of the Joint Commission on Accreditation of Hospitals (JCAH) goes back to 1913, when the American College of Surgeons (ACS) was formed. Almost immediately the ACS embarked upon a hospital standardization program when it found that more than half of the applicants for fellowship in the ACS had to be rejected because the case records they were required to submit were inadequate. ACS developed the Minimum Standard for approval, and by 1950 more than half of the hospitals in the United States met the Minimum Standard. In 1951 the American College of Physicians, the American Hospital Association, the American Medical Association, and the Canadian Medical Association joined the ACS to form the JCAH, which offered accreditation to hospitals that applied and complied with its standards. In 1959 the Canadian Medical Association withdrew to participate in its own program, and in 1979 the American Dental Association became a member of the Board of Commissioners. In 1966 the Joint Commission, in a major policy decision, changed the standards it used for accreditation from the *minimal essential* standards for proper patient care to the *optimal achievable* standards. As other health organizations developed, the Joint Commission became the accreditation body for them. In 1987, JCAH changed its name to the Joint Commission on the Accreditation of Healthcare Organizations (JCAHO). Referred to simply as the "Joint Commission," this independent, not-for-profit organization sets standards and "accredits nearly 20,000 health care organizations in the U.S. including hospitals, health care networks, managed care organizations, and health care organizations that provide home care, long-term care, behavioral health care, laboratory, and ambulatory care services" (JCAHO, 2000).

The Joint Commission is governed by a twenty-eight–member Board of Commissioners composed of nurses, physicians, consumers, medical directors, administrators, providers, employers, labor representatives, health plan leaders, quality experts, ethicists, health insurance administrators, and educators. Among its corporate members are representatives from the American College of Physicians—the American Society of Internal Medicine, the American College of Surgeons, the American Dental Association, the American Hospital Association, and the American Medical Association. Seeking accreditation is voluntary; hospitals and other health care organizations apply for accreditation and request an on-site survey. A variety of health care providers are employed by the Joint Commission to conduct the accreditation on-site surveys. The survey team assesses the extent of a hospital's compliance with the Joint Commission's standards by gathering data regarding the organization's activities.

Accreditation is not based simply on the physical environment, such as fire safety, sanitation, and bed space. It is also based on performance in functional areas, such as patients' rights, quality of care, standards for providers, patient-nurse ratios, and outcomes measures. The findings of the survey team are reported to the Board of Commissioners, which makes the accreditation decision. Site visits take place at least every three years for most organizations and at least every two years for laboratories. Accreditation categories include accreditation with commendation (eliminated effective January 1, 2000), accreditation with recommendations for improvement (accreditation with Type I recommendations as of January 1, 2001), accreditation (accreditation without Type 1 recommendations as of January 1, 2001), provisional accreditation, conditional accreditation, preliminary nonaccreditation (preliminary denial of accreditation as of January 1, 2001), and not accredited (accreditation denied as of January 1, 2001). Those organizations receiving other than "accreditation" status may have certain deficiencies to correct and a specific time period to do so in order to receive accreditation or qualify for another on-site visit (JCAHO, 2000).

Accreditation is important for health care organizations, and hospitals in particular, in many ways. Accreditation may fulfill all or part of the state licensing requirements, most health insurance company participation requirements, Medicare and Medicaid certification requirements, and managed care organization contract requirements. In addition, voluntary accreditation enhances consumer and community confidence, medical staff recruitment, quality of care, and staff education. Finally, the accreditation process provides an opportunity for organizations to assess their strong and weak features and make improvements (JCAHO, 2000).

The basic question accreditation has answered is, *Can* this organization provide quality health care? The accreditation process has traditionally focused primarily on organizational structure, processes, and equipment. Now the Joint Commission is moving beyond determining an institution's capability of providing quality care to answer the question, *Does* this organization provide quality health care? It is developing ORYX, a computerized database system, to integrate the use of outcomes and other clinical indicators into the accreditation process.

Although the Joint Commission has contributed much to the improved quality of care in hospitals, many have been critical of its activities, claiming that the organization is not inclined to publicize poor medical care or to disaccredit hospitals. The Joint Commission sees its inspections as an educational device for improving performance rather than for removing accreditation. However, Medicare and Medicaid reimbursements depend on accreditation, and the federal government expects certain standards to be fulfilled if hospitals are accredited. In the early 1990s, HCFA found that many accredited hospitals did not meet Medicare conditions of participation. Criticisms caused the Joint Commission to create an additional category of "conditional accreditation" and impose stricter timetables for improvement and the release of limited information to the federal government about those hospitals that do not meet the standards. The JCAHO Web site (www.jcaho.org) provides a directory of hospitals and their accreditation status and other general information regarding size, financial status, and the like.

Other Performance Evaluators

Hospitals have been interested in their efficiency, quality of care, and performance in relation to other hospitals for many years. In 1950 the Kellogg Foundation awarded a grant to the Southwestern Michigan Hospital Council to assist the study of professional activities in hospitals through interhospital comparisons of hospital statistical reports. The project was known as the Professional Activity Study (PAS). At the heart of PAS are the medical abstracts of all hospitalized patients in participating hospitals, which permit a hospital to review its performance over a period of time by such factors as the type of service to which the patient was admitted, final diagnosis, length of stay, type of surgery, and name of physician. Reports are prepared for hospitals monthly, semiannually, and annually. The initial PAS studies resulted in establishment of the Commission on Professional and Hospital Activities to assist in evaluating such activities.

Employers, as major purchasers of health care for their employees, compare costs for hospital care but are also interested in the quality of the care provided. Under ERISA (the Employee Retirement Income Security Act; see Chapter 3), many employers self-insure, so evaluating cost and quality becomes even a more direct issue. Many states have begun incentives to help employers, insurers, and others evaluate the performance of hospitals and other health care providers. One of the first such state incentives was the Pennsylvania Health Care Cost Containment Council (PHC4) created in 1986. The purpose of the council is to promote health care cost containment, promote the public interest by encouraging the development of competitive health care services, and ensure that all citizens have reasonable access to quality health care. PHC4 developed a computerized system for the collection, analysis, and dissemination of data. The data reflect provider quality and provider services effectiveness for specific treatment categories. Data collected and analyzed may include such information as the number of cases in the category, severity level at admission, length of stay, discharge condition (mortality), and cost of care, which are compared to expected results (benchmarking). PHC4 issues special reports developed from the data analysis and makes the raw data available to any purchaser requesting it.

Health care purchasers are enthusiastic about having such information available when contracting for care, but hospitals have mixed responses. While they find the information valuable, they also point out causes of wide variation in results that may not be captured by the data. Other states have followed through with similar outcomes measurements (Sessa, 1992). Coalitions of employers in larger communities are asking health care organizations to provide data that will help the coalition to do similar analysis.

HOSPITAL COSTS

We hear a great deal about rising health costs, and in particular about rising hospital costs—and not without cause. The American Hospital Association provides figures on inpatient expenses, adjusted per inpatient day and adjusted per inpatient stay (Health InfoSource, 1998b). In 1970, for example, the average cost of an inpatient day was $73.73, and the average cost of a hospital stay was $604.39. For 1980, the cost was $244.44 per day and $31,844.19 per stay. By 1996, the figures stood at $1,005.45 per day and $6,225.95 per stay, the decrease in cost per stay being a reflection of reduced length of stay. The increased costs have been a concern of industry because the phenomenal growth of private (voluntary) health insurance has increasingly been paid as an employee fringe benefit, forcing price increases in industrial products. The government, since the introduction of Medicare and Medicaid, has fretted over cost increases because they force politically unpopular tax increases.

Three factors account for most of the rise in hospital costs and in health costs generally. The first major factor is the increase in population. We simply have a growing population. The population is, moreover, an aging population that requires more, longer, and costlier types of care.

The second major factor is inflation. Everything costs more—drugs, linens, food, fuel, and personnel. More than half of a hospital's budget is consumed by its payroll, and because it is a heavy employer of unskilled labor, when the federally mandated minimum wage goes up, hospital labor costs jump accordingly. Similarly, hospital payroll costs overall have risen in recent years as mandated contributions to the Social Security system have risen.

The third major factor in hospital and health care cost increases is new technology and new services. As a result of scientific advances, we are able to do more things to help people than heretofore. But the price of new technology is high. Not only is the equipment expensive, but the personnel needed to operate it is also costly. A more educated population results in greater demand for health care. This does not necessarily equate to realistic demands. Technology may contribute to a belief that any disease can be cured (higher costs) rather than a commitment to healthier lifestyles, prevention, and screening (lower costs).

Every few years, there is a new controversy in the health field, a controversy that arises from new technology. The new technology permits the management of cases in new ways: lifesaving, more effective clinical management, or better diagnosis. Cardiac care advances, computed tomography (CT), magnetic resonance imaging (MRI), laser therapy, transplantation, and chemotherapy each occupied center stage at one time because of high cost and the alleged desire of all hospitals to develop the new service.

Those who are most concerned about rising health costs are quick to bemoan the "duplication" of very costly equipment and services, and they are most critical of what they perceive to be competition among hospitals to be the first with the new technology, and the desire of other institutions to keep up with the hospital that is first. This freewheeling rhetoric fails to recognize some very important points and does a disservice to hospitals. What is perceived as duplication may be simple recognition by the hospital that quality patient care and physician efficiency is enhanced by new technology. In some cases hospitals share costly medical equipment, such as an MRI scanner, by installing it in mobile vans that move from one hospital to another in order to use it efficiently, to have the technology available locally, and to contain costs.

Even when it is feasible to share facilities and high-tech equipment, a very good case can be made for duplication and the resulting excess capacity. Having technology available in the hospital where the physi-

cian practices, rather than having to schedule its use in another hospital, is very convenient. The critic may argue that this is wasteful, but it can contribute to institutional pride, which in turn can contribute to an institutional concern for excellence in medical care. In a competitive environment, hospitals are inclined to acquire technology to survive. Only the centers of excellence—the providers of comprehensive services, the full-service providers—will "win" case management (managed care) contracts. Under such exclusive contracting, some providers will win and some will lose, but all will attempt to provide a wide range of services rather than default to competitors.

Technology has spread despite the efforts of government and the health-planning agencies. These bodies slowed the process somewhat, but eventually the technology spread basically because the public wanted it, and its acquisition was facilitated historically by cost-based reimbursement to hospitals. It is fashionable to place the blame for rising costs on physicians, who are accused of providing treatment indiscriminately, and on hospitals, for their overall inefficiencies. Demand from regulators and consumers for quality care and access to all members of the community places technology development and diffusion at odds with cost control efforts.

As hospital costs rise, they must be covered if the hospital is to continue to operate. The hospital meets these costs with income from a variety of sources: gifts and endowment income, as well as occasional government grants, but mostly payments for care of patients. Some of the payments come from insurance companies such as Blue Cross and from government programs such as Medicare and Medicaid. Before the Health Care Financing Administration drastically revised hospital payments to prospective payments through DRGs, these sources of payment tended to be on the basis of hospital costs for care—frequently less than cost, but rarely, if ever, more than cost. Commercial insurers (for-profits, as distinct from the nonprofit insurers like Blue Cross) have tended to pay hospital charges for care of their covered subscribers. Typically, charges were higher than costs, enabling a hospital to cover losses in other areas and to accumulate money for the purchase of needed equipment or for other expansions.

Government and the insurance companies have been hard-pressed to continue paying upward-spiraling hospital costs. Though sometimes sympathetic to the plight of the hospitals, government is faced with a dilemma: Either it can raise taxes to pay for the increasing costs for which it is responsible, or it can shift money from another source (such as defense or education) to health. Both choices are politically explosive, so a third alternative becomes more practical—that is, trying to contain hospital costs. Insurance companies have a somewhat similar problem: Unless some way can be found to contain costs, the rates they charge must go up, and raising the rates does not sit well with the major purchasers of their policies. Very few commercial insurance companies still pay hospital charges. Increasingly the rate of payment is negotiated or fixed at what the insurance company believes is appropriate. Thus, not only are government and the insurance companies interested in containing the rise of hospital costs, but business and industry are interested because they are the principal purchasers of health insurance policies. In a growing number of urban centers, this mutual interest has led to the formation of *business coalitions* designed to develop coordinated strategies to contain costs. Certificate of need (CON) legislation, utilization review, and the shifting of more costs to the patient have also been employed, but the costs continue to rise. The federal government made the most dramatic attempt to slow the rise in hospital costs when it introduced its prospective payment system (PPS) for hospital patients covered by Medicare, with fixed payments based on assignment of each patient's diagnosis to a diagnosis-related group (DRG). Efforts to control costs are described in the sections that follow.

Peer Review Organizations

Since the advent of Medicare and Medicaid, government has assumed an increasing share of the costs of medical care, and the costs have risen rapidly. The initial legislation for Medicare in 1965 required utilization review; in 1967, this was extended to Medicaid. Peer review, in its initiation, focused on assuring medical necessity. The review process emphasized quantity rather than quality and was accomplished by ret-

rospective review of records by physicians and largely handled within the hospitals themselves. The process was ineffective in controlling costs.

The 1971 amendments to the Social Security Act mandated the development of professional standards review organizations (PSROs), an attempt by HCFA to formalize the review process and give assurance that services paid for under Medicare and Medicaid were medically necessary, of high quality, and delivered at the lowest possible cost. HCFA went on to note that these objectives, though complementary, were sometimes in conflict because the medical profession tended to stress the quality assurance element, whereas Congress seemed more interested in the cost control element.

More than 185 PSROs developed throughout the country. A major part of their work entailed preadmission review and concurrent review of hospital admissions: On the basis of physician-established criteria for hospital admission, admissions certified as appropriate were certified for a specific number of days, the number depending on the diagnosis and the norms for that area. The PSROs also reviewed admissions that went beyond the norm. The actual review of cases was largely delegated by the PSROs to the respective hospital utilization review committees.

In addition to preadmission and concurrent review activities, PSROs carried out a variety of retrospective studies on quality of care, utilization, and patterns of care that served in part as a basis for the criteria employed in concurrent review. Because the rising costs of Medicare and Medicaid were a significant problem for both federal and state governments, the emphasis on cost efficiency was increasingly impressed upon the agencies, but the results of PSRO efforts were mixed. In early 1978 the president's Office of Management and Budget (OMB) proposed that PSRO funding be deleted from the budget request to Congress because of a Department of Health, Education, and Welfare (HEW) study showing that PSROs had no significant effect on reducing costs and did not contribute significantly to increased quality of care. OMB's view did not prevail, but congressional dissatisfaction was also evident in that the appropriation for fiscal 1979 provided funds for hospital review activities but not enough for the reviews, which

Congress had earlier directed for ambulatory and long-term care.

In October 1978 the PSROs came under criticism from the General Accounting Office (GAO). The GAO criticized the salary schedules for PSRO executive directors that HEW had issued. The GAO also felt that there was room for improvement of PSRO efficiency in terms of combining some administrative staffs and functions, given the fact that in twenty-one states there was more than a single PSRO. In those twenty-one states, there were 164 PSROs. A month later, HCFA released a new evaluation that it felt demonstrated PSRO effectiveness in both cost containment and cost control. But costs were still going up, and the drive to abolish PSROs continued. In 1981 the funding for some agencies was cut off, and the administration sought again to abolish all PSROs. Congress resisted and came forth with a compromise, agreeing to replace the large number of PSROs with a much smaller number of peer review organizations (PROs) that would be responsible for quality control but would also focus more vigorously on controlling hospital costs of Medicare patients.

PROs were now required to review care of all cases in which a Medicare patient was readmitted to a hospital less than thirty-one days after the most recent discharge, as well as to review all written patient complaints (Lohr & Schroeder, 1990). If detected, unnecessary care is classified into severity levels with appropriate sanctions on the attending physician and hospital. The basics of the severity levels are as follows:

- **Level I:** without potential for significant adverse effects
- **Level II:** with potential for significant adverse effects (but none occurred)
- **Level III:** with significant adverse effects on the patient

Sanctions move from notification and education, to withholding of payment, to loss of the right to participate with the Medicare and Medicaid programs.

A PRO is an external organization that successfully bids for a contract with HCFA to carry out the required peer review functions; thus, peer review is no longer simply left to the hospital to conduct on its own. Hospitals, however, continue to maintain their own utilization review departments to monitor compliance with rules of HCFA and other regulatory bodies. Because Congress has been concerned with quality of care as well as cost, it has continually expanded the duties of PROs. By 1987, PROs were required to review the quality of care in HMOs, nursing homes, ambulatory care settings, and hospitals. New emphasis for review includes preadmission and concurrent review, a focus on variations from the standards, and education to communicate desirable processes and outcomes. As internal utilization review has become stronger, many PROs now spend more time and emphasis on data collection and evaluation to work with organizations to establish quality standards and reduce variation.

Certificate of Need

Another approach to rising health care costs has been to require health facilities to secure from state government a *certificate of need (CON)* for major capital expenditures and major expansions in services. Rising costs had been tied to duplication of services. The National Health Planning and Resource Development Act of 1974 required that states develop regulations setting a dollar amount (usually $100,000) above which a facility had to secure a CON for new services, beds, or equipment. The legislation also provided funding for new health systems agencies which were required to develop plans for health resource and health status needs for the population residing within the health services areas (Stevens, 1989). CON programs peaked in the 1970s, but their effectiveness was questioned. Organizations learned creative ways to bypass regulation, such as breaking large projects into smaller components in order to avoid CON review. Politics entered into the approval process because board members were often members of the community in which the project might be requested. Failure to approve a hospital project might mean loss of hospital administration support of other community projects. Members of the community also were hesitant to block a project that might bring more jobs into their community.

In 1987, Congress repealed the CON requirement but allowed the states to continue CON programs if they wished to use their own criteria. Many states continued CON programs; however, many hospitals opposed CON programs, stating that they should be revised to eliminate bureaucratic red tape and delays so that health care organizations can respond quickly in the current climate of increasing competition and eroding profits. In 1998, thirty-seven states still had CON programs in force (*American Health Line*, 1998). Some health care organizations oppose CON programs as being politicized, poorly managed, costly, and ineffective; advocates believe that some regulation is necessary, especially in areas where the population is growing. Whatever its merits, it is clear that the certificate of need has not been effective in controlling costs.

Payment of Hospital Costs

Hospitals have historically been paid by most insurance and government programs on a *retrospective cost,* or near cost basis; that is, they were paid after the costs were incurred. Some private insurance programs even paid whatever the hospital charged,

which could be higher than costs. These methods of payment did not encourage hospitals to operate efficiently or to economize. The very nature of these retrospective systems was an inducement to do more and keep patients in the hospital longer. Though physicians made these clinical decisions, there was no reason for them or the hospital to take into account the cost of care. As the costs of Medicare continued to rise rapidly, there was serious concern about the solvency of the Medicare program, and the federal government sought new ways to contain costs and increase its control over hospital payments.

In 1984 the federal government instituted a prospective payment system (PPS) based on diagnosis-related groups (DRGs). The primary objective of the PPS is to change the economic incentives of hospitals under the Medicare program by offering strong encouragement to reduce hospital costs. As predicted, the introduction of this system brought about important changes in hospitals, the medical profession, and the entire health care sector. For the first time in the history of Medicare, there was a decline in the number of discharges (which means that fewer people were hospitalized) and in the length of stay for hospital inpatients (see Table 7–1).

Table 7–1 Discharges, Days of Care, and Average Lengths of Stay in Short-Stay Hospitals, According to Age: United States, 1964, 1990, and 1995

Characteristics	Discharges			Days of Care			Average Length of Stay		
	1964	1990	1995	1964	1990	1995	1964	1990	1995
	Number per 1,000 population						Number of days		
Total	109.1	91.0	86.2	970.9	607.1	486.3	8.9	6.7	5.6
Age:									
Under 15 years	67.6	46.7	40.5	405.7	271.3	207.1	6.0	5.8	5.1
Under 5 years	94.3	79.9	72.2	731.1	496.4	374.4	7.8	6.2	5.2
5–14 years	53.1	29.0	24.2	229.1	150.8	120.5	4.3	5.2	5.0
15–44 years	100.6	62.6	57.6	760.7	340.5	251.2	7.6	5.4	4.4
45–64 years	146.2	135.7	122.4	1,559.3	911.5	687.1	10.7	6.7	5.6
65 years and over	190.0	248.8	266.9	2,292.7	2,092.4	1,892.4	12.1	8.4	7.1
65–74 years	181.2	215.4	235.1	2,150.4	1,719.3	1,533.4	11.9	8.0	6.5
75 years and over	206.7	300.6	311.8	2,560.4	2,669.9	2,401.9	12.4	8.9	7.7

Source: National Center for Health Statistics as reprinted in Moskowitz, 1999. © Faulkner & Gray, Inc., reprinted with permission.

Occupancy rates in both urban and rural hospitals declined as hospitals worked to discharge patients as early as possible under PPS. The total average occupancy rate for all community hospitals went from 77.3 percent in 1970 to 61.8 percent in 1997 (National Center for Health Statistics, 1999).

While it may be true that patients are discharged sicker than prior to PPS, what went along with those early discharges was a greater dependency on discharges to rehabilitation facilities, home health care, and other facilities that are less costly than hospitals. Most hospitals have employed discharge planners to facilitate the discharge of patients from acute care hospitals to appropriate posthospital services. Virtually all hospital discharge planners initially reported difficulties in placing patients in skilled nursing facilities, primarily because of restrictions in Medicare rules and regulations regarding eligibility and coverage, and because of the shortage of skilled nursing beds (U.S. General Accounting Office, 1987). Over 85 percent of the discharge planners surveyed also reported problems with home health care placement because of Medicare rules and regulations. Since the early 1980s, however, the number of nursing homes and home health agencies has increased. In additional, Medicare's payment structures have been modified (see Chapter 8). Thus, as the PPS reduces hospital costs, it exacerbates problems in other health care sectors.

Occupancy rates have also been affected by new technologies. Since the early 1980s, many procedures previously requiring an inpatient stay have been possible on an outpatient basis. Not all of these procedures are done outside of the hospital; however, outpatient care does not factor into occupancy rates. Occupancy rates consider only inpatient admissions, discharges, and beds.

The move from inpatient to outpatient therapy was not optional. Medicare, and other insurers, targeted certain procedures as payable only if done on an outpatient basis. Hospitals were compliant because outpatient payments were higher than inpatient payments and provided the hospital with a new source of revenue. Units with empty beds were consolidated and space was converted to more profitable outpatient services.

PPS and technology both contributed to a reduction in hospital admissions—from 35,155,000 in 1984 to 31,099,000 in 1996. Conversely, the number of outpatient visits increased from 211,961,000 in 1984 to 439,863,000 in 1996 (Health InfoSource, 1998b).

The average length of stay has also decreased for hospitals since the implementation of PPS—a direct cause of the decreased occupancy rates. At 7.7 days in community hospitals in 1975, the average was 6.2 days in 1996 (Health InfoSource, 1998b). The decreased length of stay was a direct result of PPS and its incentives for hospitals to operate efficiently. Patients are no longer brought into the hospital for preadmission testing as an inpatient. All preparatory care is done on an outpatient basis. Inpatient services are scheduled on a more timely basis, avoiding lags in time that provide no benefit to the patient but increase the total inpatient stay. Technology, too, has played an important role in decreasing length of stay. New surgical techniques, less-invasive therapies, and laser technology have shortened recovery and response times.

Most hospitals continued to earn profits during the first years of PPS. However, subsequent profits have been dwindling. The profits, we need to be reminded, are necessary to cover losses in other areas—for example, the losses incurred from care of the uninsured and from low Medicaid payments, as well as the purchases a hospital may need to make to improve the quality of care. As profits decline, hospitals are improving their utilization review departments to minimize unnecessary procedures and practices without affecting the quality of care, but the tensions over providing care and staying financially viable grow.

Government oversight grows with concern that hospitals are increasing their income by manipulating the diagnosis codes that are used to describe the patient's condition and treatment so that cases are assigned to DRGs for which the payment is higher (a practice sometimes referred to as DRG creep). According to the Department of Health and Human Services Inspector General's report, the coding mistakes averaged 20 percent, but most of the errors favored hospitals, creating the suspicion that some hospitals are deliberately manipulating DRGs to increase their income. Whether or not this is the case, the errors cost Medicare millions of dollars in overpayments to hospitals. Efforts have been made to help curtail deliberate overbilling through federal fraud and abuse legislation such as the False Claims Act, antikickback statutes, the Ethics in Patient Referral Act, and most recently the Health Insurance Portability and Accountability Act of 1996 (Kalb, 1999).

PPS has slowed the increase in hospital costs for Medicare patients, and it has also affected other payers for inpatient hospital services. Several state Medicaid programs are using Medicare's PPS as a model for controlling their hospital costs. Blue Cross and other private payers of hospital care are also implementing DRG-based payment systems to control their costs.

Hospitals turn to other services, particularly outpatient procedures, to bring in additional income, but that practice may soon end. Congress is establishing ambulatory payment groups similar to DRGs that pay a fixed rate according to the group (outpatient payment groups OPGs). Fixed payments should save the federal government millions of dollars, but hospitals will have to find other ways to recover losses from increasingly less profitable inpatient care and uninsured and underinsured patients.

HOSPITAL COMPETITION

A competitive market in health care developed as a result of PPS. A shorter length of stay meant lower occupancy rates. Only a greater flow of patients could counteract the short stay. In some areas, a high penetration of managed care contracting resulted in "exclusive providers," leaving those providers outside the contract to deal with an increasingly smaller patient base. Managed care also changed the emphasis of treatment from inpatient and specialty care to medical management, case management, and prevention—again decreasing the demand for inpatient care. Some areas saw an oversupply of physicians and hospital beds. Under these conditions, a buyers' market developed in the health services sector. Health services payers (insurers and employers) were increasingly able to set the prices and the conditions under which they would pay hospitals. A third operative factor in this changing environment was an administration in Washington that wanted to deregulate the health sector, to let market forces prevail to a greater extent than before, and to shift responsibilities from the federal government to the states and the private sector. These factors became even stronger after the failure of the Clinton health plan and other health care reform efforts in the mid-1990s.

In this environment, hospitals, with their decreased occupancy rates, were forced to compete for patients. They now promoted amenities such as homelike delivery rooms, improved meal service, and other "customer service" features. Strategic planning involves identifying medical services that are popular with the public (and reimbursed primarily by private insurance). Hospitals advertise on radio, television, and billboards. They affiliate with other hospitals (horizontal integration) to achieve economies of scale in supplies and services, and they contract with large purchasers of health care to provide services at a discount rate to secure a dependable flow of patients.

As profits from inpatient care decreased, hospitals expanded more profitable outpatient services into such areas as primary care, surgery, extended care, rehabilitation, home care, and occupational medicine (vertical integration). Although expanding services was necessary to survive and to provide a competitive price to purchasers of health care, it also frequently put the hospitals in the position of competing for patients with the physicians on their medical staffs, and with other health professionals and community health agencies. This situation has changed the traditional physician-hospital relationship and the hospital–community health agency relationship; in some cases in which physicians threatened to offer services on their own that would compete with those offered by the hospital outpatient department, such as in surgery and radiology, the hospitals went into a business partnership with those specialists in their freestanding enterprises. Some of the most successful diversification strategies have been freestanding outpatient surgical units, freestanding diagnostic centers, cardiac rehabilitation services, substance abuse programs, inpatient rehabilitation units, occupational medicine clinics, sports medicine programs, home health services, and women's health centers.

SUMMARY

Hospitals have undergone dramatic changes from their inception as a place for the poor sick to spend their final days before death. They have moved from being defined as a place to die to being defined as the place to be cured. But in the last twenty years hospitals have changed in both form and function—so much so that the term *hospital* has even become an inappropriate label in some cases. *Medical centers, health systems, networks, alliances*—all of these terms have been used to describe the new face of hospital care.

The community hospital, with which most of us are familiar, continues to serve many communities with short-term acute care. Chances are high, however, that the community hospital is in some way affiliated with an umbrella corporation or large chain of other hospitals.

Nonprofit institutions, governed by a board of trustees, are still the largest group of "hospital" facilities; however, many of them may have affiliations with a for-profit organization, or separate business functions that operate on a for-profit basis.

Although teaching hospitals affiliated with universities and providing high-tech tertiary care still tend to provide the bulk of medical education, physician training takes place in a wider variety of health care settings, including community hospitals, primary care clinics, rural health care settings, and public health clinics. A growing number of hospitals directly employ some of their physicians, but most medical staffs still consist primarily of independently practicing physicians.

Over the past decade, hospitals have changed from expanding institutions with little regard for cost to institutions with reduced occupancy and a great interest in cost containment. They are now more businesslike institutions that stress efficiency, and they compete for patients. The changes were caused by the efforts of government and other large health care purchasers to slow the dramatic increases in health care spending. Medicare changed its method of paying for inpatient services to a prospective payment system based on DRGs, which encouraged cost savings. Admissions and lengths of hospital stays decreased, as did the number of hospitals and hospital beds. Quality of care is increasingly important as data collection methods have enabled hospitals and health care purchasers to compare hospital performance records. Hospitals continue to search for ways to maintain or improve their efficiency and effectiveness in a climate of increased competition and cost constraints.

IN THE HEALTH CARE COMMUNITY

Pennsylvania Hospital: The Nation's First Voluntary Hospital*

During the 1700s, Philadelphia was the largest and most influential city in America. It was the third largest city in the British Empire and was famous for the Quakers (Society of Friends), who were noted for their leadership in humanitarian and scientific undertakings. The increased number of immigrants who came through the city also meant an increasing number of poor people. It was in Philadelphia that Dr. Thomas Bond, a Quaker physician who had studied medicine in London and at the famous French hospital in Paris, Hotel-Dieu, worked as a port inspector for contagious diseases and saw the need for an institution to care for the city's sick destitute. Philadelphia had an almshouse for paupers that gave some medical aid to those who were ill, but its resources were limited and its primary function was not the care of the sick. In addition, Philadelphia, like other seaports, had quarantine hospitals to keep victims of smallpox, yellow fever, and other epidemic diseases isolated. These hospitals were closed when epidemics subsided and

(continues)

*Information for this case study was obtained from historical documents and the University of Pennsylvania Health System and Pennsylvania Hospital Web sites at www.upenn.edu and www.pahosp.com

(continued)

opened again with the next outbreak. But there were no facilities for the sick poor of the city. Dr. Bond had been involved in several efforts to bring about social improvements through voluntary organizations. Therefore, it seemed natural to establish a hospital in the same way.

About 1750, Dr. Bond began soliciting financial contributions to support the proposed hospital. He was fortunate to have as a friend and adviser Benjamin Franklin, whose strong support convinced others of the need for a hospital for the destitute sick and the mentally ill. A bill to establish a provincial hospital was introduced in the Pennsylvania Assembly. It passed largely because Franklin promised to demonstrate the public's support for a hospital by raising £2,000 by voluntary subscriptions. If that amount was raised, the assembly agreed to allocate an equal amount. Thus, Franklin is thought to be the originator of the concept of "matching money" in government projects. The required amount was raised, and the governor of Pennsylvania signed the hospital bill in May 1751. The Pennsylvania Hospital was patterned after the British voluntary hospitals.

The charter of the Pennsylvania Hospital stated that the contributors to the hospital had the right to make all laws and regulations relating to the hospital and that they should meet annually and elect twelve of their group to be the board of managers. An important feature of governing the hospitals by laypeople was that it limited the physicians' control. Although in most cases the board of managers deferred to the judgment of competent physicians, it could and did overrule the physicians on some occasions.

The board of managers adopted specific rules concerning the admission of patients. It decided to refuse admission to incurables (except "lunatics") and victims of smallpox or "other infectious distemper" until proper accommodations were available. It also excluded women whose young children were not cared for elsewhere. Those admitted had to make a travel or burial deposit so that they would not become a charge to the city if they survived and the hospital would not incur a burial expense if they

died. Local authorities, philanthropists, or others often provided travel or burial deposits for the sick poor. In addition, if there was insufficient accommodation for several equally urgent cases, preference was given to those recommended by contributors to the hospital.

Although it would appear that the Pennsylvania Hospital intended to serve all of the sick poor who suffered from a curable, noncontagious illness, closer examination reveals that it was more concerned with providing for the "useful and laborious" poor rather than those who could work but would not. Both the British and Philadelphians endorsed the value of Christian charity and the potential of hospitals to increase medical knowledge and training, but they were equally concerned with how to deal with the significant increase in the number of poor people. For many, keeping the poor content and getting poor workers back on the job before their families became a public burden were major reasons for a voluntary hospital. To ensure that the "useful and laborious" poor were admitted, each prospective patient was required to have a letter describing his or her case, signed by an influential person. The sick poor who were turned away from the hospital were forced to go to the local almshouse.

The managers also made provisions to admit paying patients if there was space. Paying patients were usually servants or slaves whose masters paid the bills, paupers whose bills were paid by "overseers of the poor," and the mentally ill from middle- and upper-class families. As a result, the relatives of the insane and masters of servants or slaves often became concerned with conditions at the hospital. This concern resulted in higher standards than were likely to be found in institutions serving only the poor. Usually, paying patients were charged more than the costs they incurred, and the excess money was used to subsidize the sick poor.

The hospital opened in 1752 in a rented private home. It could accommodate twenty patients at a time with a paid matron (to take care of the house and the sick) and three part-time physicians, who

(continues)

(continued)

agreed to serve for three years without pay. It took four years before a building site several blocks beyond Philadelphia's urban population was obtained and before the first wing of the new Pennsylvania Hospital was built and ready for patients. The new building was T-shaped. There was a long hall with a consultation room, apothecary shop, and apartments for the matron and other staff. Perpendicular to the middle of this hall was the men's ward, a hall eighty feet long and twenty-seven feet wide with windows on both sides to provide ventilation. There were rows of beds on each side of the room and a wide aisle down the center. The women's ward of the same basic design was on the second floor directly over the men's ward. The second floor also contained several private rooms for paying patients and for those who, because of their condition, were not admitted to the wards. In the basement of the building, below the men's ward, were cells for the insane, baths, the kitchen, and a pantry. Apart from the main building were a wash house, a stable, and a garden. The new hospital building was the east wing of a plan for a larger H-shaped building, which would have a central building in the middle of the connecting wing. The total structure was not completed until 1804 (Figures 7–3 and 7–4).

The building was financed by the subscriptions raised of £2,000 plus the assembly's matching grant of £2,000, which was restricted to building and furnishing the hospital. Subscriptions in excess of £2,000 constituted the capital stock, which was not to be used but would generate interest to pay for the care of the sick poor. At first the interest from the capital stock could not fully support the operations of the hospital. Private parties contributed to increase the capital stock, and in 1772 the Pennsylvania Assembly made a grant of £300 to the capital stock of the hospital.

The board of managers selected physicians for the new hospital according to specific regulations. The six physicians selected (increased from the original three) had impressive qualifications (most had some medical training abroad) and served twice a week for a year without pay. Although there was no formal specialization, certain physicians tended to do the surgery, and others took a special interest in the mentally ill.

The administrator of the hospital was the matron, who was responsible for the purchasing, bookkeeping, and supervision of all staff except the apothecary. The hospital also hired a steward to assist the matron, a male cell keeper to handle the insane, two or three nurses, and several maids. The new hospital also employed a cook, a laundress, and a gardener.

The hospital could support about 70 free beds, but at times the number of inpatients exceeded 100, about one-third of them mentally ill. The number of paying patients varied. Most of the paying patients were classified as "lunatics." Because paying patients were charged more than their cost of care, every three paying patients supported one poor patient. Although the master of a slave paid for the slave's hospitalization, free Blacks were admitted as poor patients on the same basis as Whites. Another category of paying patients included those with venereal disease. The board of managers in 1763 tried to keep the number of these patients to a minimum by not admitting them unless they were in danger of dying and could not be accommodated elsewhere. The hospital also ran an outpatient department, which in the mid-1770s was treating almost 200 patients a year.

The Pennsylvania Hospital offered an important opportunity in the training of physicians. In the early years, apprentices of hospital physicians were allowed to visit patients with their mentors without charge, and those apprenticed to nonhospital physicians were charged a fee for visiting the wards. Although students followed the physicians as they attended patients and discussed individual cases, no formal lectures were offered until 1763. The hospital acquired a series of anatomical drawings and initiated lectures on anatomy for which all students paid a fee. Later, cadavers were used in the classes. The hospital also taught courses required by the College of Philadelphia's medical school (later known as the University of Pennsylvania School of Medicine). From 1762 on, the hospital had a medical library.

(continues)

(continued)

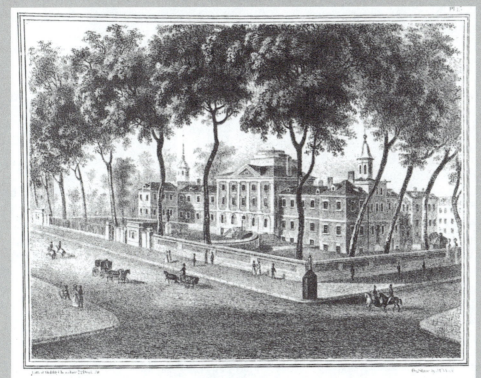

PENNSYLVANIA HOSPITAL

Wash Basin

Water Closet

Dry Room

Nurses Duty Room

Kitchen
Medical Examination

Coat Room

Parlor

Parlor

Bath Room

Water Section

Slops

Dining Room

Elevator

Ward

Ward

Clothing Room

Linen

Noisy

Office

Apothecary

Fire Proof

Ward

Ward

Figure 7–4 Pennsylvania Hospital: Original First Floor Plan, 1775.
(From *Report of the Board of Managers of the Pennsylvania Hospital,* 1897.)

(continues)

(continued)

Between 1775 and 1783 the Pennsylvania Hospital endured a very difficult period because of the impact of the American Revolution. Hostility toward the passive Quakers, the unsettled financial situation during the war, and the necessity of caring at different times for both Continental and British soldiers, resulted in decreased funding for the hospital. Conditions at the hospital deteriorated, and the mortality rate climbed.

After the Revolution, conditions at the hospital improved and the mortality rate declined, but the hospital for many years could not afford to support the same number of sick poor as it had cared for in 1775. For one thing, the public seemed to be less interested in supporting public welfare institutions than it had been before the Revolution. Another change was that the board of managers was no longer composed mainly of Philadelphia's wealthiest and most distinguished citizens, but increasingly of merchants who were wealthy but who were not part of the political leadership of the city or state. Rising costs slowed the recovery of the hospital, and maintenance work, which had been neglected during the war, was also needed.

Despite these difficulties, the board decided to complete the hospital by erecting a west wing and a central building. Although the number of sick poor patients declined, the number of insane patients continued to increase, to the point that they were often housed in the wards with other patients. Most of the building funds were obtained from the Pennsylvania legislature, the rest from private donations. By 1798 the west wing was completed, and by 1801 the center building was essentially completed. The west wing was used almost exclusively for the insane. The center building buffered the physically ill from the mentally ill and housed the administrative offices, library, apothecary shop, and living quarters for some of the staff. The operating room on the third floor of the center building was not ready for use until 1804. A skylight provided light for all but the most delicate operations. The operating room also had an amphitheater that could accommodate 300 persons. Surgery at that time was very limited because anesthesia had not yet been developed and infection was almost certain to occur, since its cause and prevention were unknown at that time. Therefore, operations in the thoracic or abdominal cavities were rare. Most surgery was related to setting of fractures and dislocations, suturing of muscles and tendons, amputations, and the removal of tumors.

The number of sick poor seeking medical care at the hospital decreased somewhat with the opening of the Philadelphia Dispensary (an outpatient facility) in 1786, but the hospital still could not accommodate all of the sick poor who applied—not for lack of space, but for lack of money to provide food and services. By 1796 the board had limited the number of nonpaying patients to thirty at one time, plus emergencies, because of limited financial resources. During that period there were twice as many mentally as physically ill patients at the hospital.

The practice of curious and sadistic visitors amusing themselves by watching and taunting the insane had begun in the colonial period and continued to be condoned by the board of managers. They charged an admission fee for such visits. The cells for the insane were damp and cold, and attempts to heat them were unsatisfactory. As the number of insane inmates increased, a two-story brick building was built in 1825 for female patients on the corner of the hospital grounds. When the number of patients with mental disorders continued to increase, the board of managers decided to separate the physically ill from the mentally ill. In 1841, all the insane patients were moved to a new building capable of accommodating 170 patients.

The main forms of therapy for the insane, as well as for many of the physically ill in the late 1700s, were bleeding and purging. At that time, physicians had little beyond their five senses and their experience to aid them in the diagnosis and treatment of medical conditions. The stethoscope and x-rays had

(continues)

(continued)

not been discovered, the clinical thermometer was not in use, and the microscope was not used for medical diagnoses.

The first specialty officially recognized by the board of managers was obstetrics. In 1803 a "lying-in" ward was opened in the east wing of the hospital. However, those were the days before aseptic procedures; puerperal (childbed) fever occurred repeatedly and forced the permanent closing of the maternity department in 1854. However, much changed for the Pennsylvania Hospital and health care in general. In 1929 a women's building opened and was considered to be one of the most innovative approaches to women's care in the country.

In the 1950s the hospital began incorporating such new technology as an intensive care unit for neurological patients, a coronary care unit, an orthopedic institute, a diabetes center, a hospice, specialized units in oncology and urology, and broad-ened surgical programs. The state's first outpatient community mental health facility was founded at Pennsylvania Hospital in 1975. Throughout the latter half of the twentieth century, the Pennsylvania Hospital continued to build new facilities and renovate existing facilities. Advances in new areas of medicine continued, particularly in fertility and reproductive technologies.

Today, the Pennsylvania Hospital is affiliated with the University of Pennsylvania Health System (UPHS), adding to UPHS a strong presence in obstetric and orthopedic services in the Philadelphia area. The hospital continues to operate under its own name, but it operates under a management contract with UPHS, which consists of the University of Pennsylvania Medical Center, Presbyterian Medical Center, six hospitals that are contractual affiliates, a network of providers known as Clinical Care Associates, multispecialty satellites at Radnor, and a managed care organization.

ACTIVITY-BASED LEARNING

- Visit the American Hospital Directory Web site at www.ahd.com. Choose a city to find the number of hospitals within that city. Look further and compare the hospitals for size, services offered, and financial statement summary. Are you surprised by the differences? Choose another city different in size from your first choice and compare the two. What are some of the interesting facts you have discovered?

- Visit the JCAHO Web site at www.jcaho.org. Visit their "Quality Check" area to determine the accreditation status of the hospitals you found in the previous exercise.

- Do any of the hospitals about which you have inquired have their own Web sites? Can you determine who are the members of the hospital board from visiting the Web site, or from other available literature about the hospital?

A QUESTION OF ETHICS

- Hospitals today are faced with many financial challenges. One method of cost containment has been to reduce the length of stay for most patients, transferring them to other locations for some of their care, such as nursing homes, rehabilitation centers, and home health agencies. Is this appropriate utilization of services, or simply a method of "patient dumping"?

- Many hospitals today are "vertically integrated": They are taking on new services in order to be able to provide a larger scope of services to patients. Should hospitals be expanding into other services in order to strengthen their financial standing? Or is this simply a method of "self-referral," reaching out for income-producing areas that are outside the realm of the mission statement of a hospital?

References

American Health Line. (1998, July 28). Certificate of need: States relax hospital restrictions. [On-line]. Available: web.lexis-nexis.com (Accessed March 17, 2000).

American Hospital Directory. (2000). *Search for a hospital* [on-line]. Available: www.ahd.com/ freesearch (Accessed March 29, 2001)

Custer, W. S., & Musacchio, R. (1986). Hospitals in transition: A perspective. *Journal of Medical Practice Management, 1*(4), 228–233.

Healthcare InfoSource. (1998b). *Hospital statistics, 1998 edition.* Chicago: American Hospital Association.

Healthcare InfoSource. (1998a). *AHA guide to the health care field.* Chicago: American Hospital Association.

Hospital's expenses for providing care to Hill-Burton patients were properly disallowed. (1996, January 16). *Medicare and Medicaid Law Bulletin.*

Joint Commission on Accreditation of Healthcare Organizations. (2000). *The Joint Commission on Accreditation of Healthcare Organizations* [On-line]. Available: www.jcaho.org/aboutjc/facts.html (Accessed March 16, 2000).

Kalb, P. (1999). Health care fraud and abuse. *JAMA, 282*(12), 1163–1168.

Lohr, K., & Schroeder, S. (1990). A strategy for quality assurance in Medicare. *New England Journal of Medicine, 322*(10), 707–712.

Moskowitz, J. (1999). *Health care almanac & yearbook, 1999.* New York: Faulkner & Gray.

National Center for Health Statistics. (1999, September 20). Facilities tables 110 through 114 [On-line]. Available: www.cdc.gov/nchs/ products/ pubs/pubd (Accessed March 14, 2000).

Rosenberg, C. E. (1987). *The care of strangers—The rise of America's hospital system.* New York: Basic Books.

Sessa, E. (1992, January). Information is power: The Pennsylvania experiment. *Journal of Health Care Benefits,* pp. 44–48.

Stevens, R. (1989). *In sickness and in wealth: American hospitals in the twentieth century.* New York: Basic Books.

U.S. General Accounting Office. (1987). *Posthospital care.* Washington, DC: Author.

Griffith, J. R. (1999). *The well-managed healthcare organization* 4th Edition. Chicago: Health Administration Press.

Yessian, M. R., & Greenleaf, J. M. (1997). The ebb and flow of federal initiatives to regulate healthcare professionals. In T. S. Jost (Ed.), *Regulation of the healthcare professions* (pp. 169–198). Chicago: Health Administration Press.

CHAPTER

8

Long-Term Care

Chapter Objectives

After completing this chapter, the reader should have an understanding of:

- The differentiation of long-term care from other types of health care services.
- The history of long-term care in the United States.
- The various payment mechanisms that influence access to and delivery of long-term care services.
- The variety of new approaches to long-term care delivery currently available.

INTRODUCTION

Long-term care refers to a range of health and social services that are needed to accommodate persons with functional disabilities. They may be persons of any age with conditions such as birth defects, spinal cord injuries, mental impairment, or other chronic debilitating conditions, but most often they are the very elderly whose ability to function independently is deteriorating. To assist these people, numerous services are provided that are based both in communities and in institutions. Long-term care services are expensive, and future costs are difficult to estimate. The government has no coherent long-term care policy, believing that the foundation of long-term care is the family and that services should not replace family efforts, but complement them. The basic policy questions for government are who should be eligible for services and who should pay for them. Questions surrounding long-term care—how it is delivered, evaluated, and financed—are among the most critical health issues facing the nation. As the population lives longer, concerns grow regarding the number of elderly living with chronic disease and disability.

The tasks of keeping individuals mobile and as self-sufficient as possible for as long as possible are the focal point of long-term care.

People of any age who are unable to cope with the tasks of daily living for extended periods of time because of physical or mental impairment need social and health care services. The risks of functional disability increase with age, however, and in the United States the number of people age sixty-five and older has increased from 8 percent of the population in 1950 to almost 13 percent in 1999 and is expected to grow to 16.5 percent by 2020 (Saphir, 1999a). After 2010, survivors of the Baby Boom generation will start to reach age sixty-five, causing a dramatic increase in that percentage of the population: An estimated 20 percent (69.4 million people) will be over sixty-five by 2030. Those eighty-five years and older are increasing faster than any other age group; this group is projected to double, from 1.4 percent of the population in 1995 to approximately 3 percent of the population in 2030 (U.S. Bureau of the Census, 1996). It is the eighty-five and older group that consumes the majority of long-term care services.

Families, friends, and neighbors help most people who are unable to cope with daily living tasks. For a growing number of others, "assisted living services" such as home care, adult day care, and other community-based services provide needed care without institutionalization. However, an increasing number of people, too frail to be left to outpatient care or left without family or friends, need some level of institutional care. This is typically available through long-term care facilities that include nursing homes, psychiatric and mental retardation facilities, and rehabilitation hospitals. The large majority of long-term care facilities are nursing homes that care primarily for the elderly. Continuing-care retirement communities and personal-care homes are newer approaches to caring for the elderly. New methods of financing care of the elderly include long-term care insurance and life insurance policies that offer accelerated or "living care" provisions allowing a portion of the life insurance benefit to be paid to a policyholder if long-term care is needed (Health Insurance Association of America, 1999). However, the poor and uninsured remain with inadequate funds to provide for any form of long-term care, leaving primary responsibility to government funding.

NURSING HOMES

The nursing home has historically represented one of the more difficult problems in long-term care. With fair regularity, scandals erupt in homes that cheat patients, physically abuse and neglect patients, provide inadequate medical and nursing care, and are fire hazards. To make matters worse, there have been an insufficient number of good nursing-home beds to deal with the growing number of aged people needing such care.

Nursing homes have their origins in the county poorhouses (or almshouses) of the eighteenth and nineteenth centuries. Local governments established these institutions to care for the poor, to provide them with shelter, food, and clothing, and with work to help pay the costs of their care. As might be expected, many, if not most, of these people were older and had no families to care for them. Being older, many were also invalids. Over time, these almshouses became the community dumps for all society's cast-offs, not only the poor and the physically ill, but also the mentally ill, the mentally retarded, and the alcoholic. There was often no place for these people to go except the local poorhouses. Generally, conditions in these homes were not good, for they had to get along on meager public appropriations and on charity. The appropriations were meager because the public had little sense of identity with these institutions or with the people in them. The inmates were poor and noncontributing to the general welfare, and many were transients without a previous history of community contributions. Why reward them with ideal facilities? Why tax the hardworking, thrifty citizenry to support those who were not that way? The politicians gave the almshouses the level of support the electorate wanted: bare minimum.

But a society gets what it pays for. Periodically scandals erupted, as they do today, and public consciences were pricked. Over time, the mentally ill and retarded were removed and sent to more appropriate institutions, most of which were state run rather than locally administered. In Maryland, the conditions in some county almshouses were so bad that the state set up a state-run chronic-disease hospital to care for the infirm in return for closing of the county almshouses. In other states, improvements were made from time to time, and these county homes, as patients were reassigned, were left mainly with the aged poor and the physically disabled who did not need hospital care but who were unable to subsist without some form of health service support.

In recent decades, the state governments have begun to regulate these homes along with church, fraternal, and proprietary nursing homes, inspecting them and setting standards for performance. But the hands of state regulation have generally been lightly applied. Few states have been prepared to close many of the county, voluntary, and proprietary homes because doing so would force the state to assume full responsibility.

As noted previously, nursing homes developed under other sponsorships. Church groups and fraternal organizations started homes for care of their members. These were mainly homes for the aged, but over time they had to develop supporting health services to meet the needs of their residents. These homes received strong support from their sponsoring bodies—not only direct financial aid but also much in-kind support in terms of gifts of equipment, volunteer maintenance, and, where there were farms, harvesting services. Sponsored homes also received a variety of volunteer, direct patient care services, such as help in feeding patients, occupational and play therapy, and social visiting. It is widely acknowledged that the quality of service in church- and fraternal-sponsored homes is high, and one rarely finds in them the shortcomings often found in local government nursing homes and in some of the proprietary nursing homes.

The proprietary private (for-profit) nursing homes emerged during the 1930s as a result of the Social Security Act of 1935, which provided welfare benefits for patients in nongovernmental institutions. The original exclusion of benefits for patients in public institutions (since repealed) apparently stemmed from congressional concern about conditions in county poorhouses and a desire to close them.

Many health professionals and civic leaders were concerned about the resulting rapid growth in the private nursing-home sector, believing that high-quality care could not be developed and maintained if the homes depended on income derived primarily from welfare recipients, because these homes not only had to provide the needed care but also had to leave enough profit to make the owner's investment of money worthwhile. Resulting scandals in the proprietary sector supported the fears of these people. Not only were the payments insufficient both to maintain quality care and to ensure a reasonable return on the owner's investment, but also the very availability of large sums of money to pay for care in facilities that were in short supply proved to be an open invitation to the unscrupulous to enter the business. As it turned

out, the poor who were chronically ill and needed nursing-home care were also often at the bottom of the list for admission to the proprietary homes. Even after the advent of Medicare and Medicaid, many of these homes gave preference to private applicants for admission, regardless of the need for care. The low payments by government programs did not permit a reasonable return on the owner's investment and still permit quality of care. Many proprietary nursing homes also restricted the number of patients they would admit who required a great amount of care, so as to avoid the greater costs of such care. In many states, as a consequence, long waiting lists developed for admission of Medicare and Medicaid patients, particularly of those who needed the most care.

Aware of these circumstances, health professionals and civic leaders encouraged the development of nonprofit nursing homes. Congress responded by amending the Hill-Burton Act in 1948 to make construction grants available for public and nonprofit nursing homes, and some states also designed new grant programs. The resistance of the proprietary sector to such grant programs was vigorous and highly political. One of the successful efforts of the proprietary sector was to get Congress to approve its eligibility for Federal Housing Authority (FHA) guaranteed construction loans.

The distribution of nursing homes and beds among the public, proprietary, church and fraternal, and other nonprofit sponsorships shifts constantly, but the proprietary sector clearly dominates. In 1997, 65.5 percent of facilities were for-profit, 27.9 percent nonprofit, and 6.6 percent government owned (Harrington, Carrillo, Thollaug, & Summers, 1999b).

The number of facilities that are owned by other organizations as part of chains is also on the increase, as is the number of hospital-based facilities (Harrington et al., 1999b). All of this is evidence of the trend toward integration that was prevalent during the 1990s. Nine of the nation's largest nursing-home chains control about 20 percent of the beds. The largest is Beverly Enterprises, with 64,100 beds (Saphir, 1999b).

The need for nursing-home beds has persisted for some years and remains of some concern. Our population is aging, and with this change comes an increased amount of chronic disease. As family units become smaller and all able persons are working, no one is at home to care for the elderly, thus further increasing the demand for facilities for care of the aged. The demand accelerated enormously with the implementation of Medicare and Medicaid, which paid for some of this care. The demand also increased as government and health insurance companies sought to reduce the lengths of stay in acute hospitals by moving patients to a less acute level of care.

With the advent of Medicare and Medicaid, the federal government established definitions for the types of institutions that would fall within the framework of those eligible for reimbursement, as well as standards to govern and ensure quality of care in those homes eligible to participate. If a home for the aged wanted to be paid under Medicare or Medicaid for care to eligible patients, the home had to meet certain standards. The federal government originally recognized two types of homes as eligible: the *skilled nursing facility* and the *intermediate-care facility*. The U.S. Department of Health and Human Services (HSS) provided the definitions:

> A *skilled nursing facility* (SNF) is a nursing home that has been certified as meeting Federal standards within the meaning of the Social Security Act. It provides the level of care that comes closest to hospital care with 24-hour nursing services. Regular medical supervision and rehabilitation therapy are also provided. Generally, a skilled nursing facility cares for convalescent patients and those with long-term illnesses.
>
> An *intermediate care facility* (ICF) is also certified and meets Federal standards and provides less extensive health-related care and services. It has regular nursing service, but not around the clock. Most intermediate care facilities carry on rehabilitation programs, but the emphasis is on personal care and social services. Mainly, these homes serve people who are not fully capable of living by themselves, yet are not necessarily ill enough to need 24-hour nursing care.

The nursing-home reform legislation that was passed as part of the 1987 Omnibus Budget Reconciliation Act (OBRA '87) created the category of nursing-home facility (NF) to describe a state-licensed facility providing skilled nursing and/or intermediate-care ser-

vices to residents on a twenty-four–hour basis. The terms *skilled nursing care* and *intermediate care* are now used to describe the two levels of care provided by most nursing facilities (Harrington et al., 1999a).

Demographics of Nursing Homes and Nursing-Home Residents

There were 15,661 certified nursing homes and 1,626,556 certified nursing-home beds in the United States in 1997. Although at one time nursing homes provided just one type of care for all residents, most now designate Alzheimer's units, AIDS units, and hospice units to care for residents with special needs.

The typical person in a nursing home is older (49.3 percent were eighty-five years or older in 1996), female (71.6 percent are women), unmarried (59.8 percent are widowed, 9.2 percent are divorced, and 14.4 percent never married), and suffering from some type of dementia (47.7 percent of the total population, and 53.6 percent of those over eighty-five years of age) (Krauss & Altman, 1998). See Table 8–1 for changes in some of the characteristics of nursing-home residents from 1985 to 1995.

The length of stay for nursing-home residents varies by the reason for admission. Those who are admitted for rehabilitation services may stay only two or three months and then return to living in the community. Those admitted because of a permanent condition may reside in the nursing home for the remainder of their lives, perhaps two or more years, depending on the age and diagnosis at admission. An average length of stay becomes misleading under such circumstances. Most nursing-home patients need unskilled care—that is, help with activities of daily living and medical oversight rather than medical treatment. Over 90 percent of nursing-home patients are sixty-five years of age or older (Krauss & Altman, 1998). The remaining are younger people who cannot care for themselves because of chronic diseases or accidents.

Occupancy rates in certified nursing homes showed a slight decline in the 1990s, from 89 percent in 1991 to 84 percent in 1997 (Saphir, 1999c). While there is much discussion about the need for long-term care with a growing elderly population, the care has

Table 8–1 Nursing-Home Residents in the United States According to Age, Gender, and Race: 1985 and 1995

	No. of Residents (%)	
	1985	**1995**
All persons		
65 years and over	1,318,300	1,422,600
65–74 years	212,100 (16.1)	190,200 (13.4)
75–84 years	509,000 (38.6)	511,000 (36.0)
84 years and over	597,300 (45.3)	720,400 (50.6)
Male		
65 years and over	334,400 (25.4)	356,800 (25.1)
65–74 years	80,600	79,300
75–84 years	141,300	144,300
84 years and over	112,600	133,100
Female		
65 years and over	983,900 (74.6)	1,065,800 (74.9)
65–74 years	131,500	110,900
75–84 years	367,700	367,600
84 years and over	484,700	587,300
White		
65 years and over	1,227,400 (93)	1,271,200 (89.4)
65–74 years	187,800	154,400
75–84 years	473,600	453,800
84 years and over	566,000	663,000
African-Americans		
65 years and over	82,000 (6)	122,900 (7)
65–74 years	22,500	29,700
75–84 years	30,600	47,300
84 years and over	29,000	45,800

Source: National Center for Health Statistics, as reprinted in Moskowitz, 1999. © Faulkner & Gray, Inc., reprinted with permission.

moved to other sites, such as personal-care homes, home care, and adult day care, all of which are discussed later in this chapter.

Hospital-Based Care

A number of hospitals have skilled nursing units (step-down units) within their facilities, developed in part to provide a more efficient use of their acute care beds. Certified hospital-based nursing homes increased from 8.7 percent of nursing facilities in 1991 to

13.6 percent in 1997. Hospital-based nursing homes may have higher-quality care because they have more Medicare patients and higher staffing levels, and are more likely to be not-for-profit (Harrington et al., 1999b).

Some hospitals are experimenting with "swing beds," which can handle acute cases one day and skilled nursing care cases the next. This allows a hospital some flexibility. It is a particularly inviting approach to a hospital that has low occupancy, and it is doubly inviting if there is a shortage of nursing-home beds in the area. Rather than close beds or keep them unoccupied, hospitals can use them to provide a stepped-down level of care, thus providing revenue otherwise lost. If the hospital is pressed for acute beds at any time, it then has the option of converting the long-term care beds back to acute beds.

Nursing-Home Costs

The costs of providing nursing-home care have exploded; costs rose from $4.2 billion in 1970 to $82.8 billion in 1997 (see Table 8–2). In 1997, Medicaid financed 47.6 percent of nursing-home costs, Medicare paid 12.2 percent, and other government sources paid about 2 percent while private insurance paid for only about 5 percent. Residents paid out of pocket for about 31 percent, and private sources other than insurance covered the remaining 2 percent (Health Care Financing Administration, 1999b; Saphir, 1999c).

Private long-term care insurance is now available, and the number of policies sold has increased from 515 in 1987 to 3.4 million in 1993. However, this is still a small percentage of the estimated 34 million Americans over the age of sixty-five in the year 2000. At the inception of long-term care policies, a typical policy paid for nursing-home care and limited home health care. Today's policies tend to include a much broader range of coverage, including both skilled and intermediate nursing-home care, personal care, home- and community-based care, and case management (Henry & Reifler, 1997). Premiums for long-term care insurance vary enormously, from $325 per year to more than $3,600 per year for an individual, depending on age, medical condition, the amount of the

Table 8–2 Expenditures and Sources of Funds for Nursing-Home Care, 1990–1997 (in Billions of Dollars)

Source	1990	1991	1992	1993	1994	1995	1996	1997
Total	50.9	57.2	62.3	66.4	71.1	75.5	79.4	82.8
Out-of-pocket payment	21.9	23.1	24.1	24.5	25.3	26.6	26.7	25.7
Third-party payment	29.0	34.1	38.2	41.9	45.8	48.8	52.7	57.0
Private insurance	2.1	2.4	2.6	2.8	3.0	3.4	3.7	4.0
Other private sources	.9	1.1	1.2	1.2	1.3	1.4	1.5	1.6
Government*	25.9	30.6	34.4	37.9	41.4	44.0	47.4	51.4
Medicare	1.7	1.9	2.9	3.9	5.5	6.7	8.0	10.1
Medicaid	23.1	27.5	30.2	32.5	34.2	35.6	37.6	39.4

*Difference between total government payments and sum of Medicare and Medicaid payments comes from other government payments.

Source: Health Care Financing Administration, Office of the Actuary, National Health Statistics Group (from www.hcfa.gov/stats).

daily benefit, and the number of days not covered when the patient is first admitted (Health Insurance Association of America, 1999). Because most long-term care patients require intermediate or custodial care, it is important to include those provisions as well as home health care in policies; it is also important that persons with mental disorders (e.g., Alzheimer's disease) not be excluded.

Unfortunately, many people cannot afford, and few have the foresight, to obtain private insurance. A few employers are beginning to offer long-term care insurance plans to employees so that they can get group rates, but the employee is usually required to pay the premium. Tax incentives (using pretax dollars for premiums or deducting premiums on tax returns) for purchasing long-term care insurance have not resulted in increased participation, except among persons in higher income brackets. Unfortunately, many Americans do not realize that Medicare does not pay for most long-term care (American Health Care Association, 1999).

Medicare will pay for nursing-home care only if the patient requires skilled nursing services or rehabilitation services on a daily basis. The care must follow a minimum three-day stay in a hospital, be ordered by a physician, and be periodically recertified as necessary for a maximum of 100 days. Because many nursing-home residents require custodial rather than skilled nursing care, Medicare is not the primary payer of their care (Medicare, 1999b).

Prior to 1997, Medicare paid for skilled nursing home care (when deemed medically necessary) on a cost-plus basis, reimbursing the facility's costs plus a small margin for profit. The Balanced Budget Act of 1997, however, changed the method of payment to a prospective payment system modeled after inpatient hospital payments. Nursing homes are now paid a flat rate per day for Medicare-eligible residents. Many nursing homes have found it difficult to maintain a high level of care under the decreased payment mechanism. However, that does not mean that the payment as calculated is unfair and totally responsible for the difficulties. Some organizations, particularly some of the large chains of nursing homes that went on a buying binge during the cost-plus payment era, simply overextended themselves and their credit lines. When skilled nursing home care was no longer lucrative, some began to divest. Others have been able to implement cost containment features while struggling to maintain quality care, just as in other areas of health care delivery.

Medicaid finances long-term care for the elderly poor and those who have exhausted their savings as private-paying residents. Unlike Medicare, most Medicaid programs pay for both skilled and custodial care for persons with long-term disabilities, but only if they are poor enough to qualify for coverage. Although funded by a combination of state and federal funds, Medicaid is run by the states, and eligibility for coverage and the services provided vary greatly among the states. Generally, Medicaid coverage is available only to persons with very low incomes. This restriction has resulted in the practice of "spending down" among some elderly, which involves paying for care out of pocket until a person becomes poor enough to qualify for Medicaid. Some elderly persons try to transfer their assets, such as real estate and securities, to trusts and relatives in order to protect the assets from Medicaid spend-down provisions. However, most states now have provisions that allow them to look back some three to five years to retrieve the value of those transferred assets. Persons who pay out of pocket for nursing-home care deplete their resources and qualify for Medicaid within a short time, since the national average cost for nursing-home care is estimated at $40,000 per year (Health Insurance Association of America, 1999). Legislation has recently been enacted to protect the spouse of a nursing-home resident from financial devastation, allowing the spouse to keep the family home and/or certain assets and income in order to continue to provide for him- or herself independently.

Quality of Care, Quality of Life

Prior to 1965, little was done to regulate nursing homes, though state governments were responsible for the licensing of nursing homes. Since the implementation of Medicaid and Medicare, Congress set minimum standards for nursing-home care under federal funding and charged the Health Care Financing Administration (HCFA) with the responsibility of monitoring, interpreting, and enforcing those standards. HCFA contracts with each state to inspect nursing homes for quality, resident care processes, staff-resident interaction, and environmental and safety standards, to become certified for Medicare and Medicaid beneficiaries (Medicare, 1999a).

At the time of Medicare and Medicaid implementation, nursing-home standards were liberally applied; that is, homes were approved even though they did not fully meet the standards. The decision by the government to apply standards liberally was political: The homes were already in business, and not to certify them and thus deny benefits to the population who thought they were getting benefits would be a political liability for the president and for the legislators who passed the legislation. However, another consideration undoubtedly operated: Getting marginal homes approved would, over time, provide an opportunity to force them to raise the quality of their services, and such improvement would be easier to bring about, the more dependent the homes were on Medicare and Medicaid payments.

Reform and improvement efforts have had little success in a "suppliers' market." As the number of people needing care rises while some states have placed moratoriums on building new facilities in order to contain costs, there are more people needing care than there are affordable beds to provide care. Meanwhile, nursing-home operators attempt to contain costs by reducing numbers of qualified staff, providing minimal activities, and regimenting care. Needless to say, many nursing homes are not cheery places in which to live or cheery places in which to work (Bryan, 1986).

Because of the concern over quality of care in nursing homes, Congress requested a study by the Institute of Medicine in 1986. The study found the quality of care "appalling," despite standards for certification and growing competition among nursing-home providers. Many residents received inadequate care, which often contributed to their deteriorating health (Bryan, 1986). The Institute of Medicine's study, among others, resulted in recommendations for new federal regulations. In 1987, Congress passed nursing-home reform legislation as part of the Omnibus Budget Reconciliation Act (OBRA '87), which called for (Harrington et al., 1999b):

- Comprehensive assessment to determine the functional, cognitive, and affective levels of residents to be used in care planning.
- Specific requirements for nursing, medical, and psychosocial services to help residents attain and maintain the highest possible level of functioning, both mentally and physically.
- Regulations protecting patients' rights.

Specific regulations enforcing OBRA '87 have brought about data collection processes that help consumers, as well as inspectors, evaluate and monitor nursing-home care. Most people dread the prospect of entering a nursing home largely because of the lack of privacy, the loss of autonomy, and the regimentation. Regulations cannot address residents' needs to have a caring environment, to have a sense of community, and to be free of loneliness, boredom, and helplessness.

The Eden Alternative

The Eden Alternative is a new way of thinking about long-term care. The concept, founded by Dr. William Thomas, transforms nursing homes into human habitats that not only shelter but also nurture those who *live and work* within them.

Dr. Thomas identifies three plagues of the elderly: loneliness, helplessness, and boredom. The treatment for these plagues is a natural environment filled with companion animals, plants, and children, as well as the spontaneity that fills most noninstitutionalized environments. When the elderly are given the opportunity to care for other living things, they respond in ways that pills and therapies cannot effect.

Adopting the Eden Alternative also means changing the approach to managing staff. Eden's premise is that "as management does unto staff, so shall staff do unto residents" (Thomas, 1998). Staff must be empowered to take part in the process of change, see residents and other staff members as part of a "neighborhood" of caring, and be able to work in a more spontaneous and natural manner. Regimentation and scheduled events give way to individual choice, opportunity, and personal growth. The Eden Alternative benefits management with lower turnover and absentee rates (Bayne, 1998).

Assisted-Living Facilities

Faced with the increasing numbers of people needing long-term care, care providers are rethinking the concept of nursing homes. New forms and combinations of care have been implemented with new residential programs and types of personnel. The Eden Alternative is one new form of care. Assisted-living facilities are another option to provide care for the elderly who cannot live independently but do not require skilled nursing care. Once referred to as personal-care homes, they allow a combination of independent residency in an apartment-like setting but provide supervision and help with some of the functional limitations of residents, such as group meals, laundry, cleaning services, and medication monitoring. Some assisted-living facilities are part of a broader "retirement community" that allows all levels of living, from independent apartments to skilled nursing care. Residents move to different levels of care as needed, with little disruption to their lives and families. Other assisted-living centers are freestanding facilities. The costs of assisted-living facilities are usually not covered by any type of insurance. Residents pay personally, as they would for rent or a mortgage, or else they qualify for government subsidy in publicly supported facilities.

COMMUNITY-BASED CARE

Many of the elderly would prefer not to go into nursing homes if necessary services were available in the community. Studies in the 1980s showed that 20 to 40 percent of the nursing-home population could be cared for at less-intensive levels if adequate community-based care were available (*Long Term Care*, 1981). However, health care payment structures encouraged people to choose nursing-home care even when community services were available. Medicaid paid for nursing-home care but not for community-based services, unless the state received a waiver from the federal government. Beginning in 1981, waivers were granted to some states to offer certain kinds of social services (e.g., help with bathing, cooking, or cleaning) to people living at home, in the hope that nursing-home care could be delayed or avoided and the high government expenditures for nursing-home care could be reduced.

The federal government financed the most extensive study of community-based care from 1982 to 1984. It involved 6,300 elderly people, whose average age was eighty, in ten states (U.S. Department of Health and Human Services, 1987b). The states were granted Medicaid waivers and funds to provide a broad base of community services to help impaired elderly to remain in their own homes rather than enter nursing homes. Comprehensive case management called "channeling" was used, whereby a person, called a case manager, identified the participating elderly person's specific problems and services needed, and developed a plan of care. The case managers helped their clients access needed services, and they coordinated community services and informal help given by family and friends. They monitored the services to be sure that they were delivered and that they met the needs of the client. The results of the study showed that the community-based programs did not reduce nursing-home costs and, in fact, increased the cost to the government. The community services had little effect on the number of nursing-home admissions. Most of the elderly studied would have remained in their own homes whether or not the community services were provided.

Mechanic (1987) points out that the reason for admission to a nursing home may be based on factors other than need, because many living in the community may have as great a need level. Rather, admission may be the result of the loss of a spouse or other significant support person(s), or a major illness or accident that makes a person lacking support unable to care for him- or herself.

The services provided in the "channeling" project did not replace the care that family and friends gave, but it complemented that care and enabled the informal caregivers to maintain their efforts rather than become overwhelmed. The channeling long-term care study "indicates that the expansion of case management and community services beyond what already exists does not lead to overall cost savings. But it does yield benefits in the form of in-home care, reduced unmet needs, and improved satisfaction with life for clients and informal caregivers who bear most of the burden. Whether these benefits are commensurate with its costs is a decision for society to make" (U.S. Department of Health and Human Services, 1987a). The results of the National Long Term Care Demonstration (as this study is called) agree with other community care demonstrations.

Kemper (1987) suggests that policy makers should move beyond asking whether expanding community care saves money and should address the issues of how much community care society is willing to finance, who should receive it, and how it can be delivered efficiently. A synthesis of twenty-seven studies of home and community care for the chronically ill elderly, including the ten-state, multimillion-dollar National Long Term Care Demonstration, concluded that the health benefits were small. Longevity and mental functioning were unaffected. Physical functioning either remained the same or decreased, apparently because the client became dependent on the home care aid. Only life satisfaction or "contentment" was favorably affected, but even this improvement was small and dissipated after several months, despite continuing care. Most of those using home care services were not at risk of entering a nursing home, and although nursing-home use was reduced in some studies, the cost of home care offset any savings from the reduced use of nursing homes.

These results make it hard to justify home care on the basis of health benefits or cost savings. However, expanding home care is still popular, not only because it is "the right thing to do" (Weissert, 1991), but also because the move to prospective payment for hospital care and the incentive to decrease the length of stay in the hospital setting has made home care available to more than the potential nursing-home population. Many patients of all ages, discharged from the acute care setting of the hospital, continue to require an intermittent level of skilled nursing care. Home care can provide that care without additional institutionalization for the patient.

Home Health Care

Home health care agencies typically provide care for the disabled in the community. They supply a combination of medical services (part-time skilled nursing care, physical therapy, speech therapy, occupational therapy, medical social services, and some medical supplies and equipment) and social services (helping clients bathe and dress, changing bed linen, and cooking) for people confined to their homes. In most cases the services supplement the care the clients receive from family and friends. Although most of the agencies' clients are elderly, there are also younger clients who are recovering from an illness or accident, or from a stay in the hospital, or have chronic medical conditions and need prolonged care but do not require hospitalization. The CDC reports that the number of persons served by home health care agencies rose from 1.2 million in 1992 to 2.4 million in 1996 (Munson, 1999).

Home care agencies operate under various names, have varying organizational ties, and offer differing services. They can be independent, hospital-operated, or health department–managed agencies. The number of home health agencies has increased from 2,242 in 1975 to 10,807 in 1997. Fifty-eight percent of home health agencies were for-profit, 29 percent nonprofit, and 13 percent government owned in 1997 (Health Care Financing Administration, 1998a).

The earliest home health care agencies were visiting-nurse agencies, which were created in the late 1800s to bring needed care to communities that had no hospital. A nurse, usually one with public health training, would visit homes to provide care to the patient and support to the family. Today, visiting-nurse agencies represent some 25 percent of all nonprofit, freestanding home health agencies in the United States, and they continue to provide care to some 10 million patients annually (Visiting Nurse Association of America, 1999).

Home health care has expanded, particularly since the 1980s, and includes such services as skilled nursing care; personal care; medication preparation and management; equipment delivery, setup, and management; respiratory, physical, speech, and infusion therapy; and even hospice care—all provided to patients in their own homes. The Joint Commission on Accreditation of Healthcare Organizations (JCAHO) accredits over 6,500 home health care organizations. Accreditation meets the organization's needs in demonstrating quality care, obtaining state licensure, and meeting certification requirements for the Medicare and Medicaid programs and other insurers (JCAHO, 1999).

Expenditures in home health care reached $13 billion in 1990 and increased to $32 billion in 1997. Public programs financed over 50 percent of the 1997 costs. Medicare paid almost $13 billion and Medicaid almost $5 billion for home health care in 1997. Patients' out-of-pocket expenditures accounted for about $7 billion, while private insurance paid only $3.7 billion (see Table 8–3). The remainder came from other private sources (Health Care Financing Administration, 1999b).

The growth in home health expenditures is a result of liberalized Medicare payments, an increase in the number of home health providers, and an increased demand for services (Medicare, 1999b). However, the 1997 Balanced Budget Act placed greater restraints on home health care reimbursement from Medicare. Services previously paid on a fee-for-service basis are now paid under a prospective payment system, just as hospital payments and skilled nursing facility payments are (Health Care Financing Administration,

Table 8–3 Expenditures and Source of Funds for Home Health Care, 1990–1997 (in Billions of Dollars)

Source	1990	1991	1992	1993	1994	1995	1996	1997
Total	13.1	16.1	19.6	23.0	26.2	29.1	31.2	32.3
Out-of-pocket payment	3.6	4.3	5.0	5.6	5.9	6.2	6.5	7.0
Third-party payment	9.5	11.7	14.6	17.4	20.3	22.9	24.7	25.3
Private insurance	2.2	2.5	2.9	3.1	3.3	3.4	3.5	3.7
Other private sources	2.2	2.5	2.9	3.2	3.4	3.5	3.7	3.9
Government*	5.1	6.7	8.8	11.1	13.7	16.0	17.5	17.7
Medicare	3.0	4.2	5.9	7.7	10.0	11.9	13.2	12.8
Medicaid	2.1	2.5	2.9	3.3	3.6	3.9	4.2	4.7

*Difference between total government payments and sum of Medicare and Medicaid payments comes from other government payments.

Source: Health Care Financing Administration, Office of the Actuary, National Health Statistics Group (from www.hcfa.gov/stats).

1999a). Tighter funding may lead to more difficult access to care, as those organizations unable to adjust through cost containment may be forced to close their doors. This comes at a time when the Agency for Health Care Policy and Research reports that nearly half of home health care clients have needs greater than the support services they receive (Thomas & Payne, 1998).

Adult Day Care

Another long-term care program that enables some elderly to remain in the community is adult day care. Adult day care programs can maintain or improve client overall functioning, increase social interactions, offer respite care for family caregivers, or even allow caregivers to remain employed. They differ from senior centers in that they serve adults who are physically impaired or mentally confused and require supervision, increased social opportunities, and assistance with personal care or other daily living activities. There are over 4,000 adult day care centers nationally, serving primarily a population of persons suffering from dementia (Henry & Reifler, 1997; National Council on the Aging, 1999).

Adult day care programs are operated by hospitals, nursing homes, and social agencies, which might be for-profit or nonprofit organizations. Adult day care is not paid by Medicare, and although some states do cover it under Medicaid, it can be a financial burden and available to only those in higher income brackets. More private long-term care insurance policies are now including "community care," including adult day care, as a covered service. As noted earlier, however, the number of the elderly covered under such policies is small. Nationally, adult day care centers charge between $20 and $40 a day, much less than the cost of nursing-home care. Utilization of services tends to mirror home health care services; that is, participants attend on average two to three days per week rather than for a full week (National Council on Aging, 1999). Transportation can be a problem that makes adult day care a much less promising investment than home care for some (Kane & Kane, 1987).

In 1993 the Robert Wood Johnson Foundation awarded a number of grants in hopes of stimulating innovation in the adult day care field. The goal of the program is to demonstrate that adult day care centers can provide beneficial services to clients and their families at affordable prices (Gunby, 1993). The grant programs recognized that high-quality activity programs help reduce depression in the participants and help them maintain function. Adult day care centers can become more responsive to caregiver needs by offering a wider range of services, such as longer hours, hours on weekends and in evenings, and overnights. However, in order for adult day care centers to be more responsive to participants' needs, reimbursement mechanisms must be willing to recognize and support those needs (Henry & Reifler, 1997).

HOSPICE CARE

Although earlier models of care for the dying existed, St. Christopher's Hospice in England is often cited as the model for hospice development in the United States. The first pilot program ran in a chronic-disease hospital in Massachusetts. The program, which emphasized symptom and pain control, focused on the psychosocial needs of both the patient and the family. In 1974 the first freestanding hospice was established, Connecticut Hospice Inc., in New Haven, Connecticut. Connecticut Hospice Inc. started as exclusively home care, but it built an inpatient facility three years later in order to deliver a full range of care (Mor & Masterson-Allen, 1987).

A number of factors contributed to the development of hospice. The late 1960s and early 1970s saw a growth in the awareness of the experience of dying. Particularly important was the influence of Elisabeth Kubler-Ross's book on the stages of dying: *On Death and Dying* (1969). It brought attention to the patient as a person and detailed the experience of dying for both the patient and the caretaker (Paradis & Cummings, 1986). Advanced technology and training in medicine as a science had produced an impersonal medical delivery system that lost sight of the patient's personhood. Although the hospital originated as a place to die, cure now became the focus. New technologies sought to defy death as a normal process. The controversial Karen Quinlan court case brought to the forefront discussion of patients' rights to terminate treatment.

Legislation in various states supported patient autonomy and decisions to withhold or withdraw treatment (Mor & Masterson-Allen, 1987). Hospice provided the palliative care and the psychosocial support needed by terminally ill patients who opted out of technological intervention near the end of life.

Hospice ideals often came into conflict with the views of established medical systems. Particularly controversial was the limited role of the physician in hospice care. Physician input was necessary for proper symptom and pain control, but this input was only part of a team effort to deliver care in the hospice environment. Nurses, chaplains, social workers, volunteers, and family all were seen as equally important. This idea was in direct conflict with the amount of power and control experienced by the physician in traditional health care settings. Particularly challenged was the role of physician paternalism. No longer was the physician expected to make decisions in the best interest of the patient. The physician was expected to communicate honestly with the patient about his or her prognosis and treatment options and allow the patient to participate fully in all treatment decisions (Abel, 1986).

Hospice also challenged traditional hospital practices that often isolated patients at a time when they most needed support. Hospice patients were allowed to have family and/or friends with them at all times, wear their own clothing, choose their meals, and encounter as few restrictions as possible. Staff spent unrestricted time with patients, delivering more spiritual and emotional care than medical care (Abel, 1986).

Hospice was first established as a nonprofit, voluntary endeavor. Volunteers provided care, and funds were secured through service organizations, philanthropies, and individual contributors (Paradis & Cummings, 1986). Earliest models were independent, providing care in the home or a freestanding facility totally separate from the hospital or established home health agency. Subsequent models have been based in a home health agency or hospital. Existing home health agencies began providing hospice care, contracting with hospitals and/or nursing homes to provide inpatient care when home-based care was no longer feasible. Hospital-based hospice might consist of separate units, scattered beds throughout the facil-

ity, or teams trained to deliver hospice care in the home (Paradis & Cummings, 1986). Variations exist even within these three major models.

As the delivery of hospice care became more widespread, securing of funds became more important. Largely through the efforts of the National Hospice Organization, efforts were made to provide funding through federal grants and third-party payers. Increased dependence of hospice on government and on private reimbursement mechanisms brought with it increased requirements to conform to certain standards and behaviors. While some hospice organizers wanted no part of the influences of regulators, even at the expense of funding opportunities, others sought integration into the established medical care system as a matter of survival. In its efforts to seek third-party reimbursement, particularly Medicare reimbursement, the National Hospice Organization worked closely with JCAHO to develop the accreditation process for hospice standards. These standards subsequently became very influential over hospice care. JCAHO now requires hospitals to accredit their hospice programs or risk losing hospital accreditation (Paradis & Cummings, 1986).

Medicare regulations, finalized by the Health Care Financing Administration in 1983, provided for payment for hospice services to certified hospice providers. It is in this set of certification requirements that the transformation of hospice takes place. Certified hospice programs are subject to the following requirements:

- A care plan must be established for each person admitted to the hospice program, and care must be provided in accordance with that plan.
- All the core services must be directly provided with hospice employees (specific regulations limit the subcontracting of services).
- All aspects of the care plan must be managed regardless of the setting in which the patient resides (the hospice manages the plan even if the patient is intermittently admitted to a hospital or nursing home) (Tierney & Wilson, 1993).
- At least 80 percent of care must be provided in the patient's home and only 20 percent in inpatient settings.

- Reimbursement was capped at $9,000 for six months of services, emphasizing the difficulty in predicting the length of a patient's life (Bulkin, Wald, & O'Brien-Butler, 1992).

Medicare reimbursement brought funding in a more steady and predictable stream than what could be provided through contributions or grants. However, it also brought about regulation that limited the availability of hospice care to some patients. The mere prospect of waiving one's rights to hospital care can be too frightening to opt for hospice care. The requirement that 80 percent of the patient's care be provided in the patient's home makes patients who have no family support structure ineligible for care (Hoyer, 1990; Jones, 1988). While Medicare funding brought hospice care into mainline medicine, it also effected change from the original conception of hospice care. But the influence worked both ways. The hospice movement encouraged physicians to discuss death with their patients and brought family and other support systems closer to the dying patient.

REHABILITATION FACILITIES

Rehabilitation hospitals or centers provide acute and/or residential care to persons suffering from traumatic brain injury, stroke, disabling diseases, cognitive disorders, and a full array of other problems resulting in functional disability. Services provided can include physical therapy, occupational therapy, speech therapy, and counseling or psychological therapy, as well as nursing care and personal care. Length of treatment might be anywhere from a few months to permanent residence in the facility. Rehabilitation centers admit persons who are otherwise medically stable, and their goal is to get the patient to the highest level of functioning possible for discharge back to the community and maintenance on an outpatient basis, or to slow the debilitation process as much as possible as the patient remains in the residential portion of the facility (Centre for Neuro Skills, 1999).

Some rehabilitation centers specialize in treatment for one category of diagnosis, such as spinal cord injury or behavioral disorders. Others provide a wide range of care. Because of the wide range of diagnoses and services provided, it is difficult to provide an average cost of care. The patient's diagnosis, variety of therapies needed, treatment response times, and comorbidities will determine costs and length of stay.

While the discussion here applies to facilities specializing in rehabilitation therapy, it is important to remember that rehabilitation services might also take place within nursing homes, acute care hospitals, outpatient facilities, and the patient's home. The term *rehabilitation facility* might also be applied to mental health and substance abuse organizations discussed elsewhere.

CONTINUING-CARE COMMUNITIES

Continuing-care communities became popular about twenty years ago as an arrangement providing for the needs of the elderly, including nursing care. These communities require a large entrance fee, of $50,000 to $100,000 or more (often obtained through the sale of a home), and a monthly payment to contribute to operating costs (often financed by pension or assets). For this fee, housing and nursing care is ensured, along with housekeeping and some meals. Persons with high-risk health problems are either excluded or required to pay more. Medicare pays for acute medical care. People are encouraged to enter after retirement while still in good health. Accommodations are usually apartments and, when residents can no longer cope in apartments, single rooms. Until recently, most communities were run by nonprofit groups, but now for-profit communities are being developed, some of which do not require a large entrance fee but charge a monthly fee according to the amount of care needed. Continuing-care communities are available only to those with adequate financial resources who want the security they provide. However, there are some government-subsidized housing complexes with facilities and services for the elderly poor who cannot manage housekeeping and personal tasks.

SUMMARY

Long-term care refers to a range of health and social services that are needed to compensate for the functional disabilities of people of any age. Although many are under sixty-five years old with chronic conditions that prevent them from functioning independently, most are the very old who are no longer able to cope with the activities of daily living without help. Nursing-home care is for those persons who are no longer able to live in the community, and its cost is financed almost entirely by Medicaid and by out-of-pocket payments of residents. Private insurance pays for only about 5 percent of nursing-home costs.

Community-based and private organizations provide home care to enable the functionally disabled to remain in the community. Home care may delay, but probably does not eliminate, nursing-home admissions; it does, however, appear to improve the quality of life of caregivers and recipient. Other long-term care services include adult day care and hospice care. The state and federal governments (via Medicaid and, to a lesser extent, Medicare) finance the majority of long-term care. The costs have risen sharply, and the demand for services continues to increase, making the question of who should pay for long-term care a prime policy issue. Many policy makers believe that neither government nor the private sector alone can provide long-term care and are seeking new ways of financing it. One approach being tested is to encourage all persons to purchase long-term care insurance just as they would health or life insurance. Financing is only one major problem; other problems include determining the appropriateness and quality of services.

IN THE HEALTH CARE COMMUNITY

The Memphis Jewish Home*

The Memphis Jewish Home (MJH) began in 1927 as the B'nai B'rith Home and Hospital for the Aged, a nonprofit institution. From its inception through the late 1980s, it continued to operate in its North Tucker location in Memphis, Tennessee, but it underwent a number of modifications to keep up with changes in nursing-home care. In 1989, in recognition that the limits of the original facility had been reached, ground was broken for a new facility able to provide new technologies and therapies.

Today the Memphis Jewish Home is a 144-bed, multifaceted, long-term care facility, licensed by the state, and Medicare and Medicaid certified. The facility, located in a 77-acre parklike setting, is the first phase of a long-term plan that will eventually include a full continuum of geriatric-specific care and services.

Services available at MJH include both skilled and intermediate long-term residential care, a special care unit for those suffering from Alzheimer's and related forms of dementia, adult day care, a children's day care center, an on-site pharmacy, and various therapy services.

Following it's mission, the Memphis Jewish Home is a not-for-profit nursing home, Jewish in character and environment, dedicated to providing the highest level of care possible with dignity, compassion, and professionalism, using the most advanced methods and resources available.

MJH accepts qualified applicants without regard to race, color, religion, or national origin, but its priority is the elderly in the Jewish community. While the board of trustees sees MJH as state of the art and having an excellent reputation, it recognizes the problems inherent in the institutional model of elder care and has voted to implement the Eden Alternative. Organizational change is seldom (if ever) easy. Although the Eden Alternative is a concept difficult for almost anyone to reject, it requires a cultural, procedural, and managerial shift that is all-encompassing.

As discussed earlier in this chapter, the Eden Alternative, conceptualized by Dr. William Thomas,

(continues)

*Information for this case study was obtained through personal interviews with the executive director and Eden Alternative coordinator of the Memphis Jewish Home and from organization documents.

(continued)

seeks to eliminate the boredom, helplessness, and loneliness that plague nursing-home residents by converting the long-term care atmosphere into a natural environment. Although some may argue that nursing homes have turned into big businesses run by those who simply seek to make a profit, most nursing homes in fact strive to provide quality care for their residents. The concept of caring *for* is simply not the same as the concept of caring *about* the nursing-home resident as a family member, individual, and valued member of society.

In the Eden Alternative mission statement Dr. Thomas says (Eden Online, 1999):

> We want to show others how companion animals, the opportunity to care for other living things, and the variety and spontaneity that mark our enlivened environment can succeed where pills and therapies fail. Our goal is to weave together that philosophy of the Eden Alternative with the practical applications and make it work in the real world of Long-Term Care.

Patricia Brown, Director of the Center for Life Span Environments and Eden Associate (1998), says of the Eden Alternative (Eden Online, 1999):

> In discussing a "Home with Spirit," the Spirit I refer to is that indefinable quality of peace, serenity and belonging you feel when you are truly connected to your surroundings. While many of us find ways to bring this sense of Spirit into our own lives through hiking in the mountains, gazing at the nighttime skies, or along the beach at dawn, think about how few opportunities our elders in nursing homes have to make this kind of connection.

The natural environment of the Eden Alternative is a combination of physical environment and the culture of the people involved. Eden brings plants, animals, and children into the lives of the elders, but it also brings a sense of family into the relationships among residents, staff, families, and volunteers. It is truly a "total" reorganization of thoughts and actions in long-term care.

In implementing the Eden Alternative™, the Memphis Jewish Home has converted its units into neighborhoods. Residents and staff join together to elect Mayors and other "officials" who plan activities and "design" the environment of their neighborhood. Bright decorations, gardens, birds, aquariums, and eventually other pets, and a variety of activities turn once institutional areas into warm and inviting human habitats. The conversion is a process—long and sometimes difficult. While the uncertainty of change frightens some staff members, it invigorates others. In the long term, the hope is for a higher quality of life for both the residents and staff of the Memphis Jewish Home.

ACTIVITY-BASED LEARNING

- The American Association of Homes and Services for the Aging (AAHSA) is a professional organization for nonprofit elder care organizations. Access the association's Web site at www.aahsa.org. Choose a state of interest to you and find out what nursing homes and continuing-care communities are listed for that state. Is there a facility nearby that you can visit?
- Log onto the Web site for the Eden Alternative (www.edenalt.com). Are any of the nursing homes in your state registered Eden facilities? Is there an Eden facility nearby? If there is, arrange to visit the facility to experience the difference.
- The American Health Care Association provides information and advocates for persons needing long-term care. Access the association's Web site at www.ahca.org to see its suggestions for choosing a quality nursing home. What are some of the points it suggests looking for in nursing-home care?

A QUESTION OF ETHICS

- Is it ethical for the elderly to pass their wealth on to their children so that they may qualify for

Medicaid coverage of nursing-home care if it is needed?

• The term *sandwich generation* has been used to describe adults torn between the responsibilities of caring for minor children while at the same time faced with caring for their elderly parents. What responsibility do children have for meeting the long-term care needs of their parents?

• Quality of life versus quantity of life issues are often discussed in relationship to the appropriateness of medical interventions in acute care settings. Quality of life is also the central theme in discussions of patient self-determination and the right to physician-assisted suicide. As the costs of long-term care rise and the numbers needing care increase, how do we decide if cost of care rather than quality of life is the driving mechanism in an individual's request to end his or her life?

References

Abel, E. (1986). The hospice movement: Institutionalizing innovation. *International Journal of Health Services, 16*(1), 71–85.

American Health Care Association. (1999, April 6). Financial preparedness: Few boomers ready for LTC costs. *American Health Line* [On-line]. Available: web.lexis-nexis.com/ (Accessed October 18, 1999).

Bayne, M. (1998, December). Spotlight on the Eden alternative. *Contemporary Long Term Care*, p. 92.

Bryan, J. (1986, June). View from the hill. *American Family Physician* [On-line serial] *33*(6). Available: web.lexis-nexis.com (Accessed October 21, 1999).

Bulkin, W., Wald, F., & O'Brien-Butler, J. (1992, May/June). Regulations vs. ideals: A case history of a hospice closure. *American Journal of Hospice & Palliative Care*, pp. 18–23.

Centre for Neuro Skills. (1999). *TBI rehabilitation* [On-line]. Available: www.neuroskills.com/rehab/ rehab.shtml (Accessed January 24, 2000).

Eden Online. (1999). *Eden alternative official website* [On-line]. Available: www.edenalt.com (Accessed May 15, 2000).

Gunby, P. (1993). Adult day care centers vital, many more needed. *JAMA, 269*(18), 2341–2342.

Harrington, C., Carrillo, H., Thollaug, S., & Summers, P. (1999a, May). *1997 State data book on long term care program and market characteristics*

[On-line]. Available: www.hcfa.gov/medicaid/ ltchome.htm (Accessed November 29, 1999).

Harrington, C., Carrillo, H., Thollaug, S., & Summers, P. (1999b, January). *Nursing facilities, staffing, residents, and facility deficiencies, 1991 through 1997* [On-line]. Available: www.hcfa.gov/ medicaid/ltchomep.htm (Accessed November 29, 1999).

Health Care Financing Administration. (1998a). *1998 data compendium.* Office of Strategic Planning. Baltimore, Maryland: US Dept of Health and Human Services.

Health Care Financing Administration. (1998b). *A profile of medicare: Chart book.* Office of Strategic Planning. Baltimore, Maryland: US Department of Health and Human Services.

Health Care Financing Administration. (1999a). *Nursing home care expenditures, Table 7* [On-line]. Available: www.hcfa.gov/stats (Accessed November 16, 1999).

Health Care Financing Administration. (1999b). *Personal health care expenditures, by type of expenditure and source of funds: Selected calendar years, 1990–97. Table 9* [On-line]. Available: www.hcfa.gov/stats (Accessed December 3, 1999).

Health Insurance Association of America. (1999). *Consumer information: Guide to long-term care* [On-line]. Available: www.hiaa.org/cons/ guideltc.html (Accessed November 29, 1999).

Henry, R., & Reifler, B. (1997). Coverage of adult day services in long term care insurance policies. *Journal of Applied Gerontology, 16*(2), 22–36.

Hoyer, R. (1990). Public policy and the American hospice movement: The tie that binds. *Caring, 9*(3), 30–35.

Joint Commission on Accreditation of Healthcare Organizations. (1999). *Home care associations* [On-line]. Available: www.jcaho.org/accred (Accessed December 3, 1999).

Jones, P. (1988, August). How has the Medicare benefit changed hospice? *Caring*, pp. 8–11.

Kane, R. A., & Kane, R. L. (1987). *Long-term care: Principles, programs, and policies.* New York: Springer.

Kemper P. (1987). Community care demonstrations: What have we learned? *Health Care Finance Review, 8*(4), 87–100.

Krauss, N., & Altman, B. (1998). *Characteristics of nursing home residents, 1996* (AHCPR Pub. No. 99-0006, Vol. 5). Rockville, MD: Agency for Health Care Policy and Research.

Long term care: In search of solutions. (1981). Washington, DC: National Conference on Social Welfare.

Mechanic, D. (1987). Challenges in long term care policy. *Health Affairs, 6*(2), 22–34.

Medicare. (1999a). *About nursing home inspections.* Available: www.medicare.gov/nursing/about.html (Accessed November 14, 1999).

Medicare. (1999b). Medicare information. In *Nursing home information site: Medicare summary* [On-line]. Available: http://members.tripod.com (Accessed October 27, 1999).

Mor, V., & Masterson-Allen, S. (1987). *Hospice care systems: Structure, process, costs and outcome.* New York: Springer.

Moskowitz, J. *1999. Health care almanac & yearbook.* New York: Faulkner & Gray.

Munson, M. (1999). Characteristics of elderly home health care users: Data from the 1996 National Home and Hospice Care Survey. *Advance Data, 309,* 11.

National Council on the Aging. (1999). *National Adult Day Services Association, Adult day services fact sheet* [On-line]. Available: www.ncoa.org/nadsa/ADS_factsheet.htm (Accessed January 21, 2000).

Paradis, L., & Cummings, S. (1986). The evolution of hospice in America toward organizational homogeneity. *Journal of Health and Social Behavior, 27,* 370–386.

Saphir, A. (1999a, September 27). Forever young: Long-term care industry must reinvent itself to keep boomers, minorities happy. *Modern Healthcare,* p. S28.

Saphir, A. (1999b, May 24). Medicare changes shake long-term care: Survey shows anticipated payment reductions prompted mergers, caused financial damage. *Modern Healthcare* [On-line].

Available: http://web.lexis-nexis.com (Accessed October 18, 1999).

Saphir, A. (1999c, July 26). Monstrous problems: Medicare's not the only bogeyman haunting the long-term care industry. *Modern Healthcare* [On-line serial]. Available: http://web.lexis-nexis.com/ (Accessed October 21, 1999).

Thomas, C. P., & Payne, S. (1998). Home alone: Unmet need for formal support services among home health clients. *Home Health Care Services Quarterly, 17*(2), 1–20.

Thomas, W. (1998). *Long term care design: Building home-ness into existing long-term care facilities.* Eden Alternative Literature.

Tierney, J., & Wilson, D. (1993, March/April). The effect of the Medicare regulations on hospice practice: Enhancing staff performance. *American Journal of Hospice & Palliative Care,* pp. 26–31.

U.S. Bureau of the Census. (1996). *Population projections of the United States by age, sex, race, and Hispanic origin: 1995 to 2050* (Current Population Reports, Vol. P25–1130). Washington, DC: U.S. Department of Commerce.

U.S. Department of Health and Human Services. (1987a). *The evaluation of national long term care demonstrations: Final report executive summary.* Washington, DC: Author.

U.S. Department of Health and Human Services. (1987b). *National long term care demonstration.* Washington, DC: Author.

Visiting Nurse Association of America. (1999). *Visiting nurse agencies* [On-line]. Available: www.vnaa.org/AVDefault.htm (Accessed December 3, 1999).

Weissert, W. (1991). A new policy agenda for home care. *Health Affairs, 10*(2), 67–77.

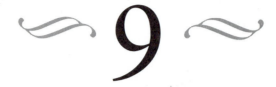

CHAPTER
9

Mental Health Services

Chapter Objectives

After completing this chapter, the reader should have an understanding of:

- The range of services encompassing mental health services.
- The history of the development of mental health services.
- The difficulties faced by the mental health sector of health care.

INTRODUCTION

The mental health system encompasses a large variety of services and service providers. As with medical care, the modern focus is on prevention and early treatment—a move away from the historical focus on isolation and control of those with mental illness. However, many difficulties still arise in the treatment of mental illness, from lack of resources to lack of understanding. Mental illness is described in many ways:

- Carrying normal fears, thoughts, emotions, and beliefs to an extreme

- Behavior dangerous to oneself or others
- Mental function resulting in unproductive activities, unfulfilling relationships with other people, and the inability to adapt to change and to cope with adversity

All of the descriptions are somewhat left to interpretation, and here lies some of the difficulty. Behavior is steeped in culture and values. Diagnosis and treatment must also be culturally based. New understandings of mental health and mental illness must be made available to communities so that those seeking care can come forward and effective treatment can be rendered without stigma and fear being attached to the recipient.

Mental illness may affect the way a person thinks (cognitive disorders), behaves (behavioral disorders), or interacts with others (emotional disorders). It encompasses a number of psychiatric disorders, including depression, anxiety disorders, schizophrenia and other psychotic disorders, substance abuse and disorders related to substance abuse, dementia, eating disorders, learning disorders, personality disorders—a variety of mental illnesses described and categorized in an official code book, *Diagnostic and Statistical Manual of Mental Disorders,* now in its fourth edition

(DSM-IV), and separate from the diagnosis codes used for physical illnesses (American Psychiatric Association, 2000).

According to the surgeon general's report (1999):

> Mental disorders (collectively) account for more than 15 percent of the burden of disease from all causes (p. 3).
>
> Approximately one in five children and adolescents experiences the signs and symptoms of a DSM-IV disorder during the course of a year, but only about 5 percent of all children experience what professionals term extreme functional impairment. A range of treatments exists for many mental disorders in children, including attention-deficit/hyperactive disorder, depression, and disruptive disorders (pp. 17–18).
>
> Anxiety, depression, and schizophrenia, particularly, present special problems in the adult stage of life. Anxiety and depression contribute to the high rates of suicide in this population. Schizophrenia is the most persistently disabling condition for young adults (p. 18).
>
> Substance abuse is a major co-occurring problem for adults with mental disorders (p. 18).
>
> Normal aging is not characterized by mental or cognitive disorders. Mental or substance use disorders that present alone or co-occur among older adults should be recognized and treated as illnesses (p. 19).

Remarkable advances have been made in the understanding of mental health and mental disorders, the function of the brain, and the relationship between mental and physical functioning of the body. But much remains to be done in converting this understanding into care and treatment of those in need.

The shortcomings of mental health services in the United States are brought forcefully to our attention by the large number of mentally ill homeless people who are seen in the streets, subways, and parks of our larger cities. It is estimated that about one-third of the homeless suffer from serious mental illness (Pardes, 1991). Less obvious is the amount of mental illness that could be prevented or controlled, but for fear of the stigma attached to mental illness. The American Psychological Association (1999) points out:

> It is a myth that mental illness is a weakness or defect in character and that sufferers can get better simply by "pulling themselves up by their bootstraps." Mental illnesses are real illnesses—as real as heart disease and cancer—and they require and respond well to treatment (p. 1).

A fragmented system of financing and responsibility has resulted in an inadequate amount of care, or care not targeted to many in need. Sufficient medical care, social support, and help with basic living needs for a prolonged period of time are not available. How this situation came about and what is being done to remedy it is the focus of this chapter.

HISTORY OF MENTAL HEALTH SERVICES

Before the 1800s, families provided the majority of care to people with mental illness; those with mental illness became a public concern only if they had no family support and were unable to care for themselves, or were violent. In the latter cases, local officials assumed responsibility for the welfare of such persons by boarding them with families or placing them in public almshouses along with the very poor, or housing them in public jails.

As the population grew and urbanization increased, there was a growing awareness of social and medical problems. Some psychiatric hospitals were established (in that era these institutions were often referred to as "mental hospitals" or as "asylums"). About this time, Dorothea Dix became very interested in the condition of almshouses and jails in her native state of Massachusetts and found, among other problems, that persons suffering from insanity (often referred to as lunatics) were held in unheated jails. She convinced the state legislature to assume direct responsibility for the care of people with mental illness. Dix also campaigned for improved conditions for people with mental illness in many other states. Her reforms led to the establishment of large state institutions in almost every state; thus, an era of "moral treatment" began, in which patients were nourished and cared for until they became well again.

The prevailing view at that time was that mental illness was the result of improper behavioral patterns that were associated with an unsatisfactory environment. It was thought that psychiatric institutions could provide a more appropriate environment, where patients could be improved physically, be treated with narcotics to calm violent behavior, and be provided with kind, individual care. Most patients were institutionalized for brief periods of time.

There were relatively few long-term or chronic cases in institutions during the nineteenth century, partly because a large proportion of people with mental illness were still kept at home or in municipal almshouses and partly because the funding of these institutions was divided between state and local governments. States provided funding to build and renovate psychiatric institutions, but local communities paid for the care and treatment of the patients admitted if their family or friends did not assume the cost. Sometimes local officials kept indigent persons with mental illness in almshouses, where the costs were less. Other times local officials pressured psychiatric hospitals to discharge patients prematurely if localities were paying for their care (Grob, 1991).

As the number of chronic patients increased, the conflicts that occurred because of the divided responsibility resulted in states assuming full responsibility for cases of mental illness. Local officials then redefined senility as mental illness and transferred poor senile and elderly patients from almshouses to state mental institutions to save even more money. As a result, state psychiatric institutions that had high turnover rates saw those rates decline with the rapid increase of long-term patients. They became institutions largely for custodial care for the aged, as well as for patients with chronic mental illness (Grob, 1991).

After 1945, psychiatrists who were associated with institutional care began to leave psychiatric hospitals and move into community and private practice. They were frequently replaced by international medical graduates with little or no training in psychiatry, and psychiatric hospitals deteriorated. Most psychiatrists in the community treated large numbers of patients with psychological problems and had little contact with the institutionalized persons with mental illness. As the links between psychiatric hospitals and psychiatrists weakened, there was a movement to strengthen outpatient care and community clinics. By the mid-1950s there were over 1,000 outpatient psychiatric clinics, most of which were state supported or state aided (Grob, 1991).

The Move to Deinstitutionalization

The support for community-based care and treatment grew steadily, on the assumption that early treatment could prevent inpatient care and that patients did better with home and family as support. At the same time a growing number of private psychiatric hospitals and psychiatric beds in community hospitals became available for short-term treatment and emergencies. The concept of community care and treatment prevailed, supported by those who did not believe in the concept of mental illness, civil rights advocates who identified people with mental illness as a group deprived of their civil liberties, and social advocates who emphasized that psychiatric hospitals are inherently repressive and dehumanizing (Grob, 1991). The Community Mental Health Act of 1963 strengthened community facilities and weakened the central role psychiatric hospitals played in the treatment of patients with mental illness.

After 1965 a number of factors contributed to the rapid decline in the number of patients in psychiatric hospitals. The introduction of psychotropic drugs enabled patients rendered dysfunctional by illness to control symptoms and function well within the community. The introduction of Medicaid, which paid the cost of nursing-home care for the elderly poor, enabled their transfer from psychiatric hospitals to nursing homes. The transfer of the elderly to nursing homes was encouraged because Medicaid was funded partly by the federal government, and this reduced the cost of elder care for state and local government.

"Prior to 1940, public policy had been focused almost exclusively on the severely and chronically mentally ill. This policy was based on the assumption that society had an obligation to provide such unfortunate persons with both care and treatment in public mental hospitals. The policies adopted during and after the 1960s rested on quite different assumptions" (Grob, 1991). These later policies created a decentralized system of services that separated care and treatment, and often focused on mild mental illness to the detriment of patients who suffered from severe mental illness, and were more difficult to treat.

In 1964, federal legislation provided construction money for community mental health centers to serve deinstitutionalized persons and others who could be treated on an outpatient basis. It was hoped that 2,000 centers would be established to meet the need throughout the nation, but the maximum number never exceeded 700. Very little money was obtained from other sources to staff and operate the centers. The federal government provided matching funds for operational costs for eight years, and after that the funds decreased and the community was to assume the financial responsibility for operational costs. That didn't happen. States were forced to provide funds, but it was not enough. Services were reduced and some centers closed. The separation of care and treatment often resulted in a lack of social services to ensure that patients had their basic living needs covered while they underwent treatment. With decreased funding for community care over time, communities had difficulty providing the volume of care required by the outpatient sector.

Many people with mental illness who lacked sufficient resources and family support experienced what came to be known as the "revolving door" concept. A patient would seek treatment in a short-term inpatient facility. Through the use of psychotropic drugs and intense counseling, the patient would be stabilized and discharged, perfectly capable of functioning in the community. But psychotropic drugs often have significant side effects. After time, as the patient feels better, the side effects become a real burden. Without continued counseling, as community centers became overburdened with many patients, not enough staff, and significant waiting lists for treatment, the patient would discontinue drug therapy. Predictably, the symptoms would recur (psychotropic drugs help control, not cure, mental illness), and the patient would experience an acute episode requiring hospitalization once again. A cyclical pattern would develop—thus the revolving door.

Even with drug therapy, outpatient therapy recognizes that patients will experience difficult periods when more intense care is necessary. Patients can be encouraged to continue drug therapy even when symptoms are minimal (a sign of the effects of the drug) and side effects continue; however, every patient has the right to refuse treatment (drug therapy), and although not desirable, it is understandable why a patient may not want to continue with the drug when symptoms go away.

Although the current state of treatment for mental illness is still largely focused on outpatient care, inpatient facilities remain available in some state institutions, private psychiatric hospitals, and specialized facilities (substance abuse facilities, children's psychiatric centers, etc.). The majority of short-term inpatient care is available through specific units in general hospitals.

Another level of care for mental disorders is partial hospitalization (or intensive outpatient care). Under this framework, patients receive treatment on an intensive basis (medications, individual and group therapy, vocational training, etc.) for some four to eight hours per day, but otherwise they remain in their own homes. This approach is an alternative to residential care, but it is more treatment oriented than regular outpatient care.

Like other areas of the health care sector, the mental health delivery system is undergoing a great deal of change. Managed care, Medicare and Medicaid, and government mandates for health insurance coverage for mental health services have affected the delivery of care—in both positive and negative ways.

CHALLENGES TO MENTAL HEALTH SERVICES DELIVERY TODAY

Mental illness is difficult enough to define; identifying a large segment of the population with mental illness—those with chronic mental illness—is even more difficult. The surgeon general's report (1999) reminds us:

> The fact that many, if not most, people have experienced mental health problems that mimic or even match some of the symptoms of a diagnosable mental disorder tends, ironically, to prompt many people to underestimate the painful, disabling nature of severe mental illness. . . Yet relatively few mental illnesses have an unremitting course marked by the most acute manifestations of illness; rather, for reasons that are not yet understood, the symptoms associated with mental illness tend to wax and wane. These patterns pose special challenges to the implementation of treatment plans and the design of service systems that are optimally responsive to an individual's needs during every phase of illness. (p. 1).

It is estimated that nearly one in five American adults has experienced mental illness of some type. About one in five children and adolescents experience diagnosable disorders in the course of a year, but only about 5 percent of all children experience "extreme functional impairment." In 1996, national expenditures for treatment of mental illness and substance abuse amounted to $79.3 billion. Treatment in community hospitals and psychiatric hospitals accounted for the largest share of expenditures (see Figure 9–1). However, most people receiving treatment live in the community. The Substance Abuse and Mental Health Services Administration reports that among persons receiving specialized hospital, residential, or outpatient care, only 4 percent of patients with mental illness and 2 percent of patients with substance abuse were receiving hospital care (Mark, McKusick, King, Harwood, & Genuardi, 1998).

Community hospitals with separate psychiatric services, private psychiatric hospitals, state and county psychiatric hospitals, and Veterans Adminis-

tration (VA) medical centers provide inpatient treatment services today. There were 653 psychiatric hospitals in the United States in 1997, 17 of which were federal hospitals and 14 of which were institutions for the mentally retarded (Healthcare InfoSource, 1998). Nursing and related care homes are also a major resource for residential care of people with mental illness (see Figure 9–1). Nearly half of the total nursing-home population has been diagnosed with Alzheimer's disease or other forms of dementia.

Few communities have a truly integrated system of treatment and social support for people with mental illness. Managed care's entry into the mental health services market has helped with coordination of medical services but has done little to enhance the types of social services needed by many people who suffer from mental illness. Reports indicate that there are more persons with serious mental illness in street shelters and prisons than in hospitals, largely because of the failure of deinstitutionalization, which resulted in the vast majority of those discharged from mental hospitals not being cared for in the community and drifting into homelessness and destitution (Hilts, 1990).

MENTAL HEALTH SERVICES PROVIDERS

Mental health services are provided by a number of different professionals, as well as in a variety of settings.

Psychiatrists are medical doctors. Like other physicians, they attend four years of medical school after receiving a bachelor's degree, complete one year of a general residency, and then complete a specialty residency. They are licensed by the state and become certified through the American Board of Psychiatry and Neurology, which issues eight types of certification in subspecialty areas such as child and adolescent psychiatry, addiction psychiatry, and forensic psychiatry, and they must be recertified every ten years (American Psychiatric Association, 2000). Psychiatrists prescribe medications and perform medical procedures with emphasis on clinical work, counseling, and research. In 1996 there were over 24,000 psychiatrists in office-based practice, up from 16,000 in 1980 and 20,000 in 1990 (Moskowitz, 1999).

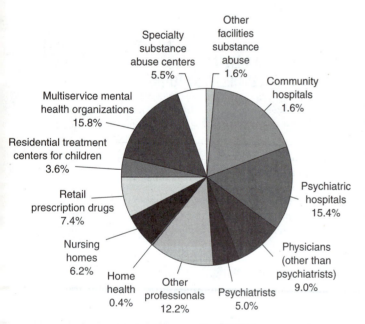

Figure 9–1 Percent Distribution of Mental Health, Alcohol, and Other Drug Abuse Treatment Expenditures by Provider, 1996 (Total=$79.3 billion)

Source: Mark, et al, 1998.

Psychologists are licensed by the states to practice after receiving an academic doctoral degree and completing a minimum of two years of supervised experience in direct clinical service. Licensure is required in all fifty states. Psychologists provide clinical care, counseling, and research. In some states, psychologists have lobbied for the right to prescribe medications, pointing to the new advances in drug therapy for such conditions as depression, anxiety, and addictions, as well as the frequency with which psychologists work with patients dealing with such conditions. Such lobbying efforts contribute to tensions that often exist between psychiatrists and psychologists as they compete for comparable treatment privileges (Moran, 1998).

The psychiatric nurse is trained beyond the RN in caring for the special needs of patients with mental illness. The range of responsibilities of the psychiatric nurse varies with the organization in which the nurse practices and the state in which the organization resides. Some psychiatric nurses conduct independent therapy sessions, while others simply provide nursing services in the psychiatric setting.

Support services are also provided by social workers and counselors. Social workers have a BS or MS degree and work with mental health facilities, providers, and patients to find housing, employment, medical care, and other support services for those in need. Counselors often have "life experience" in a given area of counseling (drug abuse, alcohol abuse, battered spouse syndrome, etc.). Counselors are not licensed by the states, but many are certified in their field. It is up to the person seeking services to inquire about the credentials of the counselor because few states exercise any control. Lack of state control is not an automatic indication of the lack of quality or efficacy of a program.

The twelve-step program, a foundation of Alcoholics Anonymous, has long been recognized as an effective way of dealing with addiction. It is a self-help approach to healing based on support among addicts facing the same or similar problems and does not rely on leadership or facilitation by mental health professionals. Many well-known programs, such as the Betty Ford Center, are based on the foundation of the twelve-step program (although the in-

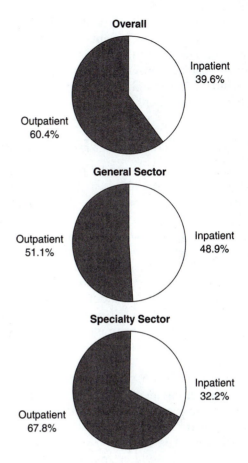

Figure 9–2 Percent of Mental Health, Alcohol, and Other Drug Abuse Treatment Expenditures by Site of Care for Overall, General, and Speciality Sectors, 1996
Source: Mark, et al, 1998.

patient portion of the program includes other therapies). Other addiction treatment programs (drug abuse, codependency, etc.) rely heavily on the principles of the twelve-step approach. Both licensed and unlicensed mental health service providers use the twelve-step approach, and again, it is left to the consumer to determine the credibility of the service.

It is important to remember that mental health services are also provided by the general medical/primary care sector of the health care community (Fig 9–2). Many family physicians provide counseling and medication to their patients with mental health problems, referring the patients to other professionals if and when necessary (Surgeon General, 1999). Community hospitals provide care in specialized units, scattered beds throughout the hospital, emergency rooms, and outpatient clinics.

FUNDING AND EXPENDITURES FOR MENTAL ILLNESS

The government paid for 54.2 percent of the care of patients with mental illness in 1996, including payments through Medicare, Medicaid, the Department of Veterans Affairs, and the Department of Defense, as well as other federal, state, and local government payments. Insurance and patient payments account for the remainder (see Figure 9–3). About 84 percent of total expenditures goes toward treatment of mental illness, while the remainder is spent on treatment of drug and alcohol abuse (see Figure 9–4).

A large portion of treatment for drug abuse takes place in special substance abuse centers, while the majority of alcohol abuse treatment takes place in the general service sector, such as community hospitals. Private-sector payments (45.8 percent of the total) include private insurance, out-of-pocket, and other private payments. Although out-of-pocket expenses decreased from 23 percent in 1986 to 16 percent in 1996, the decrease was not accompanied by an increase in

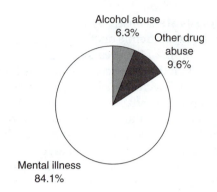

Figure 9–4   Percent of Mental Health, Alcohol, and Other Drug Abuse Treatment Expenditures by Type of Diagnosis, 1996

Source: Mark, et al, 1998.

private insurance payments, which stayed relatively stable over the same period. It is primarily an increase in public funding that is reducing the percentage of out-of-pocket expenses (Mark et al., 1998).

In 1996, almost $6 billion dollars was spent on retail pharmaceuticals for mental health and substance abuse treatment separate from facility expenditures. Only $22 million of the pharmaceutical expenditures was for substance abuse treatment (predominantly alcohol abuse); the remaining expenditures were for antipsychotics, antidepressants, anxiolytics, and other drugs used primarily for mental health treatment (Mark et al., 1998).

Private health insurance has historically been much more restrictive in benefits for mental health services than for medical services. Many people have no coverage at all for mental health services within their health insurance plan. Those that do have coverage experience higher copays and deductibles and lower maximum annual and lifetime payments. Some experience limitations on numbers of visits or numbers of days of treatment. The Mental Health Parity Act of 1996 sought to remedy the disparity in coverage. However, after a great deal of compromise over proposed legislation, the final product made only small inroads toward parity. The act mandates that health plans offering mental health services may not impose lifetime or annual limits on those services different from limits for medical services. However,

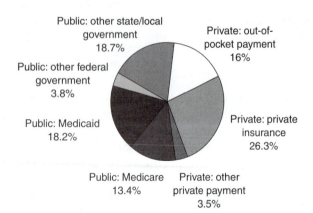

Figure 9–3   Percent of Mental Health, Alcohol, and Other Drug Abuse Treatment Expenditures by Payer, 1996

Source: Mark, et al, 1998.

any plan that can show that its premiums have increased by at least 1 percent because of the requirements can apply for a waiver (Newbould, 1998). In addition, the act does not require employers or health plans to cover or maintain coverage for treatment of mental illness, and benefits for treatment of substance abuse are excluded from the requirements (American Psychiatric Association, 1999). Additional legislation, at both the state and federal levels, has been introduced to expand parity and close loopholes. The legislation includes a call for elimination in differences in the number of inpatient days, number of outpatient visits, copayments, deductibles, and other limitations between medical and mental health benefits (American Psychological Association, 1999; Sullivan, 1997).

The growth of managed care in the medical insurance arena has also been felt in mental health services. Managed care's approach to mental health/mental illness is the case management approach. Persons seeking treatment contact their managed care provider; they are first screened for signs and symptoms and then given a referral to a professional for further screening. The screening process assures treatment at the appropriate level and for a specific term of treatment. The patient pays only a copay for each visit when receiving care from a professional in the network of providers. The approach has been instrumental in containing the costs of mental health treatment. It has, however, created tension among both consumers and providers because of the amount of paperwork required to gain approval for initial and continuing care and because of the limitations on the number of visits allowed.

SUMMARY

Mental health care needs major changes in terms of organization, financing, and services to cope with current realities. The large number of untreated and homeless people with mental illness will continue to remind us of the serious shortcomings of mental health services for a long time to come. A major problem in gaining support for the care and treatment of people with mental illness is that the diagnosis, treatment, and cure are not as precise, certain, and assured as other types of illness—the broken hip, heart disease, or cancer—which can be precisely diagnosed and definitively treated to yield a cure or an alleviation of symptoms or pain. Management of mental illness still has as a large element of simply helping patients live with their condition.

The demand for mental health services far exceeds their availability. Too few centers have been built and too few services have been provided to support the community care movement begun in the 1960s. Managed care has provided access to services formerly unavailable to some. However, many in need still have no access to care. The lack of financial commitment to mental health services by government and private insurance places pressure on mental health providers. The following story exemplifies the struggles faced by many organizations committed to providing mental health services.

IN THE HEALTHCARE COMMUNITY

Methodist Behavioral Health*

The history of Methodist Healthcare, Memphis, Tennessee, starts out somewhat like the history of the Baptist Memorial Health Care Corporation featured in Chapter 1. This should not be surprising, since hospital care was seen as a charitable function at the turn of the twentieth century. John Sherard, a North Mississippi planter, initiated the drive for a Methodist hospital in Memphis after finding his own Methodist pastor receiving charity care in a

(continues)

---

*Information for this case study was obtained through personal interviews with the administrator of Methodist Behavioral Health and the directors of each division described in the case, as well as from organization documents.

(continued)

hospital sponsored by another faith. Sherard understood that growth in the commercial area of Memphis would bring with it an increased need for medical care to a growing population. His determination resulted in the formation of a coalition of Methodist conferences from Memphis, Mississippi, Arkansas, and Alabama to study the feasibility of building a Memphis hospital. Alabama eventually withdrew because of the distance to Memphis, but the remaining coalition members approved the development of the Methodist Hospital in 1909.

This story, however, is not about the development of Methodist Healthcare, but about the struggle to maintain Methodist's commitment to mental health services in a changing healthcare environment. In its early days, mental health services consisted of simply maintaining a psychiatric inpatient unit. Outpatient care was the domain of psychiatrists and psychologists in their private offices. But the standards for mental health services changed drastically beginning in the 1950s, with the focus changing to community-based outpatient care. Methodist Hospital, and Methodist Healthcare, went through changes as government regulation, payment mechanisms, and beliefs about mental health services changed. Once a single unit within the hospital, mental health services expanded to differentiated inpatient units and multiple outpatient services; however, often these services were fragmented and not necessarily coordinated.

Methodist made a commitment to addiction services in the early 1980s. The old Crippled Children's Hospital in Memphis was purchased and opened in 1984 as a residential addiction treatment center, known as Methodist Outreach. A certificate of need approved fifty-five residential alcohol and drug treatment beds. It included facilities for both adults and adolescents, but on separate floors.

Psychiatrists at the Methodist Hospital were against the residential addiction center. They wanted the services provided at the central hospital location, where inpatient psychiatric services included a geriatric unit and a general adult unit. Outpatient services were handled primarily by psychiatrists in their private offices, however, Methodist did establish a family counseling center to provide outpatient services in a location separate from the hospital inpatient facility. The original location has changed as the services have expanded, but the current location has enough room for future expansion.

In 1992–93, the separate units were collapsed into the Behavioral Health division of Methodist Healthcare. In an effort to coordinate care, Methodist Outreach was dissolved and the location became strictly for adult day services. The adolescent services had already been closed in 1990 and moved to the central hospital. Inpatient adult addiction services also moved to the central hospital. The inpatient moves were primarily a result of restrictions on reimbursement. Nationwide, Medicare and Medicaid began to pay less for inpatient services. Government policy had changed the emphasis to outpatient care, believing that community support and the availability of psychotropic drugs made outpatient treatment more appropriate.

Private insurances also limited care with maximum lengths of stay, resulting in sicker patients and denial of payment for care for some patients. Inpatient addiction units that once treated patients over a thirty- to forty-five–day period were now sending patients to rapid detoxification in open psychiatric units. Managed care organizations contracted with hospitals for medical care at predetermined payments. However, mental health services were often carved out separately. Even if a hospital was able to win a managed care contract, it did not necessarily have a mental health contract. The organization was burdened with additional paperwork to bid for mental health services, and that meant providing a full continuum of care at reduced costs. Throughout the process, Methodist Behavioral Health survived because it sees the provision of mental health services as a part of its mission that it is not willing to abandon. Costs have been ratcheted down, but it remains a struggle to provide the full continuum of care under such restrictive payment. The focus on outpatient services has resulted in an increase in recidivism rates. In some cases, deinstitutionalization

(continues)

(continued)

has gone too far with patients with mental illness who are unable to maintain outpatient treatment, ending up on the streets and in jails.

Inpatient units at the central hospital now consist of the open general psychiatric unit and a locked adult unit. The criteria for inpatient care have become more severe. The locked unit is particularly intense, treating patients who are homicidal, suicidal, and very sick. A new unit—a pain clinic for maintenance of opiate treatment, medical management, and medical detoxification—will open in coordination with the adult addiction treatment programs.

In 1995, Methodist Healthcare bought Le Bonheur Children's Medical Center and another family center for children and adolescents. Both inpatient and outpatient child and adolescent services are now housed at the original Le Bonheur location.

Adult Addiction Services

Adult addiction services are now coordinated at the former Methodist Outreach site. Addiction treatment followed the traditional abstinence model based on the concepts of Alcoholics Anonymous.

In the early 1980s, addiction was identified as a chronic disease, but the standard treatment model was acute care. Inpatient length of stay was predetermined as detoxification plus twenty-eight days, following a teaching model—with graduation at completion of the course of treatment. The pattern was similar for adults and adolescents, although handled in separate areas of the facility (two separate floors) and with a longer length of stay for adolescents.

Through a combination of increasingly restrictive reimbursement and a number of high-profile national cases of inappropriate admission/treatment, inpatient adolescent addiction treatment services were significantly reduced throughout the 1980s. Adolescent "substance abuse" was incorporated into general psychiatric inpatient and outpatient services. As a result, in the late 1980s, Methodist Outreach phased out adolescent treatment. The Methodist Outreach location became an adult residential treatment facility, with aftercare groups provided after discharge. About 1990, the facility added partial or day treatment that consisted of all-day care but a return home overnight. Intensive outpatient treatment was also added and consisted of approximately four hours of treatment every day. Depending on their needs, clients were introduced to these modes of outpatient care after their residential treatment period.

Through the mid-1990s, the impact of managed care continued to be felt. Inpatient length of stay declined to less than two weeks, with an increased emphasis on partial hospital and intensive outpatient direct admissions. By the late 1990s, residential inpatient services were no longer financially viable. Residential services were discontinued, with inpatient detoxification incorporated into the open psychiatric unit as a separate treatment "track." The Methodist Outreach campus became an ambulatory site providing a range of flexible day and evening treatment options. Restructuring under the Methodist Behavioral Health model stresses coordination of care from detoxification to outpatient care and the provision of a full range of services while viewing behavioral health as a "product line" that needs to be financially viable.

The adult outpatient addiction center operates with a program director; three addiction disease counselors (degreed and licensed); a small nursing staff; a chaplain (who is also a counselor); and technical, medical, and clerical aids. The facility emphasizes group work with a primary counselor for each individual, and limited family work. The focus is on skill building and therapy and incorporates the twelve-step program. While clinically driven, the typical course of treatment is two weeks of the partial hospital program and/or twenty sessions of intensive outpatient services, followed by aftercare groups for one year after discharge.

Future addiction service plans include transition of inpatient detoxification to a separate twelve-bed behavioral health unit, which will also incorporate a chronic pain specialty "med-psych" track. Relocation of evening outpatient services to an East Memphis location is also planned.

(continues)

(continued)

Inpatient Mental Health Services

Methodist Behavioral Health has a certificate of need for seventy-two beds. The locked unit has twenty-five beds and runs at about a 66 percent occupancy rate. The patient population consists of persons nineteen years and older with major mental health disorders. The average length of stay is 9.2 days, after which patients move to outpatient modes of care. The open unit has twenty-seven beds and runs at an average occupancy rate of 66 percent also. The average length of stay is 7.8 days, after which patients move to other modes of outpatient follow-up.

The staff of the inpatient units consists of clinical psychologists who handle the group and individual therapy, senior mental health specialists (master's-level trained) who do much of the case management, social workers (from the medical social work department of the hospital) who do discharge planning and coordinate family activities, psychiatric nurses, a chaplain, a recreation therapist, and various aids.

Ten years ago the locked unit was more of geriatric than psychiatric unit. The elderly experience change in their mental status such as dementia and Alzheimer's. But elderly patients were eventually moved to nursing homes, and the locked unit changed its focus to intensive care, with clear admissions criteria and prognosis for improvement.

In the early 1980s a consulting management company ran the psychiatric units, but they were still under the nursing department. The hospital and the management company parted ways, but the directors stayed with the unit that remained under the nursing department. Senior administrators of Methodist Healthcare reviewed the mental health services and in the early 1990s combined the inpatient, outpatient, and addiction units into one service directly under Methodist Healthcare administration. By this time the inpatient hospital services had developed into three units: the locked unit, the open unit, and a dual diagnosis unit (mental health addiction). The inpatient services are currently under-

going restructuring to a locked unit, an open adult unit, and a pain management/detoxification/medical management unit.

The inpatient services department also runs a partial hospitalization program (intensive outpatient) for relapse prevention through the Family Health Centers. While the external health care environment seems focused on length of stay, Methodist's mission has a care focus. No patient is turned away, yet finances cannot be ignored.

Children and Adolescent Services

Child and adolescent services are also provided through Methodist Behavioral Health. The inpatient services are provided at the Le Bonheur Children's Medical Center, which joined Methodist Healthcare in 1995 and can accommodate up to fifteen patients at any given time. The service is staffed by a medical director (psychiatrist), an assistant director, a nurse, two psychiatric technicians, and a social worker. Auxiliary staff includes a recreation therapist, teacher, and chaplain. Also provided are day programs, intensive outpatient care, and individual and family counseling—some provided in the medical center and some provided at the family counseling centers. The need for mental health services for children and adolescents crosses all socioeconomic boundaries. Patients come from a centralized intake system (hotline), employee assistance programs, pediatrician referrals, managed care organizations, and the emergency room. Problems treated include depression, anxiety, behavioral problems, psychosomatic illness, major childhood psychiatric disorders, and attention problems. The Center for Children in Crisis provides multidisciplinary services to children and families in which child abuse and/or neglect has occurred or is suspected.

In child and adolescent services, too, budget issues are constant. Insurance is not covering many of the services needed by children and adolescents, or not covering services to the extent they are needed, and yet Methodist/Le Bonheur's mission is to provide care.

ACTIVITY-BASED LEARNING

The trend in mental health services is outpatient treatment. What types of services are available in your community for mental health treatment? For drug addiction? For alcohol addiction?

A QUESTION OF ETHICS

- Review your own health insurance plan. Does it provide mental health benefits? How do the benefits compare to those for medical services? In your opinion, should there be a difference in medical benefits versus mental health benefits?
- Community-based mental health services assume a level of support for the patient by family and friends. Yet many people do not have a personal support system. They cannot or do not adhere to medication regimens, have difficulty maintaining therapy and/or counseling, and so on. Should inpatient, residential care be mandated for those who are unable to maintain outpatient treatment?

REFERENCES

American Psychiatric Association. (1999). *What the new law WILL do and NOT do* [On-line]. Available: http://www.psych.org/pub_pol_adv/prity.html (Accessed November 11, 1999).

American Psychiatric Association. (2000). *What is mental illness?* [On-line] Available: http://www.psych.org/public_info/what_is_mi.html (Accessed April 28, 2000).

American Psychological Association. (1999, May–June). *APA supports full mental health parity bill.* [On-line]. Available: http://www.apa.org/practice/pf/apr99/parity.html (Accessed April 28, 2000).

Grob, G. (1991). The chronically mentally ill in America. In V. Fransen (Ed.), *Mental health services in the United States and England: Struggling for change.* Princeton, NJ: Robert Wood Johnson Foundation.

Healthcare InfoSource. (1998). *Hospital statistics, 1998 Edition.* Chicago: American Hospital Association.

Hilts, P. (1990, September 12). U.S. returns to the 1820s in care of mentally ill, story asserts. *New York Times.*

Mark, T., McKusick, D., King, E., Harwood, H., & Genuardi, J. (1998). *National expenditures for mental health, alcohol and other drug abuse treatment.* Rockville, MD: Substance Abuse and Mental Health Services Administration, U.S. Department of Health and Human Services, Office of Managed Care.

Moran, M. (1998, February 9). New twist in push for prescribing: Ballot initiative. *American Medical News,* pp. 7–8.

Moskowitz, D. (1999). *The 1999 Health care almanac & yearbook.* New York: Faulkner & Gray.

Newbould, P. (1998, February). Federal parity law takes effect. *American Psychological Association* [On-line]. Available: http://www.apa.org/practice/pf/feb98/parity.html (Accessed May 28, 2000).

Pardes, H. (1991). Problems in providing future services to the mentally ill. In V. Fransen (Ed.), *Mental health services in the United States and England: Struggling for change.* Princeton, NJ: Robert Wood Johnson Foundation.

Sullivan, M. (1997, February). State parity and licensure bills activate psychology advocates. *American Psychological Association* [On-line]. Available: http://www.apa.org/practice/pf/feb97/states.html (Accessed April 28, 2000).

U.S. Department of Health and Human Services, (1999). *Mental Health: A Report of the Surgeon General–Executive Summary.* Rockville, MD: U.S. Department of Health and Human Services, Substance Abuse and Mental Health Services Administration, Center for Mental Health Services, National Institutes of Health, National Institute of Mental Health.

CHAPTER
~10~

Managing Care by Managing Information[1]

Chapter Objectives

After completing this chapter, the reader should have an understanding of:

- Why health care organizations feel the need to develop information systems in the clinical setting, particularly a computerized medical record.
- The variety of approaches to information systems in health care.
- The difficulties encountered in adopting and maintaining health information management systems.
- The continuing need to develop health information management systems.

INTRODUCTION

Hospitals and medical practices have long used information systems for business functions such as accounts receivable, accounts payable, payroll, and electronic billing. *Clinical* applications of computerization are not as widespread. Certainly, some organizations use computer systems in specific areas, such as laboratories or patient scheduling, but their use in direct patient care is in early development, and their value has not been established. Variation in clinical practices and rapidly changing technology make standardization (which is required for any good database) difficult. In addition, as one nurse-manager phrased it, "Physicians always refer to an aversion to cookbook medicine—aversion to canned responses." Physicians often view medicine as an art and do not see inputting data into a computer as relevant to treating and caring for patients. One physician involved in the clinical use of computers suggested that not many physicians are sophisticated computer users, and they may not recognize the value of what computers can do to aid in clinical practice.

Attitudes toward health information management systems (HIMS) and specifically toward a computerized patient medical record (CMR) have changed since 1991, when the Institute of Medicine issued a

---

[1]Adapted from and reprinted with permission from *The Journal of Healthcare Information Management*®, vol. 12, no. 4, Winter 1998 © Healthcare Information and Management Systems Society and Jossey-Bass Inc., Publishers.

report suggesting three ways in which computers might help decrease health care costs (Institute of Medicine, Committee on Improving the Patient Record, 1991):

1. Improved information can reduce redundant testing and other services resulting from unavailable or lost results.
2. Administrative costs can be reduced by electronic submission of (reimbursement) claims and automatic reports.
3. The productivity of practitioners can be increased by reducing time spent waiting for missing or unavailable charts, reviewing poorly organized or illegible data, and sifting through redundant data.

Managed care's approach to delivering health care emphasizes case management and so-called cradle-to-grave patient care, providing the incentive for a single, comprehensive, computerized medical record as a natural vehicle for shared information. The paper medical record alone does not facilitate the key tasks of managed care: identifying best practices, coordinating care, ensuring compliance with established clinical pathways (protocols), and getting specialists' feedback to primary care practitioners. Advances in computer hardware and software now make possible an automated medical record that is widely accessible, comprehensive, and up-to-date and is, at the same time, capable of providing analyzable data (Institute of Medicine, Committee on Improving the Patient Record, 1991).

A CMR can enhance communication within and outside the organization. Within organizations, various departments can link order confirmation and test results directly to the patient record. Staff can clarify orders, ask and answer questions regarding patient care, and access resources. Externally, physicians can link with one another and with other facilities to share information about mutual patients. Providers can link with payers and vice versa. Coordinated care avoids duplicated efforts on the part of the patient and providers, and it decreases response time to patient care needs.

In clinical applications, HIMS must be able to meet diverse technical information–processing requirements, as well as diverse user needs. Organizations take varied approaches toward integrating HIMS into their operations, as shown in the following four examples: a midwestern *university health system*, a northeastern regional rural health system (*small rural health system*), a northeastern urban teaching health system (*urban health system*), and a northeastern statewide rural health system (*large rural health system*). The university and urban health systems developed the core of their CMRs internally (the "build" option). Both the small and large rural systems purchased vendor packages (the "buy" option). All four organizations have long-term plans of computerizing both inpatient and ambulatory patient records. However, the large rural health system began its approach with the ambulatory record, whereas the other three organizations began with inpatient records and expanded to ambulatory care. The variation in systems and approaches is the focus of this chapter.

CONTENT OF THE COMPUTERIZED MEDICAL RECORD

Although all of the organizations involved in this report do have computerized clinical records, the extent of the patients' records and the specific content area in the clinical applications vary greatly.

University Health System

The university health system began internal development of the CMR with its inpatient nursing documentation. Historically, everything that a nurse or nursing assistant did was written out in longhand and was available to care providers in the patient's chart. A small group of nursing staff responsible for

---

(Three of the organizations providing information for this chapter were conducted for a 1997 report by the Keystone Research Center entitled *Technology and Industrial Performance in the Service Sector*. The fourth is from other research.)

information systems development within the department started developing nursing documentation with a manual precursor to computer documentation (by first developing standards for handwritten documentation). Charting went from longhand narratives to "charting by exception," using flow sheets to check things off and write in values, and adding narratives only if something abnormal happened. The manual standards helped establish that there was very little unusual documentation that could not be translated into computerized values. The staff then worked to analyze needs and communicate them to programmers. Nursing orders—documentation of how the patient's plan of care was carried out, what was done, how it was done, and when it was done—were redesigned to fit a computer format. The staff started with about 3,000 orders, which they consolidated and organized into a system of core orders and subsets, producing a final set of 300 orders.

Every nursing unit in the university health system has access to all 300 orders in the system. When a nurse signs on to the CMR, the nurse can choose a category called "unit specific," which, as the name suggests, has orders that are specific to that hospital unit. All patients admitted have groups of orders specific to their condition or problem. If the nurse needs orders that are not part of the unit-specific list, he or she can retrieve the orders needed from the full list of 300. Patients with similar problems now have the same groups of orders, regardless of the unit in which they are treated. That was not always true with the paper medical record system.

Ultimately, the goal at the university health system is to include care plans (clinical pathways or guidelines) in the CMR as a guideline for care. Manual care plans are now being used in some areas, and others are in various stages of development. As a means of monitoring the quality of health care that the patient receives, case managers monitor variance of care actually received from that outlined in the care plan. Variance is not necessarily bad; it opens discussion among providers to help determine best practice and fine-tune systems or care plans. Computerizing care plans and nursing care (orders) will enhance variance tracking and systems modification.

Small Rural Health System

Clinical applications of HIMS at the small rural health system also began with inpatient nursing documentation. The small rural health system, however, purchased a software package (from one of many software developers working with health care–specific products). The health care system did not have the resources for and never really considered internally developing software. For the small rural health system, installing an on-line documentation system actually meant taking the paper-based nursing documentation, designing it for the computer (whereas the university health system could communicate its documentation needs to software programmers), and implementing it across the facility. The software does have some flexible features, however. Before implementation, people who were advocates of computerization were recognized throughout the organization, and advocates from each department helped design the flexible aspects.

The move to on-line documentation meant reevaluating documentation throughout the system. Forms used in the clinics were reviewed for commonalities so that information needed for different areas of the organization did not have to be repeated in a whole set of questions for the patient. During trial and "playtime," users helped develop many aspects of the system, but improving the flow was a more practical approach than any quantifiable measures of what takes less time, is more effective, and so on.

Like the university health system, the small rural health system moved to a charting-by-exception mode only, documenting things in the chart that were outside normal parameters. In the computerized charting and assessment module, the screen can be customized to a particular unit, the types of problems the unit nurses see most often, and the type of care they render. It does not allow for redesigning the basic screens, but it allows modification of choices on the screen. All entries (responses) can be coded as an assessment, intervention, outcome, or variance. Analysis can be done on the basis of the coding and the question. HIMS staff discourages the use of text because it is not analyzable, but text entry is an available option (the system can drop into the word-processing software WordPerfect™ for text entry). Before a nursing shift change, a printout of the current nursing notes is placed at the patient's bedside on a clipboard. A daily summary of the nursing notes is printed and placed in the permanent paper record once a day.

The small rural health system chose software from another vendor (different from the system used for nursing documentation) for its outpatient centers that it will gradually implement at individual ambulatory care sites, the first of which is a two-physician primary care site. The specifics of which components of the medical record are to be placed on-line and who will enter the information were to be determined. Physicians interviewed, however, spoke of being able to access referrals, medical records, and test and consultation results from their offices within and outside the hospital.

Urban Health System

Like the university health system, the urban health system developed the software for its patient record internally. The content, however, is quite different. The urban health system started with an order-entry system to communicate and receive results of laboratory tests, radiological studies, medication orders, and other ancillary services.

The urban health system staff saw two deficiencies in the way physicians in particular processed information. First, physicians could not remember everything, and second, they did not always remember things at the moment of impact. The staff saw information technology as a communication and notification mechanism and as a "clinical assistant" to the physician (Bates, Kuperman, & Teich, 1994).

At the urban health system, residents write most orders (16,000 on an average day, about half of them drug orders). Order entry began as an effort to reduce the errors that inevitably affect paper-based orders (e.g., when a nurse or pharmacist misreads or misinterprets the physician's handwriting, or when the transcription is faulty). An additional goal of the system was to streamline the work process, replace the flow of paper with computer communications, and allow physicians to write orders remotely.

The order-entry system provides interactive warnings and reminders to physicians and has led to reductions not only in adverse drug events but also in the prescription of ineffective and unnecessarily expensive drugs. The system issues reminders of alternative therapies or tells the physician that for one reason or another the order is not a good idea. Warnings and reminders exist for laboratory tests, radiography, and even repeated surgery. Much of the value of the system is in the timing. Warnings and reminders pop up when the physician is placing the order, permitting immediate modification.

The HIMS staff at the urban health system also developed programs to help track inpatients and match them with the provider responsible for their care. The system allows hospital staff to identify the attending physician when families make inquiries into the patient's care, allows notification to primary care physicians when patients arrive at the emergency room for care, and also is a mechanism to identify providers responsible for signing incomplete orders in the medical record.

Large Rural Health System

Like the small rural health system, the large rural health system purchased a software package when it approached a computerized patient medical record. Unlike the other three sites, the large rural health system began its CMR efforts in its ambulatory care sites. The CMR encompasses all aspects of the medical record and is designed eventually to replace the paper system. It is also designed to link with other computerized functions, such as patient scheduling, laboratory systems, and demographics/billing functions. The large rural health system implemented the CMR in selected pilot sites (several sites ranging from two-physician to seven-physician practices were on-line at the time of this report) in an effort to determine a protocol for systemwide implementation. Although going paperless is a long-term goal, it is not a primary consideration in the early implementation sites.

The CMR system chosen by the large rural health system is graphical and allows users to "point and click" but also requires keyboard of patient information (data) entry. Screens document the results of nurses' examinations (including the reason for the visit, vital signs, and so on), physician encounters (progress notes), orders (laboratory tests, medications, radiological studies, referrals), and patient history (family history, social history, allergies, medications, immunizations). The system provides warnings for drug allergies and drug interactions and reminders for continuous care (both chronic and preventive care), but both warnings and reminders are highly dependent on the availability of an accurate patient history in the system.

Both nursing examination and physician encounter screens contain a combination of data fields for systematic entry and text area for preformatted or free-form text. Preformatted text capabilities facilitate the incorporation of clinical pathways into the CMR system. Only a physician can "close" an encounter, and once closed, the encounter cannot be modified. Additional notes must be entered through an addendum to the record. Closing the encounter requires entry of procedure and diagnosis codes. Various printouts can be generated if documentation is to become part of the paper medical record or if records are requested for other providers not on the CMR system.

One of the long-term goals is to allow each of the large rural health system's ambulatory sites to link to one another and to the main campus. Patients would then be able to move throughout the health care system with one comprehensive medical record. Providers would have immediate access to all care received by their patients within the system. Security levels ensure that providers not involved in a patient's care would not have access to that patient's information. The systemwide record, however, is not one of the immediate results of implementation because there are over sixty ambulatory sites to be converted on an incremental basis and inpatient documentation may require a different software system.

DATA ENTRY

Just as the content of the CMR varies between organizations, the "who, when, and where" of data entry differs across facilities.

University Health System

At the university health system, terminals are at the bedside for easy access by the clinician in about half the patient rooms. Terminals are also in other service areas where paper documentation was previously done. The goal is to have terminals in every room. Nursing documentation is printed from the computer and placed in the paper record once a day for a permanent medical record. Development and reorganization of the nursing orders is an ongoing process as feedback is received from users and new functions are added to the system. Although nurses do the actual data entry, physicians can view the nursing notes on-line. The physicians' progress notes are not currently on-line.

Nurses received formal classroom training before implementation, as well as support during it. The implementation process was really controlled. The staff initially did some electronic charting and some paper charting. The thinking was that if problems arose, it would be easier to fix them on a small number of patients than to correct something on a whole unit.

Anxiety was high; almost everyone felt somewhat intimidated by the computer, but most were able to learn that there was nothing they could do to the computer that the HIMS people could not undo. The anxiety may not have been only computer anxiety; this was a whole new way of charting, in addition to a move to a computer system. In postimplementation observation, nurses indicated what they did not like about the system. However, when asked if they would want to go back to the manual system, only a small minority said yes. They recognized problems but did not want to eliminate the system.

Small Rural Health System

Each patient room at the small rural health system is equipped with a lockbox containing a laptop computer. Additional computer terminals are also available at the nurses' station, where nurses may enter information rather than at the bedside if they prefer. The system appears to be menu driven and focuses on lists. It is not a highly graphical system or a so-called point-and-click system, and it does not appear to be particularly easy to use.

The information systems department conducts training for use of the nursing notes. One nurse manager mentioned that getting nurses comfortable with computer use is not as big an issue as it once was because the small rural health system has had information systems in various degrees since the early 1980s. Training for the nursing notes system takes place in the units as systems are implemented, but it also becomes an ongoing process as new staff members join the hospital.

Because the small rural health system has limited resources, formal evaluation of the system on a cost benefits level is impossible. A registered nurse, talking about his experience with the system, believed that it takes him longer to do data entry because he does not know how to type; nevertheless, he did not appear to be strongly averse to using the system. The amount of time spent on computer documentation rather than paper documentation seems to depend on the user, as does the quality of the documentation. As the medical director observed, "Most reports indicate that computers don't necessarily save time and money, but at the same time everyone who uses them can't imagine going back to a manual system."

Urban Health System

The order-entry system at the urban health system requires direct data entry by the ordering physician. At first, many physicians resisted the system. The HIMS staff tried to be responsive to user needs by addressing reasonable requests for changes or corrections and by having staff available to offer help and give hints to ease system use. It is important to remember, however, that the primary users of the system are residents—hospital employees in relatively subordinate positions who are somewhat powerless to change administrative decisions.

Nurses receive about three hours of training on any new system being placed. New hires are given training during their orientation activities. Physicians get an hour of training but are given the option to spend more time through open sessions that allow more individual practice with the system. One information systems nurse described the system as "designed to be intuitive, so not much training is neces-

sary" but also said that she would like to see more time devoted to training.

Formal analysis indicates that the urban health system has experienced significant cost savings by preventing adverse patient reactions to drugs and by reducing the number of orders for ineffective or unnecessarily expensive drugs. However, some physicians claim that they now spend an extra ten to twenty minutes a day in the hospital because of order-entry requirements. No one seems to doubt that nurses, pharmacists, and clerical workers spend less time tracking down physicians to verify incomplete or illegible orders than in the past, but these areas have not been systematically studied.

Large Rural Health System

The CMR system adopted by the large rural health system requires direct data entry by all personnel, including clinicians. Physician data entry is by far the most controversial of the issues surrounding implementation. Even for those clinical personnel who are computer savvy and proficient typists, documentation in the system appears to take longer than handwritten or dictated notes. Reaction by physicians to the use of computer terminals in the examination room is somewhat mixed. Some find it intrusive and do most of their documentation outside the examination room; others use it to share information with their patients (Barsukiewicz, 1998).

Implementation is in the early stages, and it remains to be seen if long-term experience with the system will alleviate some of the time demands inherent in system use. Training started with formal classes two to four weeks before implementation. All staff—clerical, clinical support, and physicians—receive training on all aspects of the CMR, even though the live setting would limit access to certain areas determined by job description. Training involves scenarios emulating actual patient encounters, as well as structured moves through various screens. Before the implementation date, dress rehearsals attempt to provide a more realistic concept of how the system works. Support training staff is on-site for two to three weeks during the implementation period. Plans for ongoing training for new personnel and for upgrades in the system are determined on an as-needed basis and are not yet formalized as a training strategy.

IMPACT ON COST AND QUALITY ANALYSIS

Cost and quality analysis is highly dependent on the data available for analysis. Comparing data within an organization over time or between organizations requires standardization of input (information available for comparison). Although there seems to be a universal belief that HIMS can control and access data, the approach toward data capture (what information will be entered into the computer and in what format) varies greatly across organizations. Each of the approaches holds promise for a more comprehensive medical record that may enhance the quality of care for the patient. Adoption of HIMS thus far, however, leaves little evidence of a health care delivery system universally moving closer to comparable cost containment data and outcomes measurement data. (See Chapter 11 for more information on outcomes analysis.) Although technologically capable of handling the array of information generated by health care organizations, information systems still present difficulties not easily handled by all organizations, especially those with limited in-house information systems staff.

Each organization made a choice between building its own system or buying a vendor system as prepackaged software, and each had its own reasons for the decision it made. During an interview, one chief information officer (CIO) offered the following reasons for his organization's decision to develop software internally:

- The organization's people believed they could do it better.
- Internal development confers competitive advantage. If other health care institutions buy vendor systems, they have no way of differentiating themselves through their information systems.
- Vendor systems often fail to deliver the promised performance.
- If you do it yourself, you learn from the process and build on the experience.

Although organizations may want to provide quality measures that are directly comparable with those of others, the desire to have some sort of competitive edge from computer applications is an obstacle in the trend toward universal computerization. But competition is not the only reason why organizations seem to be reinventing the wheel. Not all are at the same starting point. Some have various components of clinical information systems in place and are not starting from scratch. Over time, organizations build up certain conventions—for example, for patient identification and documentation requirements—and they continue down that path. Developing software that allows for those unique conventions or trying to change those conventions are equally difficult projects.

Whether implementing internally developed or vendor-provided software, organizations emphasize systems that are user-friendly. That term often implies the use of some graphics, minimal training requirements, and flexibility to allow easy transition from a manual system. Flexibility is often the number one criterion for organizations choosing software and the number one sales point for vendors marketing their software. Yet too much flexibility contributes to the difficulties in analyzing data for true outcomes analysis. More than one of the systems discussed here allow flexibility in the way data are entered or the way screens are presented. Although certain aspects of the system may be structured for data retrieval, such as vital signs or laboratory or medication orders, progress notes remain the least structured aspect of the systems. In fact, in all but one case, physician progress notes are not part of the system. Yet progress notes may contain truly valuable information about the patient's outcomes or cost of treatment.

Some organizations incorporated *International Classification of Diseases*, ninth revision (ICD-9) and *Current Procedural Terminology* (CPT-4) coding into their physician documentation processes (Krall, Chin, Dworkin, Gabriel, & Wong, 1997); others advocate using Systematized Nomenclature of Medicine (SNOMED) (Weber, 1997); and ICD-10 is on the horizon as a new standard for billing. Nursing does not have a standard language similar to the diagnosis and procedure codes used in medicine. Indeed, nursing care is often completely invisible in current health care payment policies and outcomes analysis. Nursing classification systems are currently under development at a number of major research sites, and it is difficult to project when one system may be adopted universally (Delaney, Mehmert, Prophet, & Crossley, 1994; Prophet, 1994).

A remaining concern is cost. There are questions about whether major HIMS implementation is worth the dollars invested. Each of the organizations presented here admitted to difficulties involved in "justifying" their HIMS investments. The CIO of the urban health system described administration as willing to support and encourage HIMS development. Gains are seen in cost, efficiency, accuracy, and quality, but management decisions are made on the basis of evaluation combined with "gut reaction." One CIO said, "As a member of the executive team, I have a responsibility to lay out what it is going to take to have the information management capabilities that I think they need. And yet it's a huge price tag at a time when they are thinking about reducing everything else. In order to come up with it [dollars], they have to pull it out of someone else's pocket and that's tough."

Few health care organizations have the resources to conduct the research that helps determine the value of HIMS implementation. The CIO of the university health system stated, "In order to get administration to spend more, I have to prove that what they've spent so far is worthwhile, but they won't give me the staff to really look at that." The hard numbers are therefore difficult to get. Much of the decision making about values gained must come from anecdotal accounts or from generalizing research results from other institutions to the local setting.

SUMMARY

Health care organizations adopt health information management systems to manage the large amount of data available in the patient medical record. The computerized medical record, however, must be more than a mirror image of the paper record to yield analyzable data necessary to answer the consumer's questions about cost and quality of care. Although organizations strive to achieve standardization of medical recording required for analysis, they must also be attuned to factors necessary to achieve user comfort with entering information into the computerized record. The closer organizations move to ease of conversion to computerized medical records, the further they may be moving away from data integrity—standardized input of information to make it comparable within and across organizations. What is more, the optimal balance point between flexible systems and standardized entry may be different for each organization.

While a CMR eliminates costs involved in locating medical records and makes the records accessible to more than one person and/or department at a time, it brings with it many questions. Is the cost of the CMR justifiable? Is the CMR more or less confidential than a paper medical record? Does the CMR standardize information so much as to lose personalized information that is often valuable to the physician in developing a strong physician-patient relationship and therefore more individualized care? These are questions that cannot be addressed in this text but are vital for further study.

The following story is another organization's experience with computerization. This time, the organization provides strictly outpatient care; it is a group medical practice.

IN THE HEALTH CARE COMMUNITY

Esse Health: The Essence of Health Care*

Esse Health is an independent physician practice with over sixty-five physicians and twenty locations in the St. Louis area. Physicians from two parent organizations, Health Key Medical Group and Beacon Health Care, formed Esse in 1996. Their goal was to strengthen their ability to deal with the insurance industry and manage the care of their patients without a high degree of outside intervention.

Esse Health has long had a commitment to state-of-the-art information systems. While many medical groups, large and small, have invested in computerized systems to do billing, financial management, and scheduling, few actually formed information systems (IS) departments. Most medical practices purchase software systems developed by vendors specializing in health care applications and rely heavily on those vendors for maintenance and upgrades of their computers with little, if any, thought of data management.

Organizations owned or managed by corporate structures, such as managed care organizations or integrated health systems, have felt the pressures of cost control and addressed these pressures through utilization review and the establishment of best practices. It is the corporate entity, however—not the physician practice—that invests in information systems to gather such data. Although physicians have remained aware of the need to demonstrate the quality of their services, independent practices have been limited in developing better information systems by the costs of equipment and personnel and their limited capital resources. Esse Health, however, wanted to take its own steps toward data management—steps that would allow physicians (rather than managed care corporations or utilization review panels) to define best practices and provide evidence of quality health care delivery. The process would begin with the collection and analysis of data regarding their own patients' care.

The data management process began with the development of an information systems department. Initially, Esse Health linked practices together for centralized services, including billing and insurance contracting. In 1997 the group connected all physicians with e-mail and provided Internet access. The long-range plan, however, included plans for an electronic medical record (EMR). The EMR would open doors to data analysis but would provide other advantages as well:

- More legible and organized patient records
- Immediate access to the records
- Sharing of information with patients and other providers
- Reduction of medical errors

Esse Health works with a variety of payers—from fee-for-service payers, preferred providers, and HMOs to fully capitated plans. Although the group's initial software system managed this variety of billing processes, it fell short on accounts receivable follow-up. The system also was not Y2K compatible. The selection criteria for an EMR vendor included a solid financial management component as well. Computer-based appointment scheduling, another feature of the existing system, was an additional requirement for any new system.

Because Esse Health manages fully capitated contracts, the group focused on data needed for outcomes management (how the patient responds to specific treatment). Because the full capitation included outpatient medications, research on medication efficacy would help control costs. Esse Health hired research pharmacists (PharmD's) to act as consultants to the physicians and to pursue grants from pharmaceutical companies for drug trials and outcomes research. In 1998, Esse Health established the Esse Research Institute to pursue these objectives.

The search for EMR software was not without risk. Esse had one false start in narrowing the field to two vendors—having one drop out, and then

(continues)

*Information for this case study was obtained through personal interviews with the administrator and physicians of Esse Health and from organization documents.

(continued)

dealing with a fair amount of unresponsive behavior from the remaining vendor. The organization chose to "start over" by looking at a vendor that had not previously been considered. The selected vendor was a new company, and Esse knew the risks: to suffer through testing the system in order to have greater input into modifications and upgrades. It was a risk Esse was willing to take.

As in all other organizations, the change to an EMR at Esse Health has not been easy, and it is by no means total and complete. While all sites have been wired and equipped, each site and each physician within the sites make use of the EMR to a varied degree. A pilot site for the initial implementation of the EMR was determined by the location's size and the attitude of that location's personnel. This was not going to be an easy task, and it was important to start with those who were most willing to deal with a high level of frustration in the beginning stages. Dr. Charles Willey, the current president of the organization, reduced his clinic hours in order to lead the EMR efforts. His clinic location was also the first to implement the EMR, although that was not the initial plan.

Preparation for the EMR included a needs assessment; an overview of the existing processes, staffing, and office layout; and training. Physicians receive one-on-one training; staff members receive group training. Records preparation includes summarizing the existing paper record and transferring pertinent information into the EMR system. This was, as in other case reports, the most difficult of the issues faced in EMR implementation. Time is a critical issue. Physicians and other health care providers have faced increasing pressures to work with their patients in a timely manner, provide personalized care, and yet be as efficient and productive as possible. The time required to convert the patient's paper record into the electronic format is significant. Dr. Willey found himself working evenings and weekends to accomplish the transition—not a desirable prospect for any physician when faced with the desire to implement the EMR.

The EMR's scanning capability has been helpful. Information from outside sources (referrals, diagnostic tests, etc.) can be integrated with the data entered in-house. Although the scanning quality was questionable at early stages, Esse's input to the vendor improved the process and quality. The convenience of having medical information "at one's fingertips" is a significant advantage in triaging the patient. Nurses staffing the telephones can view the patient's information at a moment's notice and advise the patient or contact the physician accordingly.

Flexibility has also been a key feature of the system and the organization's approach to implementation. Dr. Willey has chosen to have computer terminals in each of his exam rooms, where he directly views and inputs data. Other physicians have chosen to view and enter data at centrally located terminals outside the exam room. The EMR system allows exam information to be added to templates (more organized, retrievable data) or to be transcribed from dictation and uploaded to the EMR. Some physicians do their own input of orders (requests for tests, medications, etc.); others ask their medical assistants to do the input.

In the brief one and a half years since Esse Health began its conversion to an EMR, technological advances have changed the way doctors and patients deal with information. In the early months of 2000, some physicians in the group began "beta testing" a handheld device to enter data into the EMR. Originally conceived and developed by Esse Health's leaders as a method for managing prescription drug costs in fully capitated contracts, this device is rapidly developing into an integral component of the EMR. By adding decision support software, the handheld device makes it more convenient for physicians to enter diagnoses and drug information. Esse Health, working with the Pearl software company Medpearl.com, plans to expand the capabilities of the handheld device into ordering laboratory tests and capturing other data.

Conversion to an EMR at Esse Health is by no means total. There is additional work to be done in interfacing the in-house laboratory information. There is much work to be done in building Web site capability for interaction with patients, allowing

(continues)

(continued)

patients to view their own information while maintaining data integrity and confidentiality. There is also much to be done in working within the diverse culture of an independent medical practice. Not all physicians are committed to the EMR implementation at this time. Some use portions of the system; others use none, waiting for the "bugs" to be worked out before taking the plunge.

A paperless medical practice within and across sites is a long way into the future for Esse Health. However, Esse has made the commitment and is seizing a leadership role in using technology to advance the quality of health care delivery.

ACTIVITY-BASED LEARNING

• Use your favorite Web browser to locate software companies marketing computerized medical record systems. Work your way through two or three of the Web sites to learn more about their particular CMR systems. Do the sites have a demonstration or at least a view of some of the screens available? What is your opinion of the system(s)? Would you find the CMR a useful way of documenting medical records?

• Do any of the health care organizations in your area use a CMR? Try to arrange to see a demonstration of how it is used.

A QUESTION OF ETHICS

• Given the focus of cost containment in health care delivery, is it appropriate for health care organizations to be spending millions of dollars on acquiring, adopting, and maintaining computerized medical record systems?

• Consider the paper medical record in any health care organization—its storage, access to care providers, and source of your medical information. Is it more, or less, confidential than a proposed computerized medical record? What steps should be taken to ensure the confidentiality of a medical record? How accessible should a patient's medical record be to payers of health care services, providers of health care services, and the patient whose information it contains?

References

Barsukiewicz, C. (1998). *Computerized medical records: Physician response to new technology.* Unpublished doctoral dissertation, Pennsylvania State University.

Bates, D., Kuperman, G., & Teich, J. (1994). Computerized physician order entry and quality of care. *Quality Management in Health Care,* 2(4), 18–27.

Delaney, C., Mehmert, M., Prophet, C., Crossley, J. (1994). Establishment of the research value of nursing minimum data sets. In S. J. Grobe and E. S. P. Playter-Wenting (Eds.), *Nursing informatics: An international overview for nursing in a technological era.* (pp. 169–173). Amsterdam: Elsevier.

Institute of Medicine, Committee on Improving the Patient Record. (1991). *The computer-based patient record: An essential technology for health care.* Washington, DC: National Academy Press.

Keystone Research Center. (1997). *Technology and industrial performance in the service sector* (field research report). Washington, DC: U.S. Department of Commerce, Technology Administration Office of Technology Policy.

Krall, M., Chin, H., Dworkin, L., Gabriel, K., and Wong, R. (1997). Improving clinician acceptance and use of computerized documentation of coded diagnosis. *The American Journal of Managed Care,* 3(4), 597–601.

Prophet, C. (1994). Nursing interventions classification (NIC). In S. J. Grobe and E. S. P. Playter-Wenting (Eds.), *Nursing informatics: An international overview for nursing in a technological era,* (pp. 692–696). Amsterdam: Elsevier.

Weber, J. (1997). Improving health care through clinical documentation. *Healthcare Information Management,* 11(2), 59–66.

CHAPTER

11

New Approaches to Health Care Delivery

Chapter Objectives

After completing this chapter, the reader should have an understanding of:

- The importance of quality of care.
- The need for outcomes measurement.
- Innovative approaches that organizations take to address issues of quality of care and outcomes measurement.
- The challenges that health care delivery organizations continue to face.

INTRODUCTION

The discussion of quality of health care services is evident in every aspect of health care delivery. Although we would all hope that quality has always been at the forefront of concern, we are more aware of quality when working in an environment of very strong cost containment. Is it possible to provide high-quality care while striving to reduce the costs of health care delivery? The managed care market rose to the forefront because of its promise to deliver care cost-effectively without reducing quality. Certainly,

the fee-for-service environment and cost-plus reimbursement mechanism for reimbursing hospitals fostered a system that paid little attention to efficiencies. However, spending more money does not automatically translate into higher quality of care. Therefore, greater efficiency *could be applied* to reduce costs while still maintaining the quality of care provided. However, quality is an intangible. Because it is difficult to define, it is difficult to measure, yet measuring quality has been the thrust of health care policy in recent years.

MEASURING OUTCOMES TO DEFINE QUALITY

In the 1980s, Dr. Aredis Donabedian made a significant impact on the discussion of quality in health care. Donabedian's model of quality specifies three criteria: structure, process, and outcomes (Donabedian, 1980). *Structure* focuses on the attributes of the setting. The facilities and equipment must be adequate in size and safety. The human resources should include a good patient-provider ratio, certified providers, and continuous training. The organization should have a functional structure of goals and communication, and a solid financial base.

191

Process focuses on the delivery of care. Medical care should be delivered within certain standards of care following medical guidelines and should be properly documented as delivered. The comfort of the patient, both physically and emotionally, should be considered. More closely tied to the patient are the *outcomes* measures, including patient status, patient satisfaction, and population status.

Evaluating structure and process is less problematic than evaluating outcomes. From the perspective of the provider, quality of care may be measured by the appropriateness of the care provided and the technical skill with which it is provided. From the consumer's perspective, the concern is the interaction with the health care professional, particularly regarding the amount of information received about the medical treatment considered. From the perspective of a health care plan (or the employer purchasing a plan), the concern is the health of the population and access to care (Blumenthal, 1996b).

Variation in the process and outcomes of medical practice has long been the norm because of the complexity of medicine and the complexity of the conditions with which each patient may present. New advances in clinical epidemiology and in computer technology, however, have spawned the opportunity to learn from variation and determine those processes that produce the best outcomes defined as patient status (Blumenthal, 1996a). It is now possible to accumulate and analyze multiple types of data from billing records, patient encounters, and even computerized medical records. Such data will make it possible to identify the variations in practice that provide the best outcomes (Blumenthal, 1996a).

In the short term, outcomes measurement provides health plans and employers with information regarding hospital performance and, in some cases, individual physician performance. Outcomes measurement in the long term may provide more standardized care. Consumers will have access to information on the appropriate regimen of care for a specific group of common afflictions. Variations will still exist, mainly because of the variations in patients' conditions (age, comorbidities, lifestyle, etc.). However, patients will be more informed about options for care and about the expected outcomes of each option.

One of the first efforts to collect and disseminate data reflecting health care provider quality and service effectiveness was the creation in 1986 (through the Health Care Cost Containment Act) of the Pennsylvania Health Care Cost Containment Council (PHC4). From its data collection efforts, PHC4 has published reports for the public that compare hospital performance on specific medical procedures (Pennsylvania Health Care Cost Containment Council, 1992). For example, a report on open-heart surgery may contain such information as number of cases performed, expected mortality rate, actual mortality rate, length of stay, and average cost per case. The report allows consumers to compare their local area hospitals and to ask questions prior to admission to a hospital for that particular condition or disease.

On a national level, the National Committee for Quality Assurance (NCQA) was created in 1991 to accredit and review health maintenance organizations. Through its process of evaluating HMOs, it provides objective information on sixty measures in the areas of quality, access to care and patient satisfaction, membership and utilization of services, financial performance, and general management for over 450 HMOs (Prager, 2000). The data come largely from the Health Plan Employer Data and Information Set (HEDIS), created by employers and health plans to standardize information for comparative purposes. Although this information consists of performance data regarding HMOs, it says much about the providers who are part of the HMO network. HMOs are compared for their childhood vaccination rates, diabetic eye exam rates, use of beta-blocker treatment after heart attack, postpartum visits after a live birth, asthma control, cholesterol screening, and so on.

Outcomes are important measures for employers to consider when choosing health plan options for their employees and important measures for consumers to consider when choosing a health care provider. However, outcomes are not the only measure of quality.

SERVICE AS A QUALITY MEASURE

Standardized treatment makes it more difficult for health care providers to differentiate themselves in a competitive environment. Certainly, in very specialized care, some providers come to mind almost immediately. Sloan-Kettering Cancer Center, Johns Hopkins Hospital, and the Mayo Clinic are but a few of the names that most of us readily recognize. However, not all of us have access to these specialized centers because either geographic location or our personal situation does not lend itself to seeking treatment at such institutions. Most of us choose from a more local selection of providers. If all hospitals provide nearly the same spectrum of care (general surgery, diagnostic imaging, laboratory tests, therapies) with similar health outcomes, what criteria help determine the hospital we choose? If all physicians follow similar protocols for care, how do we choose a particular physician? Health care providers are beginning to pay more attention to *how* they provide treatment—not just the treatment itself—and have become more aware of the service component of health care delivery as a means of attracting patients in a competitive environment.

The Service Component of Physician Practices

Prior to the 1980s, when there was little recognition of competition among physicians, medical offices and clinics often operated on a schedule convenient to the physicians rather than the patients. Patients often found themselves taking time off from work or taking their children out of school to accommodate the office hours of the practitioner. Competition has changed much of that. Physicians' offices are now open longer hours to provide evening and sometimes weekend appointments. Amenities such as convenient parking, proximity to referral physicians, on-site laboratories, and prescription dispensing have become the norm for medical practices—all as a service to the patient. Comfortable waiting rooms, patient education materials, television, playrooms, and a wide variety of magazines await the patient's arrival.

Perhaps the largest service incentive, however, has been the focus on quality management. Employees now go through continuous quality improvement seminars to learn to *service* patients rather than treat patients. Management, too, learns to work with, rather than supervise, employees. Mentoring, nurtur-

ing, encouraging creativity and autonomy, and encouraging personal growth are tools that managers learn as leadership skills to build a better environment for employees in health care organizations. As management learns to treat employees in a more caring and involved manner, staff learns to treat patients in a more caring manner.

Chapter 10 provided information on how health care organizations are implementing computer systems, and computerized medical records (CMRs) in particular, to streamline medical record keeping and to provide comprehensive information regarding patient care. The CMR, however, also offers a new opportunity for service to patients through links to patient education. The physician, on the basis of a particular patient's diagnosis, can link to appropriate Web sites or internal files to print information that the patient can take home. The educational material may include important follow-up instructions, background information on a particular illness/disease, and important notes on preventing recurrence and/or further progression of the problem. Patients, who often find verbal instructions and information overwhelming at the time of an encounter with the physician, find the take-home materials invaluable (Barsukiewicz, 1998; Watson, 2000). The CMR may also allow patients to interact with their provider via e-mail or other electronic forms of communication.

The Service Component of Health Services Organizations

Chapter 8 discussed efforts in long-term care to bring a more natural and spontaneous environment into the nursing-home setting through implementation of the Eden Alternative. Eden is not the only approach to bringing a better quality of life to long-term care residents. Another approach is the Pioneer Network, which "embraces resident-centered care including an environment of neighborhoods instead of nursing units and schedules determined by residents" (Trocchio, 2000, p. 1). In the Pioneer Network approach, residents live a more natural lifestyle, determining for themselves when they want to get up, what and when they want to eat, and what they want to do for the day. There is anecdotal evidence that the Pioneer

Network approach, as with the Eden Alternative, reduces dependency on drugs, reduces staff turnover, and contributes to a healthier and happier environment for both residents and staff.

Hospitals, too, are seeking a better environment for their patients, whether in the inpatient or outpatient setting. Chapter 1 told the story of the Baptist Memorial Health Care Corporation. One of its facilities in particular—Baptist Memorial Hospital in Collierville—was *built* with a service focus in mind. Although the hospital provides inpatient and outpatient services, the physical structure of the facility is such that the two types of services are somewhat separated for patients receiving care. Patients and others visiting the facility are greeted by a large, airy central lobby with a beautiful fountain, foliage, skylights, and comfortable seating. Immediately adjacent to the central lobby is a dining room, a community medical library open to the public, and a cardiac rehabilitation center. Surrounding the central lobby area are the diagnostic services and the outpatient surgery area. What is not immediately evident is the fact that this central lobby area serves as the waiting area for each of the services surrounding it.

Inpatient services are provided on the second floor in self-contained twelve-bed nursing wings, each containing a dedicated nursing station, supply room, and equipment. In the maternity wing, large and comfortable birthing rooms are actually labor, delivery, recovery, and postpartum rooms all in one. Physicians' offices are on the second and third floors of the hospital, providing for integrated care. The hospital was built with patient comfort and convenience in mind. Inpatients essentially are cared for in dedicated areas separate from outpatient activities. Outpatients move through the facility without having the feeling of being in a hospital. The beauty of the setting is a "therapy" in itself.

One might question the cost of a beautiful setting with fountains and restful, peaceful décor. In building a new facility, however, materials costs were very much a part of the strategic plan, and efforts were made to use materials and space in an aesthetically pleasing, efficient, and cost-effective manner (R. Lassiter, personal communication, February 28, 2000). The result is a facility (use of the word *hospital* no longer seems appropriate) that is patient centered and reflects the changes taking place in health care delivery today.

The incentive to change hospital care into a more patient-centered process in more pleasant surroundings is not limited to new construction. Facilities can be found in many areas that have made changes to incorporate a service focus into health care delivery. Many hospitals have developed means of providing more patient-friendly care, from greeters at the main entrance to escorts who help patients find needed services. Preregistration to cut down on waiting times and paperwork is now the norm for most inpatient and outpatient services. Some hospitals in busy and congested areas have incorporated valet parking into their patient services.

A more formal program dedicated to transforming hospital care into a natural, comforting, and homelike environment is known as the Planetree project. Planetree was founded in 1978 on the concept that a homelike environment, encouraging family involvement and integrating a more holistic approach to care, enhances the healing process (Planetree, 2000b). As described in its Web site (www.planetree.org) and brochure:

> Planetree's approach is holistic and encourages healing in all dimensions—mental, emotional, spiritual and social, as well as physical. It seeks to maximize health care outcomes by integrating complementary medical therapies such as mind-body medicine, therapeutic massage, acupuncture, yoga and energy therapies . . . with conventional medical therapies . . . and recognizes the importance of architectural and environmental design in the healing process.

Planetree facilities are designed with spaces for patients and families to have both quiet places when they desire solitude and inviting meeting places when they want to socialize. The conventional hospital room is not always conducive to either. Planetree incorporates lounges, kitchens, libraries, chapels, and gardens into the facility. Music, storytelling, and art complement the warmth of the environment, and humor is incorporated to "create an atmosphere of serenity and playfulness" (Planetree, 2000a). Although Planetree has not become the majority form of inpatient care, it is more than just a dream. Some nineteen organizations are official Planetree affiliates at the writing of this text (see the story of Windber Medical Center at the end of this chapter). Perhaps the most difficult aspect of implementing a concept such as Planetree is the cultural change that must take place. Staff training, education, and commitment to the concept are long-term processes, much like commitment to Total Quality Improvement projects that focus on customer service and increasing quality in any organization.

SUMMARY

Not all organizations are successful in implementing quality incentives. A successful organization is one with strong and dedicated leadership. Health care organizations in particular have been slow to change, and the turmoil caused by cost containment, the move to managed care contracting, a high degree of government regulation, and increased competition have left organizations struggling to find new ways to differentiate themselves yet hesitant to take on long-term, major projects in an era of uncertainty.

IN THE HEALTH CARE COMMUNITY

Windber Medical Center*

Windber Medical Center opened in 1906 as the Windber Hospital and Wheeling Clinic mainly to provide services to the miners of the Berwind-White Coal Company, which had developed the town of Windber, Pennsylvania. Since that time, the range of services has grown, as has the hospital to a 102-bed, full-service community hospital. In the late 1980s, the changes that affected the rest of the health care market also affected Windber Hospital. As a small community hospital, Windber was forced to take a hard look at its future. To adapt to managed care contracting and price negotiations, in 1997 Windber joined the Conemaugh Health System, an affiliation of four independent hospitals. It was also in 1997 that the medical center embarked on developing a strategic plan.

The CEO and the board of directors recognized the Planetree project as a kinder, gentler approach to inpatient care, and although it would take major changes to the culture and structure of the organization, it could be the long-term answer to both budget and image problems of the medical center. Windber

Medical Center made an investment of about $100,000 in adopting Planetree's concepts and has seen returns in high patient satisfaction rates and a rising patient census. These are key positive indicators in a facility with competition from much larger hospitals sharing the same market area. Prior to implementing Planetree, Windber struggled with a "hometown coal region" image, which allowed the larger hospitals to draw patients who felt that larger meant better. The CEO, Nick Jacobs, even today feels it is much harder to change the image in the local community than outside the community. Community members who have not experienced the changes at Windber still feel it is better to go outside the local area to the larger hospitals to get quality care, yet Windber has developed partnerships with the U.S. Department of Defense for programs in heart disease reversal, prostate cancer reversal, the development of a genetic breast care center, and developing postpolio syndrome research. Health care administrators from different areas of the United States and the rest of the world have come to Windber to see Planetree in action.

(continues)

*Information for this case study was obtained through personal interviews with Mr. Nick Jacobs, CEO of Windber Medical Center, and from organization documents.

(continued)

In the strategic planning phase, Windber was able to define key initiatives, including establishing centers of excellence. One such initiative was establishing the area's first hospice center. Hospice and respite care have been part of Windber's commitment to care for over twenty years and were offered through the palliative care unit. The brand new hospice center in a new wing of the facility is built into a natural setting with attractive rooms and a more homelike environment. Physicians were able to support the Planetree project as an opportunity to take the *caring* of hospice into all areas of inpatient care. Hospice provides the opportunity for physicians, patients, and families to experience the advantages of holistic care of the patient's body, mind, and spirit.

Another initiative from Windber's strategic plan was recognizing the role the medical center needed to play in working with the aging population. Developed through a partnership with the Area Agency on Aging, Windber Medical Center has become the community center, encompassing a senior activity center with a workout center, indoor walking track, outdoor trails, and a transportation system. The workout center offers memberships to the Area Agency on Aging to hand out to persons as they see fit. An exercise physiologist and physical therapist are on site for consultation for members, in addition to supervised care. The workout center, however, is not limited to use by the aged.

The Coronary Artery Disease (CAD) Reversal Center offers the Ornish program of diet, stress management, exercise, meditation, and support programs. Those who have CAD and those who are at risk for but wish to avoid CAD, are welcomed into this progressive program that empowers patients to live a higher quality of life.

Windber Medical Center continues to improve its entire campus and infrastructure to provide more patient-centered care. It also continues a commitment to staff training and empowerment to making the atmosphere a warm, friendly, and comfortable place—not just for patients, but also for all who work within the medical center. Many of the physical improvements made to existing structures have come about through the excitement and commitment of the internal maintenance staff. Small changes, such as bread makers on each unit providing homemade bread to patients, visitors, and staff twice a day, and aromatherapy throughout the hospital, make some of the most significant contributions to change.

The difference was apparent on a walk through the medical center. The "hospital smell" was nonexistent, yet aromatherapy was light enough not to be apparent until the entire ambience of the facility was apparent. Inviting yet unobtrusive décor said, "Welcome." Three pianos strategically placed allowed comforting music to filter through the units. Perhaps most obvious, however, were the comfortable conversations that took place between patients, staff, and administration. The tour of the facility took a long time simply because of the frequent stops for Mr. Jacobs to converse with patients and staff—all part of the new Windber culture.

ACTIVITY-BASED LEARNING

• Access the Planetree Web site (www.planetree.org) and find the list of affiliates. Are any of them in your area? Is it possible to visit a Planetree site? If not, access the Web site of one of the affiliate organizations. Do you see a difference in the Planetree organization compared to your local health care organization(s)?

• Hospitals and medical centers try very hard in promotional materials and advertising to differentiate themselves. Pick a local hospital or medical center and investigate new services or facilities that they have incorporated into their organizations in order to attract consumers and differentiate themselves in the realm of providing quality health care.

A QUESTION OF ETHICS

- Given the struggles in containing the costs of health care and given the increasing numbers of Americans who find themselves without health insurance, should organizations be investing in physical changes to their facilities to attract new patients through a more comfortable environment?
- Are holistic medicine and the incorporation of alternative medicine with traditional medicine, in your opinion, good medicine?

REFERENCES

Barsukiewicz, C. (1998). Computerized medical records: Physician response to new technology (Doctoral dissertation, the Pennsylvania State University, 1998). *Dissertation Abstracts International, 59,* 08B:3996.

Blumenthal, D. (1996) Quality of care: What is it? *New England Journal of Medicine, 335*(12), 891–894.

Donabedian, A. (1980). *Explorations in quality assessment and monitoring: Vol. 1. The definition of quality and approaches to its assessment.* Ann Arbor, MI: Health Administration Press.

Pennsylvania Health Care Cost Containment Council. *Background information about the Health Care Cost Containment Council* [author]. Harrisonburg, PA: Brochure.

Planetree Project. (2000a). *Dedicated to the healing of the mind, body & spirit by leading in the development of a new model of health care delivery.* Derby, CT: Griffin Health Services Corporation.

Planetree Project. (2000b). *Welcome to Planetree* [On-line]. Available: www.planetree.org (Accessed July 12, 2000).

Prager, L. (2000, September 24). Managed care sees large gains in key quality areas. *American Medical News,* pp. 14, 16.

Trocchio, J. (2000). Pioneer Network seeks innovation, culture change in long-term care. *Catholic Health World, 16*(13), pp. 1, 5.

Watson, M. (2000, October 15). Doctors plan paperless practice. *The Commercial Appeal,* pp. C1, C4.

APPENDIX

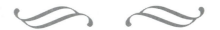

Acronyms in Common Use

AA Alcoholics Anonymous

AACOM American Association of Colleges of Osteopathic Medicine

AAFP American Academy of Family Physicians

AAMC Association of American Medical Colleges

ABMS American Board of Medical Specialties

ACEHSA Accrediting Commission on Education for Health Services Administration

ACGME Accreditation Council for Graduating Medical Association

ACME Accreditation Council for Continuing Medical Education

ACS American College of Surgeons

ADA American Dental Association; American Dietetic Association; American Diabetic Association

AFDC Aid to Families with Dependent Children

AHA American Hospital Association

AHCPR Agency for Health Care Policy and Research; succeeded by AHRQ

AHRQ Agency for Health Care Research and Quality; formerly AHCPR

AMA American Medical Association

ANA American Nurses Association

AOA American Osteopathic Association

APHA American Public Health Association

APA American Psychiatric Association

AUPHA Association of University Programs in Health Administration

BC/BS Blue Cross/Blue Shield

BSN Bachelor of Science in Nursing

CAT Computerized Axial Tomography; See CT

CBO Congressional Budget Office

CCU Critical Care Unit

CCME Coordinating Council on Medical Education

CDC Centers for Disease Control and Prevention

CHAMPUS Civilian Health and Medical Program of the Uniformed Services

CHAMPVA Civilian Health and Medical Program of the Veterans Administration

CLIA Clinical Laboratory Improvement Act

CME Council on Medical Education; Continuing Medical Education

CMR Computerized Medical Record

CON Certificate of Need

CPR Cardiac Pulmonary Resuscitation; Computerized Patient Record

CPT-IV Current Procedural Terminology, 4th Ed

CQI Continuous Quality Improvement

CRNA Certified Registered Nurse Anesthetist

DC Doctor of Chiropractic
DDS Doctor of Dental Surgery
DHEW Department of Health, Education, and Welfare; succeeded by the DHHS
DHHS Department of Health and Human Services
DMD Doctor of Dental Medicine
DSM-IV Diagnosis and Statistical Manual of Mental Disorders, 4th Ed
DO Doctor of Osteopathy
DPM Doctor of Podiatric Medicine
DRG(s) Diagnosis Related Group(s)

ED Emergency Department
EENT Eye, Ear, Nose and Throat
EMR Electronic Medical Record
EMS Emergency Medical Services
EMT Emergency Medical Technician
ENT Ear, Nose, and Throat
EPA Environment Protection Agency
EPSDT Early and Periodic Screening Diagnosis and Treatment
ER Emergency Room
ERISA Employee Retirement Insurance Security Act
ESRD End Stage Renal Disease

FDA Food and Drug Administration
FHA Federal Housing Authority
FLEX Federal Licensing Examination
FMG(s) Foreign Medical Graduate(s)
FMGEMS Foreign Medical Graduate Examination in Medical Sciences
FSMB Federation of State Medical Boards
FTC Federal Trade Commission

GAO General Accounting Office
GDP Gross Domestic Product
GNP Gross National Product
GP General Practitioner
GYN Gynecology

HCFA Health Care Financing Administration
HEW Health, Education, and Welfare; succeeded by HHS

HEDIS Health Plan Employee Data and Information Set
HHS Health and Human Services
HIMS Health Information Management Systems
HIAA Health Insurance Association of America
HMO Health Maintenance Organization

ICD-9 International Classification of Diseases, 9th Ed
ICF Intermediate Care Facility
ICU Intensive Care Unit
IHS Indian Health Service
IMG International Medical Graduate
IPA Individual Practice Association
IS Information Systems
IOM Institute Of Medicine

JAMA The Journal of the American Medical Association
JCAH Joint Commission on Accreditation of Hospitals; Succeeded by JCAHO
JCAHO Joint Commission on Accreditation of Health Care Organizations

LCCME Liaison Committee on Continuing Medical Education
LCGME Liaison Committee on Graduate Medical Education
LCME Liaison Committee on Medical Education
LCSB Liaison Committee for Specialty Boards
LPN Licensed Practical Nurse

MCAT Medical College Admission Test
MD Doctor of Medicine
MH Mental Health
MR Mental Retardation
MRI Magnetic Resonance Imaging

NBME National Board of Medical Examiners
NCHS National Center for Health Statistics
NCQA National Committee for Quality Assurance
NEI National Eye Institute
NHI National Health Insurance
NIA National Institute on Aging
NICU Neonatal Intensive Care Unit

NIH   National Institutes of Health
NLN   National League of Nursing
NLRB   National Labor Relations Board
NMA   National Medical Association
NRMP   National Residency Matching Program
NP   Nurse Practitioner

OB   Obstetrics
OBRA   Omnibus Budget Reconciliation Act
OD   Doctor of Optometry
OMB   Office of Management and Budget
OR   Operating Room
OSHA   Occupational Safety and Health Administration
OT   Occupational Therapy

PA   Physician's Assistant
PCP   Primary Care Physician; Primary Care Practitioner
PET   Positron Emission Tomography
PHC4   Pennsylvania Health Care Cost Containment Council
PHO   Physician Hospital Organization
PharmD   Doctor of Pharmacy
POS   Point of Service
PP   Preferred Provider; Participating Physician
PPO   Preferred Provider Organization
PPS   Prospective Payment System
PRO   Peer Review Organization

PSRO   Professional Standards Review Organization
PT   Physical Therapy

RFP   Request For Proposal
RN   Registered Nurse
RBRVS   Resource Based Relative Value Scale

SAMHSA   Substance Abuse and Mental Health Services Administration
SMI   Supplementary Medical Insurance
SMSA   Standard Metropolitan Statistical Area
SNF   Skilled Nursing Facility
SNOMED   Systemized Nomenclature of Medicine
SSI   Supplementary Security Income
STD   Sexually Transmitted Diseases

UCR   Usual, Customary, and Reasonable
UR   Utilization Review
USIMG   U.S. International Medical Graduate
USMG   United States Medical Graduate
USMLE   United States Medical Licensing Examination

VA   Veterans Administration

WHO   World Health Organization
WIC   Women, Infants, and Children

INDEX

3